Lecture Notes of the Institute for Computer Sciences, Social Informatics and Telecommunications Engineering   55

James C. Lin   Konstantina S. Nikita (Eds.)

Wireless Mobile Communication and Healthcare

Second International ICST Conference
MobiHealth 2010
Ayia Napa, Cyprus, October 18–20, 2010
Revised Selected Papers

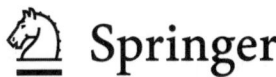 Springer

Volume Editors

James C. Lin
University of illinois at Chicago (M/C 154)
Chicago, Illinois 60607-7053, USA
E-mail: lin@uic.edu

Konstantina S. Nikita
National Technical University of Athens
Electrical and Computer Engineering Faculty
15773, Athens, Greece
E-mail: knikita@ece.ntua.gr

ISSN 1867-8211   e-ISSN 1867-822X

DOI 10.1007/978-3-642-20864-5

Springer Heidelberg Dordrecht London New York

CR Subject Classification (1998): C.2, H.5.2-3, J.3, K.4.2

Typesetting: Camera-ready by author, data conversion by Scientific Publishing Services, Chennai, India

Printed on acid-free paper

Springer is part of Springer Science+Business Media (www.springer.com/mycopy)

Preface

MobiHealth 2010 the International ICST Conference on Wireless Mobile Communication and Healthcare is now history and we hope that it was a successful experience for all participants. During its course, we had the privilege to attend keynote lectures by leading experts as well as invited and contributed paper presentations which uniquely revealed the rapidly changing face of healthcare delivery services facilitated by wireless communications, mobile computing and sensing technologies.

In his keynote address, Guang-Zhong Yang outlined the advances in wireless healthcare services by considering the increasing sophistication and miniaturization of wireless sensor technologies. The talk focused on the provision of "ubiquitous" and "pervasive" monitoring of physical, physiological, and biochemical parameters in any environment without activity restriction and behavior modification. Maria-Teresa Arredondo, in her keynote address, outlined the need for novel solutions to the problems faced by the European health systems in handling chronic diseases. The talk focused on the major role of patient-centered health systems in chronic disease management, prevention and cost reduction in the medium–long period, and outlined the increasing active role of patients and families in self-care, health promotion and disease prevention.

New research, applications and case studies were featured within the framework of MobiHealth 2010. A number of highly timely mobile communication systems that can be used for public health, home and chronic disease monitoring were presented. Recent advances in e-health were discussed, and the potential of integrating leading-edge networking technologies, such as cloud-based services and mobile communications, with personal health records in order to offer healthcare services over the Web was investigated. Interoperability issues in e-health were examined and the current challenges, directions and recommendations toward an e-health interoperable framework were presented. The field of wireless medical devices was also explored. Novel implanted and wearable sensory devices were proposed, and the performance of protocols which are widely used for biomedical telemetry was investigated. Moreover, signal processing techniques for healthcare monitoring systems were proposed. A series of projects in the field of wireless communications in healthcare were presented, providing telehealth and telecare platforms for ambient assisted living, elderly monitoring and chronic disease management.

Several open issues and technical challenges were identified as key factors for revitalizing health care delivery and assisting the shift toward preventive, personalized and citizen-centered care. These include a new generation of less obtrusive, energy-efficient pervasive and non-invasive sensors for body area networks and large-scale screening purposes. Furthermore, as more and more data are gathered, thanks to increased sensing capability, data processing and interpretation become more crucial. Expert systems and intelligent, self-adaptive, disease-specific and predictive algorithms based on a combination of data acquired from different sensor types have to be developed, capable of turning acquired data and information into knowledge to support medical decision making and action. Emphasis should be placed on usability, user acceptance, standardization and interoperability towards ubiquitous and pervasive healthcare delivery services. Emerging applications were identified, which include lifestyle and general well-being monitoring, monitoring and management of neurodegenerative diseases, computer-assisted rehabilitation and therapy and social networking of relatives and peers for the monitoring of elderly.

The conference organization was the combined effort of many people working as reviewers, authors, committee members and support staff and we want to thank all of them for their contribution.

We hope all conference participants enjoyed both the scientific and social programs, established new friendships and partnerships and experienced Mobi-Health 2010 as a memorable event that stimulated their thinking and refreshed their motivation and energy.

Konstantina S. Nikita
James C. Lin

Organization

Steering Committee Chair

James C. Lin   University of Illinois at Chicago, USA

Steering Committee Members

Janet Lin   University of Illinois at Chicago, USA
Arye Nehorai   Washington University, St. Louis, USA
Konstantina S. Nikita   National Technical University of Athens, Greece
George Papadopoulos   University of Cyprus, Cyprus

General Chair

James C. Lin   University of Illinois at Chicago, USA

Technical Program Chair

Konstantina S. Nikita   National Technical University of Athens, Greece

Local Arrangements Chair

George Papadopoulos   University of Cyprus, Cyprus

Publications Chair

Irene Karanassiou   National Technical University of Athens, Greece

Web Chairs

Maria Christopoulou   National Technical University of Athens, Greece
Asimina Kiourti   National Technical University of Athens, Greece

Publicity Chair

Konstantinos Michmizos   National Technical University of Athens, Greece

Conference Coordinator

Gabriella Magyar   ICST

Technical Program Committee

Konstantina S. Nikita	National Technical University of Athens, Greece
Robert Allen	University of Southampton, UK
Pantelis Angelidis	University of Western Macedonia, Greece
Paolo Bernardi	La Sapienza University of Rome, Italy
Nikolaos Bourbakis	Wright State University, USA
Gouenou Coatrieux	ENST Bretagne, France
Thomas Falck	Philips Research Europe, Eindhoven, The Netherlands
Dimitrios I. Fotiadis	University of Ioannina, Greece
Osamu Fujiwara	Nagoya Institute of Technology, Japan
Maysam Ghovanloo	Georgia Institute of Technology, USA
Robert S.H. Istepanian	Kingston University, London, UK
Irene Karanasiou	National Technical University of Athens, Greece
Mohan Karunanithi	Australian E-Health Research Centre, Australia
Ilkka Korhonen	VTT Information Technology, Finland
Stavros Koulouridis	University of Patras, Greece
Luis Kun	National Defense University, DC, USA
Niels Kuster	ITIS Foundation/ETH, Switzerland
Efthyvoulos Kyriakou	Frederick University, Cyprus
Norbert Leitgeb	Graz University of Technology, Austria
James Lin	University of Illinois at Chicago, USA
Janet Lin	University of Illinois at Chicago, USA
Dimitrios Lymberopoulos	University of Patras, Greece
Ilias Maglogiannis	University of Central Greece
Garik Markarian	Lancaster University, UK
Arye Nehorai	Washington University, St. Louis, USA
George Papadopoulos	University of Cyprus
Constantinos Pattichis	University of Cyprus
Agnette Peralta	Department of Health, Philippines
Nada Philip	Kingston University, London, UK
Andriana Prentza	University of Piraeus, Greece
Laura Roa	University of Seville, Spain
Georgios Sakas	Technical University Darmstadt, Fraunhofer-Institut fur Graphische Datenverarbeitung IGD, Germany
Dan Schonfeld	University of Illinois at Chicago, USA
Min-Yi Shih	Physical Optics Corporation, California, USA
Koichi Shimizu	Hokkaido University, Japan
Toshiyo Tamura	Chiba University

Table of Contents

Session 4: Interoperability in e-Health

Session 5: Signal Processing Techniques for Monitoring Services

Session 6: Implantable and Wearable Biomedical Devices

Session 7: Ambient Assistive Technologies

Session 8: Mobile Health Technologies, Applications and Integrated Systems for Chronic Disease Monitoring and Management

Session 9: Emergency and Disaster Applications

Session 10: Mobile Devices and Wireless Technologies for Patient Monitoring

Poster Session

Session 1

Intelligent Public Health Monitoring Services

Tele-psychiatry: Socioeconomic Results and the Way Forward

Markela Psymarnou, Athanasia Karanasiou,
Eleftheria Vellidou, and Pantelis Angelidis

Vidavo S.A., 9th Klm Thessalonikis Thermis Av.,
57001, Thessaloniki, Greece
{markela,support,projects,pantelis}@vidavo.gr

Abstract. Over the past years, the scientific community has witnessed a tremendous growth of applications in heath care telematics. The adoption rate of web based practices was not the same for all medical specialties. Others such as cardiology were fast adopters mainly due to the "electric" nature of the standard diagnostic tools (electro-cardiographer) but others such as psychiatry are still lagging from adopting new methodologies. Now that ubiquitous broadband Internet access is here to stay the time has come to explore the potential of mental care services that could be offered over the web.

Keywords: tele-psychiatry, health telematics, web based, electronic health record, AMC, direct costs, effectiveness.

1 Introduction

From the early introduction of voice telephony, patients in distress and frustration used to call their physicians urgently seeking for consultation. These phone calls did not follow any clinical protocol and though efficient in terms of crisis management they did not qualify as a treatment method. Later on, suicides and crises intervention hotlines staffed with trained volunteers provided a more organized form of telephone counseling.

It was back in 1959 when the first tele-psychiatry system was set in operation in Nebraska, U.S.A. 2-way closed circuit microwave television was used to transmit demonstration of neurologic patients from the State mental hospital to Nebraska Psychiatric Institute 112 miles away in Omaha as part of the education of first year medical students [1].

Although tele-psychiatry has a long history, its practical consequences in every day mental health care practice have been limited. Development, construction and operation and maintenance costs have been prohibitively high. The majority of "on line time" was spent either on medical education as well as on administration purposes.

2 Identifying the Beneficiaries of Tele-psychiatry

Telemedicine is defined as the delivery of healthcare services, where distance is a critical factor, by all healthcare professionals using information and communications

J. Lin and K.S. Nikita (Eds.): MobiHealth 2010, LNICST 55, pp. 3–10, 2011.
© Institute for Computer Sciences, Social Informatics and Telecommunications Engineering 2011

technologies for the exchange of valid information for diagnosis, treatment and prevention of disease and injuries, research and evaluation, and for the continuing education of healthcare providers, all in the interest of advancing the health of individuals and their communities [2]. If this definition were explicitly adapted for psychiatry it abides by the WHO definition on health that it is a state of complete physical, mental and social well-being and not merely the absence of disease or infirmity [3].

Obvious applications for preserving population's health status include psychiatric care for people living in remote and isolated areas. The uneven distribution of medical practitioners between rural and urban areas is well documented even for the well developed countries. Tele-psychiatry makes it possible to provide universal access to the same quality level mental health care services regardless of the limitations imposed by geographic locations.

However it is not only the inhabitants of rural areas who are underprivileged regarding the accessibility to these particular services. Certain populations amongst them the elderly and people with disabilities find it really hard to cope with public transportation due to general poor health, specific mental condition e.g. agoraphobia and deprivation from financial affluence in order to finally visit the appropriate health care Institution and the specialized psychiatrist. Many are the cases when the mentally ill even lack the required family support and they are left either alone or in the care of the community with the fear of social stigmatization being the rationale behind the abandonment.

Finally offenders of all ages, races, religion etc feature the highest rates of mental disorders. In UK alone, only one in ten prisoners has no mental disorder [4].

Tele-psychiatry could enable patients to be examined, assessed and receive the benefits of specialized psychiatric services in their preferred surroundings and acting complementary to the primary care physician thus ensuring the continuity of care.

NHS or any form of private care today cannot afford to staff every single hospital or nursing home with specialized psychiatrists. When primary care physicians undergo the critical task of dealing with treatment resistant patients they would either deliver suboptimal care or refer the patient to very expensive tertiary hospital care away from his/her family and preferred surroundings jeopardizing their overall stability and well being.

It is not only the patients who benefit from the new tools such as remote consultations. The physicians could now have an incentive to remain in rural areas as geographic distance from the sources of knowledge (e.g. prestigious health care Institutions) is not synonymous to professional isolation.

3 Contemporary Means of Tele-psychiatry

Psychiatry is not a specialty that requires touch during examination of the patient. Sessions are mostly in the form of interviews where interviewer and interviewee have agreed to meet in a predefined location such as a nursing home, a hospital, private clinic or even at the patient's home and physical contact is limited to a mere handshaking at the beginning or the end of the session.

Even duration is not predefined. The sessions could last for as long as the involved parties consider it helpful or efficient. Number of involved people is not standardized either. Group therapies have gained momentum especially when participants form a group sharing experiences and seeking guidance for dealing with issues ranging from substance abuse to mourning and providing care to the chronically ill.

Broadband internet has made video-conferencing through standard tools such as Windows Live Messenger (MSN), Skype etc available to all. Even if the patient cannot configure his or her environment to enable such a facility, social services could cater for such a need at a "care at home" level. Practically what video-conferencing offers is a simulation of the consultation session between the psychiatrist and the patient rendering location insignificant provided that broadband internet access is established in the concerned region. Multi-party sessions could also be supported simulating group therapeutic consultations.

One of the numerous advantages of tele-psychiatry is that allows for immediate recordings that could be stored in relevant fields of the patient's electronic health record and reviewed later on by the same physician or sent to another colleague for second opinion and further evaluation. Medical research depends heavily on easy to process digitalized data and these recordings combined with coded history and diagnostics constitute a very promising combination for breakthrough results not only in the field of psychiatry but also in the adjacent field of neurology and its subspecialties, neurobiology and neurophysiology.

An important study by Steffens and others [5] has demonstrated the added value of the video recordings taken while demented subjects were participating in research interviews. The overall gestalt of the patient in the environment is a very important contributor to diagnostic assessment which is the basis for an adequate cum effective treatment of the subject's disorder.

Privacy and confidentiality are better addressed in the closed confines of the digital world. There are numerous techniques these days to prohibit eavesdropping on video conferencing and data storage from heterogeneous sources is safer than ever through the use of cryptography and smart cards throughout the health care network of professionals thus allowing access to data for only the authorized practitioners.

4   Pilot Assessment: The Key to Global Acceptance

Many mental care practitioners insist that tele-psychiatry is just another gimmick. They appear to be reluctant to use a technology considered unproven. Despite its long history, clinical studies establishing accuracy, reliability, ease of use and clinical utility are not that many though their number is fast increasing [6].

A recent study that took place in Greece evaluated the tele-psychiatric process used for assessing and preparing patients who could potentially leave the institution and transferred to boarding homes as part of the national deinstitutionalization program. The study used video-conferencing as the tool to connect University of Athens Psychiatric Clinic and Tripoli's (city of central Peloponnese) Psychiatric hospital [7].

The results of the study were very encouraging. The project has been evaluated through the use of questionnaires given to patients and mental health professionals to fill in. ADSL connection was used and the bandwidth exceeded a lot the sufficient bandwidth for examining and making decisions concerning most mental disorders according to the Telepsychiatry Project of the Consolidated Department of Psychiatry of Harvard medical School (128kbits/sec) [8].

The majority of the patients have accepted the new method of examination without problems and the level of satisfaction from the method appears to be high. The health practitioners' acceptance is at the same level and they also claim to have found the video conference system very easy to use and efficient in their everyday routine.

5   Financial Considerations: The Cretan Way

One of telemedicine's many promises in general is increased effectiveness i.e. provision of health services with better clinical results at the same or reduced cost when comparing them with existing practices. Effectiveness is always measured comparatively to other clinical interventions applied to treat the same condition as shown in Figure 1:

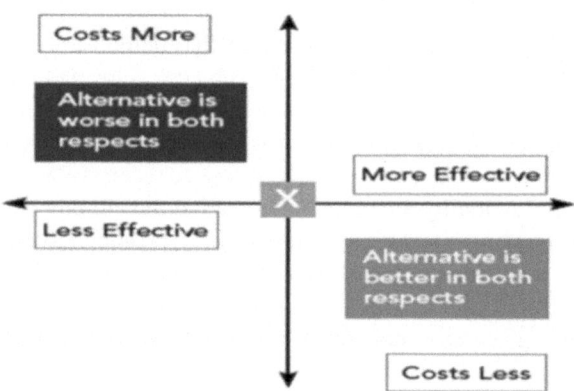

Fig. 1. Comparing alternatives to a given health intervention [9]

The conventional means of providing psychiatric care in geographically isolated areas consist of a mobile unit staffed with at least one psychiatrist, one psychologist and a nurse. The visits of the unit are periodical of a fixed frequency; the routes they follow are predefined in order to reach patients who more than likely are recently deinstitutionalized hence are already diagnosed with a mental condition.

This scheme was followed for years by the Mental Health Centre of Chania in Crete, Greece till its management [10] decided to install a tele-psychiatry platform that allows the Centre's treating psychiatrists to connect over the web with three rural

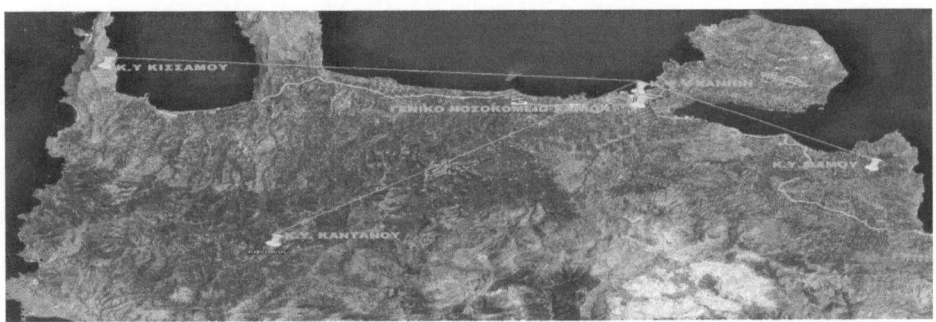

Fig. 2. Map of Chania Prefecture showing the locations where the pilot is in operation

surgeries in Vamos, Kasteli and Kandanos respectively in order to monitor the progress of their patients.

Taking into consideration the findings of other pilots such as the one described in the previous paragraph where the conclusion was that over the web consultations offer the same qualitative results as the conventional face to face sessions then the other parameter that is under scrutiny is the financial viability of the new service.

The dedicated study targeting the Chania case reached the conclusion that one mobile unit was approximately 5.000 € more expensive to run on a yearly basis than the tele-psychiatry web platform. Only in Chania Prefecture, the mobile units are 3 while Crete has a total of 14 units in operation. A simple multiplication yields a yearly profit for the National Health System of approximately 70.000€ that could be reinvested in other facilities to improve the characteristics of health provisioning in deprived areas.

6 Assessment Methodology for the Chania Tele-psychiatry Platform Effectiveness

The first step for assessing the effectiveness of any given clinical intervention is identifying the costs involved. The complete assessment framework consists of the following:

1) What we compare: In this case is psychiatric treatment over the web (tele-psychiatry) with the conventional face to face sessions with the use of a mobile unit staffed with adequate health professionals
2) Cost Categories: Usually we are discussing direct costs corresponding to the value of resources available for the health service provisioning. The metric used is the Annual Mean Cost (AMC) and what is important in the assessment is the definition of Delta – Difference (Δ) between the AMCs of the two clinical interventions.
3) Time schedule that the evaluation will take into consideration
4) Perspective: Costs are perceived differently from various actors e.g. society, the physicians, the patients or the National Health System all have their own

views when assessing a practice. The NHS perspective was used in the Chania case as the costs involved are easily identifiable.

5) Discount Interest Rate: It is connected to the time schedule of the evaluation as the money costs change every year and the clinical implementations have a time schedule of more than 3 years.

The cost categories for installing the tele-psychiatry application between two points (the Mental Health Centre and the rural surgery of Kandanos) are tabulated below:

Table 1. Tele-psychiatry Direct Costs

	Cost Category	Value
1	Equipment Costs (2 LCD 20 ' monitors, 2 PCs one to be used as file server, 2 Web Cameras, 2 Laser Printers, 1 Rooter) with a life span of 4 years	3.500 €
2	Connection fees for 2 IP lines at 20 € each per month for a year with a life span of 4 years	480 €
3	Technical support and maintenance fees (software) 300 € per month for a year with a life span of 4 years	3.600 €
4	Web application development costs with a life span of 10 years	25.000 €

After calculating the surcharges of the discount interest rates applied according to the application's life span we have reached the calculation of the Annual Mean Cost (AMC) for tele-psychiatry tabulated below:

Table 2. Tele-psychiatry AMC

Cost Category	Annual Mean Cost (AMC) for tele-psychiatry (in €)
1	984,82
2	0
3	517,09
4	3.878,22
5	3.359,79
TOTAL AMC : 8.739,92 €	

The cost categories for the set up of a mobile unit commuting between the Mental Health Centre of Chania and the rural surgery of Kandanos are tabulated below:

Table 3. Mobile Unit Direct Costs

	Cost Category	Value
1	Car purchase with a life span of 10 years	15.000 €
2	Car maintenance fees at 7% of the purchase cost per year and for 10 years	1.050 €
3	Fuels costs for twice per week covering a distance of 140 klm (both ways) for 50 weeks and for a life span of **10 years** (1.1 € gasoline per liter consumption of 8 € per 100 klm)	1.352 €
4	Driver's salary	7.020 €
5	Relocation Expenses for 4 people (psychiatrist, social worker, nurse, driver), 10 € per visit (4 people x 10 € x 50 weeks)	2.000 €

Following the same methodology as for the tele-psychiatry the AMC for the mobile unit has been calculated and it is presented below:

Table 4. Mobile Unit AMC

Cost Category	Annual Mean Cost for the mobile unit (in €)
1	2.015,87
2	1.098,70
3	1.414,71
4	7.345,64
5	2.092,776
	TOTAL AMC : 13.967,70 €

Finally, the comparison will result in the following formula:

$$\Delta \text{ (AMC mu – AMC tp)} = 13.967,7 \text{ € - } 8.739,92 \text{ € = } \mathbf{5.227, 78 \text{ €}}$$

hence proving that tele-psychiatry is more effective than the traditional means of mental health care provisioning to remote areas with the use of a mobile unit.

7 Conclusions

Currently, video-conferencing offered at ADSL connection speed is the main enabler of tele-psychiatry. This technique used in conjunction with a patient's electronic health record can successfully simulate and substitute the in vivo consultation and deliver to the mentally ill the same quality of service regardless of their location.

The burden of dealing with treatment-resisting patients will be lifted from the shoulders of primary health care practitioners since they can afford to electronically refer the patients to a specialized psychiatrist.

The trauma of moving the patients away from their families and familiar surroundings can be avoided and their recovery can take place in an environment in which they feel safe and well adjusted.

Last but not least there are substantial evidences that the increased effectiveness of telepsychiatry in comparison to conventional methods of treatment will be of paramount importance for the decision makers when dealing with the implementation of mental health services in clinically underserved areas.

References

1. Liebson, E.: MD Assistant Professor of Psychiatry at Tufts New England Medical Centre in Boston MA U.S.A Telepsychiatry: 35 years' experience by,
   http://www.medscape.com/viewarticle/431064_1
2. International Society for Telemedicine and eHealth – NGO in Official relation with WHO, Glossary of Telemedical Terms (WHO 1998),
   http://www.isft.net/cms/index.php?q_-_z
3. Preamble to the Constitution of the World Health Organization as adopted by the International Health Conference, New York, June 19-22 (1946); signed on July 22, 1946 by the representatives of 61 States (Official Records of the World Health Organization, no. 2, p. 100) and entered into force on April 7 (1948)
4. Mental Health Foundation, Statistics on Mental Health,
   http://www.mentalhealth.org.uk/information/
   mental-health-overview/statistics/
5. Steffens, D.C., Welsh, K.A., Burke, J.R., et al.: Diagnosis of Alzheimer's disease in epidemiologic studies by staged review of clinical data. Neuropsychiatry Neuropsychol. Behav. Neurol. 9, 107–113 (2002)
6. Zarate, C.A., Weinstock, L., Cukor, P., et al.: Applicability of telemedicine for assessing patients with schizophrenia: Acceptance and reliability. J. Clin. Psychiatry 58, 22–25 (1997)
7. Zacharopoulou, C., Konstantakopoulos, G., Tsirika, N., Vavourakis, P., Lymperaki, G., Tempeli, A., Valma, V., Panagoutsos, P., Katsadoros, K.: Evaluation of a tele-psychiatry pilot project,
   http://www.klimaka.org.gr/newsite/downloads/
   telepsychiatry.pdf
8. Baer, L., Elford, R., Cucor, P.: Telepsychiatry at forty: what have we learned. Harvard Review of Psychiatry 5, 7–17 (1997)

A Citizen Telemonitoring Strategy
as Envisaged for Central Greece

George E. Dafoulas[1], George Gorgogetas[2], Kalliopi Liatou[2],
Kostas Karampoulas[2], George Vallas[3], and Pantelis Angelidis[4]

[1] Faculty of Medicine, University of Thessaly, Greece
[2] e-trikala SA, Municipality of Trikala, Greece
[3] Cities Net SA, Digital Municipal Community of Central Greece
[4] Faculty of Engineering Informatics and Telecommunications,
University of Western Macedonia, Greece
{gdafoulas,ggorgogetas,kliatou,kkarampoulas}@e-trikala.gr,
gvallas@citiesnet.gr, pantelis@vidavo.gr

Abstract. Renewing Health, a Pilot A, CIP/PSP project, funded from the European Commission, aims at implementing large-scale real-life test beds for the validation and subsequent evaluation of innovative telemedicine services using a patient-centric approach and a common rigorous assessment methodology. The services offered are designed to give patients a central role in the management of their own diseases, fine-tuning the choice and dosage of medications, promoting compliance to treatment, and helping healthcare professionals to detect early signs of worsening in the monitored pathologies. The current paper discusses the telemonitoring strategy as envisaged for Central Greece in the framework of the Renewing Health project.

Keywords: telehealth, telehomecare, telemedicine.

1 Introduction

The world population is growing while in Europe it is decreasing due to ageing. The number of people over 65 will rise nearly 40% between 2010 and 2030 and the number of people over 80 will have doubled by 2050 [1]. Associated with this ageing demography, the cost of healthcare is rapidly increasing while the tax base in increasingly at stake. People over the age of 65 receive four times the number of medical tests as others [2]. There will be even fewer economic "producers" to support the social and health costs related to Europe's population of retirees.

Health spending is rising faster than GDP and it is estimated to reach 16% of GDP by 2020 in OECD countries [3].

Recent research has suggested that the health ICT industry has the potential to be the third largest industry in the health sector with a global turnover of €50-60 billion, of which Europe represents one third [3]. By 2010, a double digit growth rate of up to 11% is foreseen as driven by a search for more productivity and performance [4]. However, this potential growth might not occur if the existing barriers to the market are not removed together with more evidence of its effectiveness.

J. Lin and K.S. Nikita (Eds.): MobiHealth 2010, LNICST 55, pp. 11–16, 2011.
© Institute for Computer Sciences, Social Informatics and Telecommunications Engineering 2011

It is not only ageing which matters, but also the pattern of disease is changing. 60% of all deaths are due to chronic diseases [5]. This imposes even greater workload on healthcare providers and resources at a time when mobility and individualism have diminished the traditional family carer's potential. Without actions to address these causes, deaths from chronic diseases will increase by 17% over the next years. In the USA, 85% of all hospital costs and 69% of all physician costs are spent on treating chronic diseases. In Europe, chronic diseases are estimated to amount to over 70% of healthcare costs. But today, chronic diseases are not yet managed appropriately. According to the World Health Organisation (WHO), at least 80% of all cardiovascular disease and type II diabetes and over 40% of cancer could be avoided.

Telemedicine and homecare is the segment with the greatest potential for financial and clinical impact [6] and is due for immediate expansion. Homecare telehealth moves beyond the hype and is considered a serious solution by healthcare purchasers. Protocols and technologies to help implement and provide advanced mobile tele-homehealth care applications are under development.

Nevertheless, these applications-telemedicine and free movement of electric health data – poses a series of open questions regarding: a clear definition of telemedicine services, legal framework and liability issues , harmonization of diagnosis related groups that can be treated by telemedicine, accreditation of health professionals who provide telemedicine applications, interoperability issues,   cost effectiveness, and reimbursement for telemedicine services [7,8].

2   Initiatives on European Level to Deal with Challenges of Telehomecare

In 2010, the European Commission, via its Competitiveness and Innovation Programme, issued a call [9] to support a large-scale telehomemonitoring pilot project for up to 7 M€ of EU contribution. This will include a network of procurers and payers of healthcare services.

The main outcomes of the pilot should:

- Provide patients with the means to manage their health conditions outside traditional care settings, by using innovative Personal Health Systems and integrated telemedicine services.
- Provide health professionals with more comprehensive monitoring and diagnostic data for decision making, thus facilitating personalised care for chronically ill patients
- Enable, on a large scale, continuity of care through enhanced interaction between patients and primary care settings as well as secondary care settings.

The pilot intents to develop sustainable business models, which will eventually harness the benefits of the targeted innovative eHealth set of tools and services. It will produce large scale, measurable, comparable and statistically significant results, regarding the effectiveness of the solutions tested, using a commonly agreed and scientifically sound assessment methodology.

The consortium of 9 Regional Health Authorities was selected to implement this large-scale pilot (called Renewing Health, www.renewinghealth.eu) for the validation of innovative telemedicine services using a patient centric approach and a rigorous assessment methodology common to all the pilot sites. Pilots will be carried out in nine of the most advanced regions of the European Union belonging to 9 different Member States and will make use of advanced Personal Mobile Health Systems which follow the chronic patient wherever he/she is and which are integrated with the other clinical information systems already in place. The Project will give birth to a new paradigm for the deployment of innovative telemedicine services and will include a Randomised Control Trial with more than 8.000 patients. The Project is supported by the Health Authorities of the participating regions which have responsibility for the healthcare budget and which are fully committed to deploy the telemedicine services in their territory, once they have been validated and to co-operate among them to promote the uptake of the services at pan-European level.

RENEWING HEALTH, will use the evaluation MethoTelemed Guidance [10] (developed by study sponsored by the EC) which will be applied to measure the impact of the eHealth service deployed on a number of indicators which refer to Health Related Quality of Life, user satisfaction, clinical outcome and healthcare spending. This means the project will be able to build a convincing business case to be presented to National, Regional and Local Health Authorities, and stimulate them to speed up the deployment of patient-centred eHealth service solution. The deployment in other regions will be substantially eased by the openness of the Consortium to share with other regions the results of the Project and to assist them in implementing the services, maximising the chances of success and reducing time scales and costs.

MethoTelemed is a benchmark document, on how and to what extent telemedicine applications have been deployed in healthcare systems and it will provide a structured framework to assess the effectiveness of telemedicine applications and their contribution to quality of care.

3   Description of the Telehealth Project of Central Greece

Telemonitoring services of the Digital Community of Central Greece (11 Municipalities of Central Greece, representing more than 1.000.000 citizens), will be provided to individual citizens with chronic heart failure, chronic asthma, diabetes, arrhythmias, dementia and hypertension.

The equipment includes tele-electrocardiographs, tele-spirometers, tele-GPS trackers, tele-scales, tele glucose-meters and blood pressure meters.

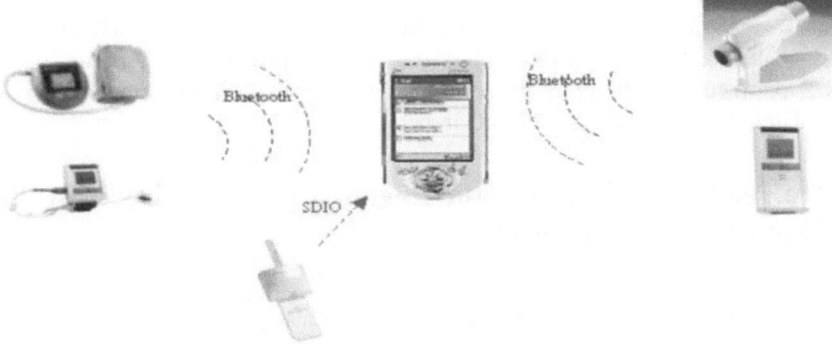

Fig. 1. Operational diagram

The infrastructure and services will be operational within 2010 and are partly funded by the 4th Community Framework Support (CSF).

In particular, the Telehealth centre will provide telemonitoring services to chronic patients and the elderly as well as social services to the patients participating in the project. Novel telemedicine devices will be used, for the wireless transmission of vital signs to a web-based platform. Individual citizens will be equipped with light-weight handheld devices and record their vital signs at home which will then be transferred (via the telehealth centre) to the municipality hospital over internet or GPRS for review and feedback by the experts.

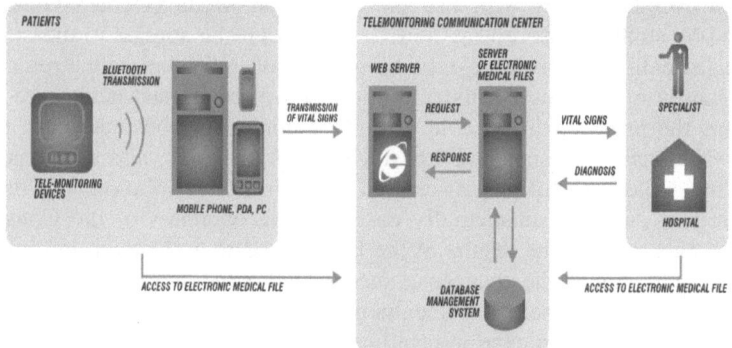

Fig. 2. Data flow Diagram

Through these Personal Health Systems and innovative types of telemedicine services, medical staff can monitor the health status of patients anywhere and anytime.

The service will therefore allow enhanced interaction between patients and primary care settings (i.e. GPs) as well as secondary care settings (hospitals and/or specialists) The 5th Regional Health Authority (5th RHA), a beneficiary of the project, will ensure proper monitoring of the patients by specialists and it will provide support to the everyday clinical effort. In addition, the 5th RHA's HIS is under completion (Nov 2009 - 12 Hospitals + 1 University Hospital + 33 Health Centres) which will provide the means and infrastructure for putting innovative services to the task, performed by IT aware specialists.

The Telehealth Centre is located in the Municipality of Trikala, which has run a local telehealth service already for 3 years, partly funded by the 3rd Community Framework Support (CSF). Therefore the Municipality of Trikala is the Competence Centre for the Digital Community of Central Greece.

4   The Telehealth Project of the Region of Central Greece in the Renewing Health Project

The goals of the Telehealth Project of the Region of Central Greece align with the concept of RENEWING HEALTH project and with the Objective 1.1: ICT for patient-centred health service, of the call for proposals 2009 for Pilot Type A, Theme 1: ICT for health, ageing and inclusion.

The specific telehealth services to be included in the context of the RENEWING HEALTH project will focus on the major chronic diseases and specifically on Cardiovascular Diseases (CVD) - like Chronic Heart Failure, Hypertension and Arrhythmias; Chronic Obstructive Pulmonary disease (COPD) and Diabetes.

4.1 Interoperability / Ethical Issues

The service will fully respect the fundamental right to the protection of personal data, and in particular of personal data related to health, in line with the relevant EU and national legislation. Use of existing European, International or commonly agreed standards will ensure the interoperability of the service.

4.2 Health Technology Assessment

Chronic diseases management with telehomecare can introduce cost savings while improving quality of life and prognosis for the patient.

The validation and deployment of the service will be carried out in real life settings and using the same methodology for all cities of the Digital Community of Central Greece.

The evaluation of the pilot will be carried out using the MethoTelemed assessment model in all the participating regions/partners of RENEWING HEALTH project, including the telehealth services in Central Greece. The objective is to achieve a systematic and multidisciplinary assessment of the impact of the integrated telemedicine services, and to produce convincing and reliable results in accordance with scientific guidelines.

Apart from the difference in the clinical effectiveness, Health-related Quality of Life score between the Intervention and the Control Group will be also measured with the generic and diseases specific quality of life questionnaires. Patient Satisfaction with the telehealth service will be evaluated as well.

Difference in number of annual admissions to hospital between the Intervention and the Control Group, together with the difference in number of consultations with GPs between the Intervention and the Control Group, will be evaluated.

Through the above a cost–utility analysis will be performed in order to evaluate the prospective of the ability of the telehealth services as an alternative to the standard medical treatement of chronic diseases.

In order to achieve, measurable, comparable and statistically significant results, regarding the effectiveness of the telehealth solutions tested, the principles of clinical evaluation with use of the randomized clinical trial or controlled trial with intervention and control groups, will be used:

Table 1. Pathologies and patient basis of Renewing Health in Greece

Pathology		Patient basis
Diabetes	Intervention group (number)	100
	Control Group (number)	80
COPD	Intervention group (number)	100
	Control Group (number)	80
CVD	Intervention group (number)	100
	Control Group (number)	80
Total		540

Table 2. Economical evaluation of telehealth in patients with CHF/COPD and Diabetes type 2

Objective	To assess the cost-effectiveness and cost-utility of telehealth compared with usual care.
Perspective	Societal (alternatively, national health system).
Methodology	Cost-utility, cost-effectiveness analysis.
Primary outcome of economical evaluation	cost per quality adjusted life year (QALY) gained.
Secondary outcomes	total cost of the intervention, cost per clinical event avoided, cost per improvement in other clinical outcomes.
Discounting rate	3% for clinical and economical outcomes. Differential Timing of expenditure. Since the trial will last more than one year, two main adjustments must be considered , related to the inflation for cost and time preference for cost and effect (discounting). According to the US Public Service Panel on Cost-Effectiveness in Health and Medicine, suggest 3% is the most appropriate , discount rate for economic evaluation. However , any past studies have used 5% rate , that makes it also acceptable.
Sensitivity analysis	one-way and two-way for all assumptions made.
Data collection	A trained nurse will collect both clinical and economical data monthly, using Case Report Forms (CRFs)

References

1. OECD, Health at a Glance, OECD INDICATORS (2005)
2. Health Information Network Europe (HINE) report – European eHealth forecast (2006)
3. Price, Waterhouse, Coopers study, HealthCast 2010: Creating a Sustainable Future (2006)
4. Accelerating the developmet of the e-health market in Europe, e-health task report (2007)
5. WHO report, Building foundations for eHealth (2006)
6. Gartner study: The potential of telemedicine applications (October 2006)
7. Telemedicine for the benefit of patients, healthcare systems and society. COM (2008)689 Final (November 2008)
8. Tran, K., Polisena, J., Coyle, D., Coyle, K., Kluge, E.-H.W., Cimon, K., McGill, S., Noorani, H., Palmer, K., Scott, R.: Home telehealth for chronic disease management [Technology report number 113]. Ottawa: Canadian Agency for Drugs and Technologies in Health (2008)
9. ICT PSP Objective identifier: 1.1: ICT for patient-centred health service
10. Official Journal 04.06.2008 - 2008/S 107-142555 - Tender SMART 2008/0064

Estimation and Analysis of Thermal Response of Human Tissue during EM Exposure

M. Prishvin[1], L. Bibilashvili[1], R. Zaridze[1], A. Mohammod[2], and R. Islam[2]

[1] Laboratory of Applied Electrodynamics, Tbilisi State University, Tbilisi, 0128, Georgia
[2] University of South Carolina, USA
prishvin@gmail.com

Abstract. During last decades, the environment has undergone serious changes from EM point of view. An objective of this paper is to analyze realistic exposure scenarios by means of numerical computations. Our aim is to determine peak values of SAR and temperature rise in various scenarios. This paper contains results of computer simulations performed on a human model [1] with and without consideration of detailed blood perfusion in the model [2].

1 Introduction

The recent results of the study on numerical simulations of electromagnetic (EM) exposure of human body by wireless transmitters are discussed in this paper. To date, a large number of dipole, monopole, and PIFA antennas were studied at different frequencies and distances to quantify the SAR level produced in the human body. The present study expands this work by simulating the temperature rise in human body related to those exposure conditions. The thermal simulations were conducted using the proprietary program package, which was developed in our Laboratory – FDTDLab [3-5] in cooperation with Motorola Inc (2002-2008). Validation of FDTDLab was proved for EM and thermal solutions part using different ways [4, 5]. The software package was enhanced with several new features including the calculation of peak values in selected tissue regions and/or tissue, and most importantly the consideration of directional blood flow in the tissue capillary and its effect on the special distribution of the temperature and temperature rise in the Human model [1].

Part of this work was conducted within MMF Phase II project. Our aim was to investigate EM exposure and determine peak SAR and temperature rise values in various scenarios without consideration of directional blood flow. Modified bio-heat equation and vascular structure generation algorithm is introduced for more advanced simulation method currently under development [2]. The task included: use of the Finite Difference Time Domain (FDTD) method and anatomically based human head models; computation the peak 1-g and 10-g averaged SAR [6-9] and the temperature rise in the tissue for canonical dipole antennas of various length ($\lambda/2$, $\lambda/4$, $\lambda/8$ and at 300, 450, 900, 1450, 1900, 2450, 3700 and 6000 MHz and at distances of 5, 10 and 20 mm from the head model. The 1-g and 10-g averaged-SAR distributions were subsequently computed on the basis of the algorithm specified in IEEE C95.3-2002 standard (IEEE, 2002) (2002) [7-9].

J. Lin and K.S. Nikita (Eds.): MobiHealth 2010, LNICST 55, pp. 17–24, 2011.

2 Materials and Methods

The simulations were conducted using the FDTD method. Temperature increase in tissue was simulated due to RF exposure from antennas placed at different distances from the head models. The EM and thermal coupled solver FDTDLab, developed at TSU [4, 5], was used. As it is shown in [5] the thermal solver is tested against an analytical solution for a simplified case. At the initial phase of the project various standard antenna and phantom orientations were simulated. Along with the SAR the conventional bio-heat model was used to compute temperature rise and then more advance thermal model that includes the directional blood flow information and then newly developed method that generates vascular structure geometry and blood flow velocity field was also used for heat exchange simulations in those conditions. The difference between the conventional and advance model has been observed and analyzed.

A new algorithm for construction of realistic vessel networks, blood flow velocity vectors and a new approach to simulate heat exchange in tissue during EM exposure considering heat convection by blood was implemented in FDTDLab software. Heat exchange in tissue is calculated according to the modified Pennes equation [2]. The distinctive feature of the new approach is that the blood perfusion and temperature is not constant through the model. Blood flow velocity vector field is defined together with the geometry and remains unchanged during simulations while blood temperature is calculated at every point in the model based on approximated heat exchange mechanism with tissue. As a result a non-constant blood temperature is obtained during simulations and new tissue temperature and temperature rise has been produced which appear to be slightly lower than the tissue temperature computed using conventional Pennes bio-heat model. The new blood flow model also produces different temperature rise distribution with the hot spots at slightly different locations compared to the conventional model.

3 Dipole Antennas

On Fig. 1 dependencies of peak 10g SAR and temperature rise on frequency are shown. As it can be seen from Fig. 1a and Fig. 1b minimal SAR and temperature rise for dipole antennas are observed around 900MHz. Due to complexity of the model and frequency dependent material properties, points of maximal SAR and temperature rise are located in different parts of the head and may not correspond to each other (Fig. 2). As a result graphs are not smooth and it is harder to make conclusions based on them. Since at lower frequencies field penetration depth is significantly deeper, peak values of SAR and temperature rise for inner parts of the model (e.g. brain, eye, etc.) are much higher for lower frequencies.

Starting from 1450 MHz the penetration depth of EM field is small and biggest part of radiated energy is absorbed at the surface, which in the studied model in most cases is the ear.

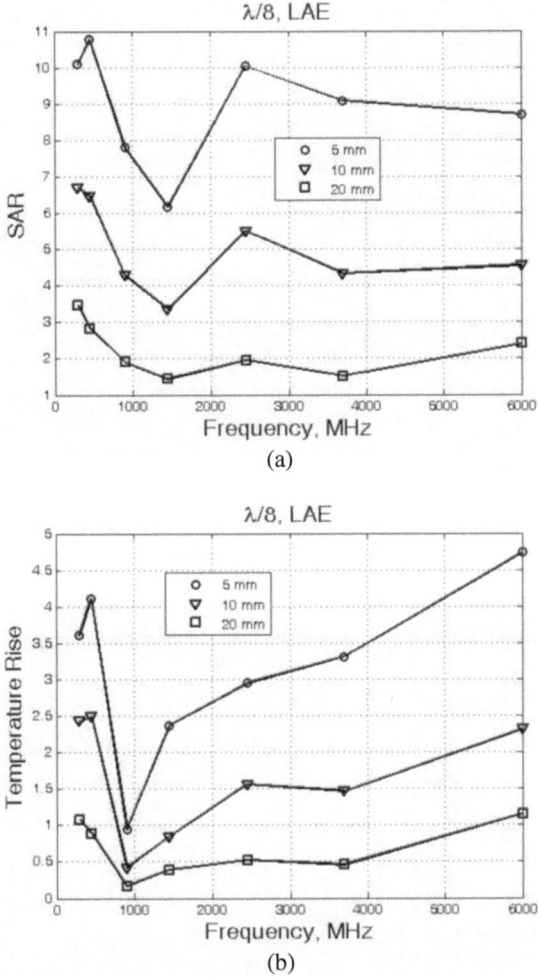

Fig. 1. (a) SAR on frequency. All data normalized to input power, (b) Temperature rise on frequency. All data normalized to input power.

As it can be seen from Fig. 2 location of peak temperature rise and SAR depend on particular case and may not correspond to each other. In this case match only locations of peak 1g SAR and temperature rise while the location of peak 10g SAR is in another part of the model. The geometry of the antenna and its placement can drastically affect resultant distributions of SAR and temperature rise.

The complexity of the geometry makes hard to predict the location of peak values and compare their values. When the field penetration depth is comparable with the linear dimensions of the model, a focusing effect can be observed Fig. 3.

As a result in order to obtain correct results the location of the dipole should be chosen in order to avoid focusing effects. But, if the position of device is changed during the communication process, the peak values are washed out and the impact could be smaller.

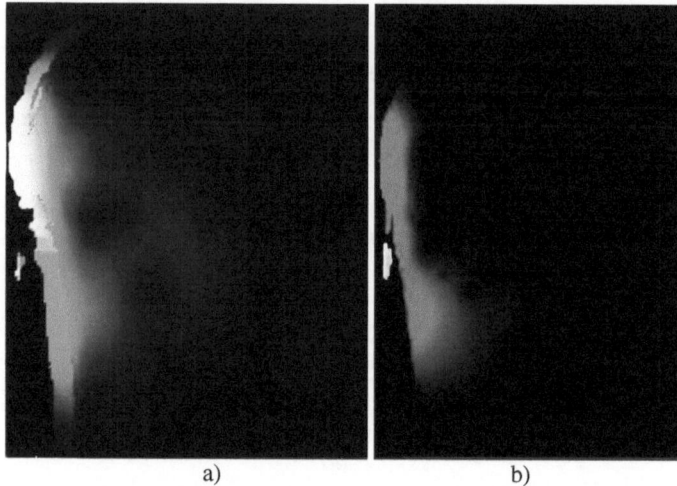

a)   b)

Fig. 2. Locations of peak a) 10g SAR =6.7w/kg b) temperature rise ΔT=0.36°C of λ/8-th Dipole Antenna for frequency 300 MHz, at 10 mm distance

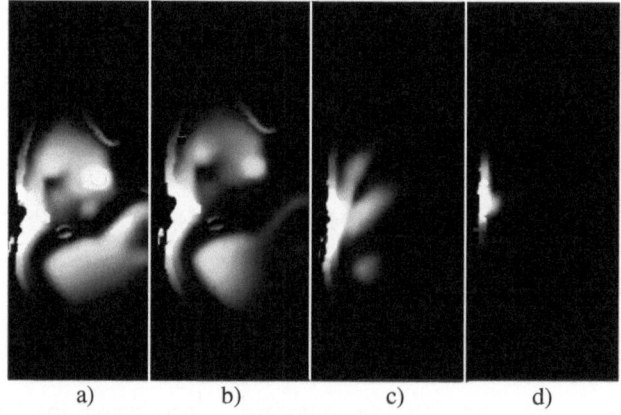

a)   b)   c)   d)

Fig. 3. Field penetration depth for λ/2-th dipole antennas. 1g SAR with frequencies: a) 300 MHz b) 450 MHz c) 1450 MHz and d) 3700 MHz.

4 Monopole Antennas

Resonant monopole antennas operating at (300, 900, 1450, and 1900) MHz were investigated in terms of this project. Temperature rise and SAR was the subject of study in all calculations. Antennas were placed at distances of 10 and 20 mm from the Duke Head model [1]. Three types of monopoles namely; the straight, the helical and the meander were mounted on top of a metal box. Simulations at 900 and 1900 MHz were done using XFDTD (at USC) while those at 300 and 1450 MHz were done using FDTDLab (at TSU).

A 1 mm uniform discretization was used. Each monopole was excited using a 1 mm gap excitation with a continuous wave sinusoidal source at corresponding frequency. All SAR and temperature rise data were normalized to 1W of power. The SAR and temperature rise data reflect the maximum absorption of power by the specific antenna under consideration. In XFDTD eight layers of PML were employed as absorbing boundaries in FDTDLab seven layers were used.

As it was expected, both SAR and temperature values decrease with the increase of distance. Since tissue thermal parameters like specific heat, heat conductivity, blood perfusion etc. are independent of frequency the temperature rise depends only on SAR. At fixed frequency SAR and temperature rise are in good correlation. Peak temperature rise values induce by different antennas may appear in different parts of the model (e.g. some are located in the earlobe while other may appear above the ear or in its middle). The maximal temperature rise $\Delta T=0.99°C$ and maximal 10g SAR=10.5 W/kg were observed at 1900 MHz for 10mm helical monopole. The minimal temperature rise $\Delta T=0.21°C$ was observed at several frequencies. Minimal peak 10g SAR was observed at 300MHz for straight monopole located at 20mm distance from the model.

It was noted the due to the complexity of the geometry and a asymmetrical radiation pattern of the antennas location of peak temperature rise and peak 10g SAR may not match. This fact makes analysis of SAR and T-rise correlation harder (Fig.2).

It was observed that in some 20mm the points of maximal temperature rise and 10g SAR match while at 10mm they do not. In such cases it is hard to expect good correlation between temperature rise and SAR.

5   PIFA Antennas

The second task consisted in examination of planar inverted-F antennas (PIFA) operating at, 1900 , 3700, and 6000 MHz. Antennas were placed at distances of 10 and 20 mm from the Duke head model. Two different orientations of the PIFA namely the conventional and the flipped were used. Simulations at 1900, 3700 and 6000 MHz were conducted using FDTDLab (at TSU). The distance „d" is calculated as the separation between the outer edge of the compressed ear and the surface of the metal box facing the metal strip of the PIFA. The time step for thermal calculations was 0.5 second for all antennas. The basal body temperature was considered as 37°C. Air at 23°C with a thermal conductivity of 0.026 Watt/meter/°C was used as the immersive medium.

The maximal temperature rise $\Delta T=4.68°C$ and maximal 10g SAR = 8.41 W/kg were observed at 6000 MHz 10mm PIFA antenna with flipped orientation. The minimal temperature rise $\Delta T=0.21°C$ was observed at 1900MHz for PIFA antenna with conventional orientation located at 20mm distance from the model.

Good correlation between SAR and temperature rise was observed at all frequencies. Although the temperature rise of 4.68 °C is high enough the resultant maximal temperature does not exceed 37°C. While conducting the calculations it was noted that antenna position may drastically affect resultant peak values of SAR and temperature rise and corresponding distributions.

The maximum ΔT exhibits a strong correlation with both peak 1-g avg. SAR and peak 10-g avg. SAR. Fig. 4 shows the peak ΔT values for the 1900, 3700 and 6000 MHz PIFAs plotted against the 10-g avg. SAR. Similar dependency is observed for 1g SAR. [10-12].

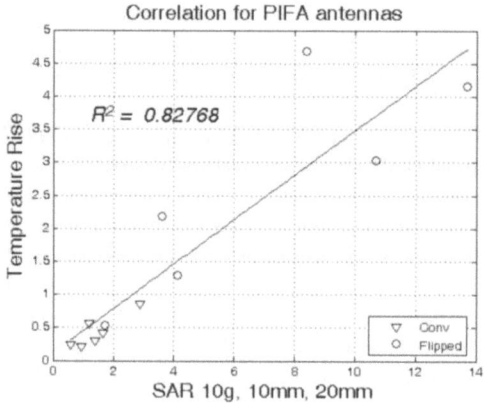

Fig. 4. Correlation between 10g SAR and temperature rise at 1900, 3700, 6000 frequencies

6   Additional Notes

The software package FDTDLab was enhanced with several new features. A new model of blood perfusion with directional capillary blood flow [2] taken into account was added to it along with such features like analyzing peak values for temperature rise and SAR for selected tissues and regions.

While the difference produced by two models was noticed, the thorough analysis is needed to quantify it. As an example the Fig. 5 shows the difference in temperature rise distribution computed for the same exposure condition using the conventional and new heat-exchange model.

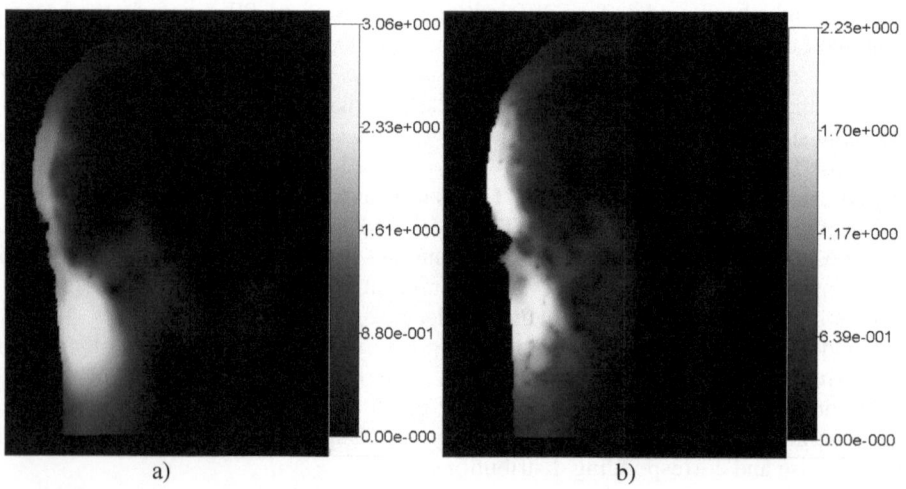

Fig. 5. Temperature rise for: a) Pennes model and b) modified model with new vascular structure model. SAR normalized to 1W input power.

Both models considered in this study are restricted to low power exposure conditions but may be extended to higher power levels by introducing reported in literature approximations of the basic thermal regulation mechanisms.

The modified model [2] is linear, and there is good correlation between peak 10g SAR values peek temperature rise values calculated according to it. At Fig. 5 calculations according to the modified model are presented. Fig. 5a shows temperature distribution according to conventional bio-heat equation, Fig. 5b distribution obtained according to the modified equation [2].The darker parts correspond to venous endings while the lighter areas to arterial endings where the blood penetrates into examined volume.

In addition to the described calculations using the Visible Human Model [1] a simplified model has been studied. [10],[11]. It appeared that presence of a hand affects the radiation pattern and the resultant SAR and temperature distributions.

7 Conclusions

Dipole, monopole, planar inverted-F antennas operating at 1900, 3700 and 6000 MHz were investigated. Peak values of specific absorption rate (SAR) and induced temperature rise in the Duke Head model were presented. Peak temperature rise ranged from 0.1°C to 4.7°C for all the antennas considered. Antennas in the flipped orientation in general induced much higher temperature rise than in the conventional. It was shown that geometry of the model and antenna radiation pattern drastically affects the resultant distributions of SAR and temperature rise [11]. In some cases peak values of SAR and/or temperature rise may change by 70% if antenna is shifted by 10mm in a plain parallel to the surface. This fact makes analysis much harder and in order to obtain valuable results each antenna at each distance should be studied separately.

References

1. Kuster, N.: IT'IS Foundation, http://www.itis.ethz.ch/
2. Prishvin, M., Manukyan, L., Zaridze, R.: Vascular Structure Model for Improved Numerical Simulation of Heat Transfer in Human Tissue. In: 20th International Zurich Symposium on Electromagnetic Compatibility, Zurich, Switzerland, January 12-16, pp. 261–264 (2009)
3. Bijamov, A., Razmadze, A., Shoshiashvili, L., Zaridze, R., Bit-Babik, G., Faraone, A.: Software for the electro-thermal simulation of the human exposed to the mobile antenna radiation. In: Proceedings of VIII-th International Seminar/Workshop on Direct and Inverse Problems of Electromagnetic and Acustic Wave Theory (DIPED 2003), Lviv, Ukraine, September 23-25, pp. 173–176 (2003),
http://www.ewh.ieee.org/soc/cpmt/ukraine/
4. Zaridze, R.S., Gritsenko, N., Kajaia, G., Nikolaeva, E., Razmadze, A., Shoshiashvili, L., Bijamov, A., Bit-Babik, G., Faraone, A.: Electro-Thermal Computational Suit for Investigation of RF Power Absorption and Associated Temperature Change in Human Body. In: 2005 IEEE AP-S International Symposium and USNC/URSI National Radio Science Meeting, Washington DC, USA, July 3-8, pp. 175–178 (2005)

5. Shoshiashvili, L., Razmadze, A., Jejelava, N., Zaridze, R., Bit-Babik, L.G., Faraone, A.: Validation of numerical bioheat FDTD model. In: Proceedings of XIth International Seminar/Workshop on Direct and Inverse Problems of Electromagnetic and Acoustic Wave Theory (DIPED 2006), Tbilisi, Georgia, October 11-13, pp. 201–204 (2006)
6. Islam, M.R., Razmadze, A., Zaridze, R., Bit-Babik, G., Ali, M.: Computed SAR and Temperature Rise in an Anatomical Head Model by Canonical Antennas. In: BEMS Annual Meeting, BEMS 2009 Congress Centre, Davos, Switzerland, June 14-19 (2009), http://bioem2009.org/technical-program/
7. Zaridze, R., Razmadze, A., Shoshiashvili, L., Kakulia, D., Bit-Babik, G., Faraone, A.: Influence of SAR Averaging Schemes on the Correlation with Temperature Rise in the 30-800 MHz Range. In: EUROEM 2008 European Electromagnetics, Swiss Federal Institute of Technology (EPFL), Lausanne, Switzerland, July 21-25, p. 120 (2008)
8. Bernardi, et al.: Specific Absorption Rate and Temperature Increases in the Head of a Cellular-Phone User. IEEE Trans. Microwave Theory Tech. 48(7), 1118–1126 (2000)
9. Razmadze, A., Shoshiashvili, L., Kakulia, D., Zaridze, R.: Influence on averaging masses on correlation between mass-averaged SAR and temperature rise. Journal of Applied Electromagnetism 10(2), 8–21 (2008), http://jae.ece.ntua.gr/JAE (December 2008/SAR and temperature rise Zaridze Paper 2.doc.pdf)
10. Mazmanov, D., Manukyan, L., Kakulia, D., Razmadze, A., Shoshiashvili, L., Zaridze, R.: MAS based software for the solving of diffraction and SAR problems on unbounded objects. In: Proceedings of XIth International Seminar/Workshop on Direct and Inverse Problems of Electromagnetic and Acoustic Wave Theory (DIPED 2006), Tbilisi, Georgia, October 11-13, pp. 11–16 (2006)
11. Zaridze, R., Prishvin, M., Tabatadze, V., Kakulia, D.: Hand Position Effect on SAR and Antenna Pattern in RF Exposure Study of a Human Head Model. In: BEMS 2009 Congress Centre, Davos, Technical Program, Switzerland, June 14-19 (2009), http://bioem2009.org/technical-program

Session 2

Mobile Health Technologies, Applications and Integrated Systems for Chronic Disease Monitoring and Management

A Logic Simplification Based on Expert System Application for TBC Diagnosis

Harun Sümbül[1] and Fatih Başçiftçi[2]

[1] Department of Electric and Electronic Engineering,
Gümüshane University 29100 Baglarbasi/Gümüshane, Turkey
harunsumbul@gmail.com
[2] Department of Electronics and Computer Education,
Selcuk University Alaeddin Keykubat Campus 42003 Selcuklu/Konya, Turkey
basciftci@selcuk.edu.tr

Abstract. Tuberculosis (TBC), caused by the bacterium My tuberculosis (Mtb), is a growing international health crisis [1]. TBC is one of the main causes of death produced by infectious illness and is responsible for almost 3 millions deaths every year [2]. In this study, a controlled Expert System (ES) have designed to diagnosis of TBC and truth table have created by considering the probabilities of TBC (12 symptom, $2^{12}=4096$ different cases). According to the probabilities of TBC, 6 different cases have accepted as output values and reduced rule bases have obtained. These output values have been processed by an ES and have tried to diagnosis of TBC with help to ES. We obtained very good results and the results of analyses carried out indicated that controls performed with ES provide less time, less probability, reliable and consistent diagnosis and that are feasible in real life.

Keywords: Logic Simplification, Logic Synthesis, Reduced Rule Bases, Expert System, TBC.

1 Introduction

TBC remains a global emergency with estimates of 1.8 millions deaths worldwide in 2008 and over 9 million cases. According to the World Health Organization (WHO) worldwide, disease mortality was approximately 1.5 million people, with 5 million new and relapse cases in 2005 [3]. In 2008, estimated global incidence rate fell to 139 cases per 100,00 population after reaching its peak in 2004 at 143 per 100,00. However, this decline was not homogeneous throughout WHO regions, with Europe failing to record a substantial decline, but rather appearing to have reached a stabilization of rates [4]. Despite effective antimicrobial chemotherapy, TBC remains a leading cause of death from an infectious disease [5]. Newly, infected persons may be identified by investigation of close contacts of an infectious case. The Centers for Disease Control and Prevention recommend identifying and offering therapy to all close contacts of persons with active TBC [6]. Twenty-two countries in the European Union (EU) and European Economic Area (EEA) reported treatment outcome monitoring

J. Lin and K.S. Nikita (Eds.): MobiHealth 2010, LNICST 55, pp. 27–34, 2011.
© Institute for Computer Sciences, Social Informatics and Telecommunications Engineering 2011

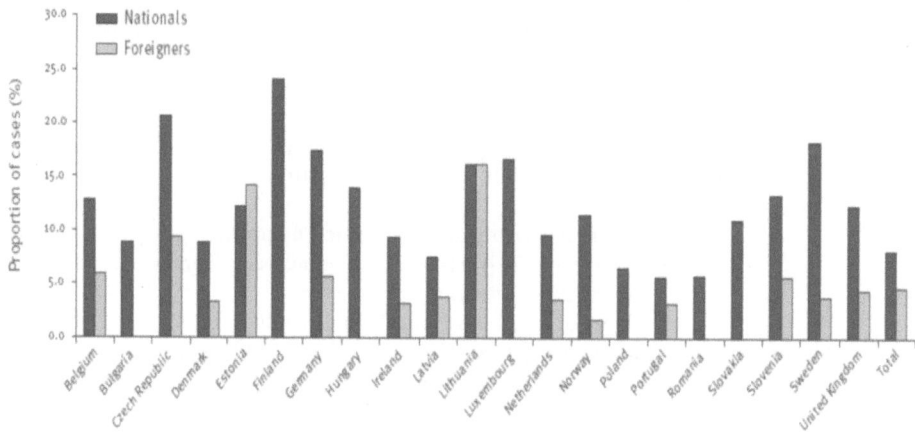

Fig. 1. Proportion of TBC death by geographic origin, EU/EEA countries, 2007 (EAA: European Economic Area; EU: European Union) [7]

data for culture-confirmed pulmonary TBC cases reported in 2007 [7]. We can see proportion of TBC deaths by geographic origin at Fig. 1.

As can be seen at Fig.1, TBC is a serious threat. Excluding countries at Fig.1 that did not or not in all years report cases. Worldwide there are roughly 12 million new active cases annually, and of those about 2 million will die every year [8].

2 Materials

TBC is one of the most common infectious diseases worldwide. In developing countries, TBC is associated with high morbidity and mortality rates. The disease is increasing in Western countries especially among immune compromised individuals such as patients who are HIV (Human Immunodeficiency Virus) infected [9].

Attention to TBC control in the EU, EEA and in the world has been raised in recent years through a number of initiatives, including the launching of a Framework Action Plan to Fight TBC in the EU. Among the key issues underlined in the Action Plan is the need to achieve and sustain acceptable levels of treatment success among all TBC patients [10].

2.1 TBC's Symptoms

- A cough that lasts (for more than 3 weeks)
- High fever (systematic symptom)
- Sweat (specially during night)
- Come out sputum and blood as coughing
- Loss of appetite
- Weight loss
- Weakness

- Weariness
- Hemoptysis
- Thorax, back and flank aches
- Shortness of breath (respiratory symptom)
- Hoarseness (in the future)

Special symptoms;

- Cough, Sputum, hemoptysis,
- Thorax, back and flank aches
- Heartbeat

2.2 Similar Diseases

There are some diseases like TBC because of symptoms and specialties. These diseases are; Primary TBC, Post Primary TBC, Sarcoidosis, Pleuritis and Mumps. These diseases have been explained detailly in resources [11–13, 14].

2.3 Expert System and Architecture

Expert Systems (ES) is a branch of Artificial Intelligence (AI). AI is the capability of a device such as a computer to perform task that would be considered intelligent if they were performed by a human [15]. An ES is a computer program that attempts to replicate the reasoning processes of expert and can make decisions and recommendations, or perform tasks, based on user input [16].

Rule-based ESs should contain, at the very least, the three components of an AI production system: the knowledge base; the database; the rule interpreter. You can see that structure at Fig. 2.

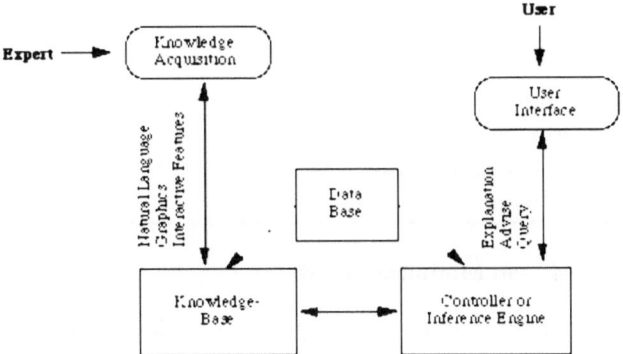

Fig. 2. An Expert System Structure

The knowledge base holds the set of rules of inference that are used in reasoning. Most of these systems use IF-THEN rules to represent knowledge. Typically systems can have from a few hundred to a few thousand rules. The database gives the context of the problem domain and is generally considered to be a set of useful facts. These are the facts that satisfy the condition part of the condition action rules as the IF THEN rules can be thought of. The rule interpreter is often known as an inference engine and controls the knowledge base using the set of facts to produce even more facts. Communication with the system is ideally provided by a natural language interface. This enables a user to interact independently of the expert with the intelligent system [17].

3 Method

To prevention of TBC, there are a lot of method, for instance a circuit-based simulation, using an antibody-based piezoelectric biosensor, fuzzy logic, image processing and neural computing, lazer therapy and so forth.. However, our used method that Logic Simplification Method is considerably a new method to diagnosis of TBC, including truth table, input and output values, reduced rule bases. In function, 4096 different cases evaluated for each one output function. Table 1 show below input and output values for function.

Table 1. Input, output cases and symbols

Input Symbols	Input Cases	Output Symbols	Output Cases
x1	A long lasting cough	y1	TBC
x2	High fever (systematic symptom)	y2	Primary TBC
x3	Sweat (specially during night)	y3	Post Primary TBC
x4	Come out sputum and blood as coughing	y4	Sarcoidosis
x5	Loss of appetite	y5	Pleuritis
x6	Weight loss	y6	Mumps
x7	Weakness		
x8	Weariness		
x9	Hemoptysis		
x10	Thorax, back and flank aches		
x11	Shortness of breath (respiratory symptom)		
x12	Hoarseness (in the future)		

3.1 Logic Synthesis and Minimization Method

Two-level logic minimization is a basic problem in logic synthesis [18, 19]. The minimization of Boolean Functions (BFs) can lead to more effective computer programs and circuits. A wide variety of Boolean minimization techniques have been explained in [18, 19, 20 and 21].

In order to simplify the formed function, Exact Direct Cover Minimization Algorithm has been developed. This algorithm is explained in [21]. Exact Direct Cover Minimization Method algorithm is given in below;

```
Minimization Algorithm (S_ON, S_OFF)
Begin
   start:
      if (S_ON =∅) then goto end
      TM ← select any On minterm from the S_ON set
      Call S_PI(TM) procedure
      if |S_PI(TM)|=1 then goto result
      Select PI which is cover the most minterm from
           the S_ON set
   result:
      S_EPI(TM) ← selected S_PI(TM)
      set of result ← S_EPI(TM)
      Call cover procedure
      goto start
   end:
End


Determination of S_PI(TM) Procedure
Begin
   1) Expand the elements of SOFF set by the TM X
   2) Remove from a result the non maximal cubes
   3) Subtract the result from the n-cube
      S_PI(TM)←(x)^n#(step 2)
   4) Return (S_PI(TM))
End


Cover Procedure
Begin
   S_ONi ← S_ON(i-1) # S_EPI (TM)
   S_EPI ← S_EPI ∪ S_EPI (TM)
   Return (S_ONi and S_EPI)
End
```

4 Results

TBC will continue to be the public health problem with more than one crore of patients at one time. The main hurdle in the control of TBC is poor cure rate (35%) due to high drop out because of long duration of treatment. With present strategy of treatment, the control of TBC is a far cry for several decades. In near future the situation will further deteriorate due to AIDS (Acquired Immune Deficiency Syndrome) and during resistance, unless and until some new methods of treatment are not used [22].

In this study; all the probabilities of the 12 symptoms which are the general symptoms of TBC and simplified output values have been evaluated (12 symptom, 2^{12}=4096 different cases and 6 different cases). In function, 4096 different cases evaluated for each one output function. In the reduction of symptoms, Logic Simplification Method has been used. By this method, reduced functions for each output have been obtained in Table 2.

The mean of 0, 1 and x which shows like simplification function at Table 2 is: For 0; there is not symptom For 1; there is a symptom. For x; it is not importing for symptom of represent disease who is ill person. For example; Disease probabilities and results for y3 have been given in table 3.

Table 2. Simplification output values

Output Symbols	Output Cases	Simplification funcion			
y1	TBC	010100000010	111x11011010	1111xx0xxxx1	1111xxxxx00x
		1111xxxxx1x0	1111xxx0xxxx	1111x0xxxxxx	1111xx1xxx1x
		11111xxxxxxx	1111xxxx1xxx		
y2	Primary TBC	1010x1101000	10101x101101	xx1x11xxx0x0	xx1x111xxxx1
		xx1x1101xxxx	xx1x11x0x1xx	xx1x11xxxx0x	xx1011xxxxxx
		x11x11xxxxxx	xx1x11xx1xxx	1x1x11xxxx1x	
y3	Post Primary TBC	101010101100	111xx11x1111		
y4	Sarcoidosis	1011101001x1	1011x01x0010	101000110x1x	1x101x10001x
		101x011x011x	101xxxx1x01x	1111xx1xxx1x	1x1xxxx1xx11
		1x1x0xx0xx1x	1x1xx00xxx1x	1x1xxxx0x11x	1x11xxxxx11x
		1x1x11xxxx1x	1x11xxxx1x1x	1x1xxxxx111x	110xxxxxxx1x
		11x0xxxxxx1x			
y5	Pleuritis	xxxxxxx111xx			
y6	Mumps	101010101010	111110111x11	xxxx1x1x11xx	xxx0xx1x11x1
		0xx1xx1x11xx	x0xxxx1x11x0	xxxxx11111xx	11xxxx1x11xx
		xx0xxx1x11xx	xxxxx01x11xx	xxxxxx1x111x	

Table 3. Symptoms, Output Cases and results for y3

Output Symbols	Cases	Symptom and Output Cases											
		x1	x2	x3	x4	x5	x6	x7	x8	x9	x10	x11	x12
y3	Post Primer TBC 101010101100	1	0	1	0	1	0	1	0	1	1	0	0
y3	Post Primer TBC 111xx11x1111	1	1	1	x	x	1	1	x	1	1	1	1

According to Table 3, the mean of 101010101100 output values; we can say Post Primer TBC a person which has x1, x3, x5, x7, x9, x10 probabilities and has not x2, x4, x6, x8, x11, x12 probabilities. Furthermore, if we want to see the result (for 101010101100) in a ES;

Rule: *IF* x1 is 1 and x3 is 1 and x5 is 1 and x7 is 1 and x9 is 1and x10 is 1 and x2 is 0 and x4 is 0 and x6 is 0 and x8 is 0 and x11 is 0 and x12 is 0 *THEN* patient is Post Primary TBC.

Table 4. Rule table for y3 output

IF	input												THEN	output
	x1	x2	x3	x4	x5	x6	x7	x8	x9	x10	x11	x12		Y3
	1	0	1	0	1	0	1	0	1	1	0	0		Primary TBC

In conclusion, we thing that use logic simplify method might be used as a reliable in ascertain for TBC.

References

1. May, E., Leitao, A., Faulon, J.L., Joo, J., Misra, M., Oprea, T.: Understanding Virulence Mechanisms in TBC İnfection Via a Circuit-Based Simulation Framework. In: 30th Annual International Conference of IEEE, pp. 4953–4955 (2008)
2. Lenseigne, B., Brodin, P., Hee Kyoung, J., Christophe, T., Genovesio, A.: Support Vector Machines For Automatic Detection Of Tuberculosis Bacteria In Confocal Microscopy Images. In: 4th IEEE International Symposium on Biomedical Imaging: From Nano to Macro 2007, pp. 85–88 (2007)
3. World Health Organization, Global Health Atlas,
   http://www.who.int/globalatlas/
4. Global tuberculosis control: a short update to the 2009 report, Geneva: World Health Organization (2009),
   http://www.who.int/tb/publications/global_report/
   2009/update/tbu_9.pdf
5. Ferebee, S.: Controlled chemoprophylaxis trials in TBC. A General Review 26, 28–106 (1970)
6. Tuberculosis elimination revisited: obstacles, opportunities, and a renewed commitment. Advisory Council for the Elimination of Tuberculosis (ACET). MMWR Morb. Mortal Wkly Rep. 48(RR-9), 1–13 (1999)
7. Manissero, D., Hollo, V., Huitric, E., Ködmön, C., Amato-Gauci, A.: Analysis of tuberculosis treatment outcomes in the European Union and European Economic Area Report (2010)
8. Chakrabarti, P.: Early, Easy, Inexpensive Diagnosis An Urgent Need for Global TBC Control. In: Frontiers in the Convergence of Bioscience and Information Technologies, FBIT 2007, pp. 241–244 (2007)
9. Mehta, S., Gilada, I.S.: Global Tuberculosis Control Surveillance, planning, financing. WHO Report 13, 87–89 (2005)
10. Fernandez de la Hoz, K., Manissero, D.: On behalf of the Tuberculosis Disease Programme. A Framework Action Plan to Fight Tuberculosis in the European Union 13(12), 74–80 (2008)
11. Erbaycu, A.E., Güçlü, S.Z.: Sarkoidozve Tüberküloz: Benzerlikler Farklılıklar, Sarkoidoz Etyolojisinde Mikobakterilerin Rolü. İzmir Göğüs Hastalıkları ve Tüberküloz Kliniği 16, 95–101 (2005)
12. Hendee, J.C.: An expert system for marina environmental monitoring in the Florida Keys National Marine Sanctuary and Florida Bay. In: Brebbia, C.A. (ed.) Proceedings of the Second International Conference on Environmental Coastal Regions, pp. 57–66. Computational Mechanics Publicationas/WIT Press, Southampton (1998)
13. http://www.cs.cf.ac.uk/Dave/AI1/mycin.html
14. Demircan, S., Uzar, A., Topçu, S.: Tüberkülozda cerrahi endikasyonlar. Solunum Hastalıkları Dergisi 8, 643–650 (1997)
15. Mockler, R.J., Dologite, D.G.: Knowledge-Based Systems. In: An Introduction to Expert Systems. Macmillan Publishing, New york (1992)

16. Zengin, K., Taksin, M., Cicek, Y., Unal, E., Ferahman, M., Dogusoy, G.: Primary Gastric Tuberculosis Mimicking Gastric Tumor that Results in Pyloric Stenosis Eur. Surg. 35, 220–221 (2003)
17. FitzGerald, J.M., Mayo, J.R., Miller, R.R., Jamieson, W.R., Baumgartner, F.: Tuberculosis of the thymus. Chest 102, 1604–1605 (1992)
18. Sasao, T.: Worst and Best Irredundant Sum-of–Product Expressions. IEEE Transactions on Computers 50(9), 935–947 (2001)
19. Mishchenco, A., Sasao, T.: Large-Scale SOP Minimization Using Decomposition and Functional Properties. In: IEEE CNF, Design Automation Conference, Proceedings, pp. 149–154 (2003)
20. Kahramanli, S., Başçiftçi, F.: Boolean Functions Simplification Algorithm of O(N) Complexity. Journal of Mathematical and Computational Applications 8(4), 271–278 (2002)
21. Başçiftçi, F.: Local Simplification Algorithms for Switching Functions. PhD Thesis, Graduate School of Natural and Applied Sciences, Selcuk University (2006)
22. Anand, A.L.: Role of laser therapy in management of "treatment failure" cases of pulmonary tuberculosis as an adjuvant to chemotherapy. In: Engineering in Medicine and Biology Society, 1995 and 14th Conference of the Biomedical Engineering Society of India, pp. 4/111–4/112. IEEE, Los Alamitos (1995)

On Assessing Motor Disorders in Parkinson's Disease

Markos G. Tsipouras[1], Alexandros T. Tzallas[1], Evanthia Tripoliti[1], Georgios Rigas[1],
Panagiota Bougia[1], Dimitrios I. Fotiadis[1], Sofia Tsouli[2], and Spyridon Konitsiotis[2]

[1] Unit of Medical Technology and Intelligent Information Systems, Department of Material Science and Engineering, University of Ioannina, 45110 Ioannina, Greece
[2] Department of Neurology, Medical School, University of Ioannina, 45110 Ioannina, Greece
{markos,evi,rigas,fotiadis}@cs.uoi.gr
{atzallas,pbougia,skonitso}@cc.uoi.gr

Abstract. In this paper we propose an automated method for assessing motor symptoms in Parkinson's disease. Levodopa-induced dyskinesia (LID) and Freezing of Gait (FoG) are detected based on the analysis of signals recorded from wearable devices, i.e. accelerometers and gyroscopes, which are placed on certain positions on the patient's body. The signals are initially pre-processed and then analyzed, using a moving window, in order to extract features from them. These features are used for LID and FoG assessment. Two classification techniques are employed, decision trees and random forests. The method has been evaluated using a group of patients and the obtained results indicate high classification ability, being 96.11% classification accuracy for FoG detection and 92.59% for LID severity assessment.

Keywords: Parkinson's disease motor symptoms assessment, Levodopa-induced dyskinesia, Freezing of Gait, accelerometer, gyroscope.

1 Introduction

Parkinson's disease (PD) is a disorder that affects nerve cells in a part of the brain that controls muscle movement. Symptoms of PD may include resting tremor, bradykinesia, rigidity, forward stopped posture, postural instability and freezing of gait (FoG) [1]. Levodopa is highly effective in reducing the symptoms of the disease and remains the standard drug for patients suffering from PD [2]. However, long-term levodopa treatment is often complicated by significantly disabling fluctuations and dyskinesias, referred as levodopa-induced dyskinesias (LIDs).

FoG is a paroxysmal phenomenon commonly seen as an advanced symptom in PD. The FoG events are transient, generally lasting for a few seconds, tending to increase in frequency as the disease progresses [3]. The management of FoG is difficult and often ineffective [4]. Clinical assessment of FoG is largely based on subjective patient reports, such as the Unified Parkinson's Disease Rating Scale (UPDRS). Only a few computerized methods, for the detection of the FoG symptoms, have been presented in the literature. These can be grouped into two basic categories: a) those which are based on the analysis of electromyography signals, and b) those which are based on motion signal analysis [3, 4].

J. Lin and K.S. Nikita (Eds.): MobiHealth 2010, LNICST 55, pp. 35–38, 2011.
© Institute for Computer Sciences, Social Informatics and Telecommunications Engineering 2011

LID is a disabling and distressing complication of chronic levodopa therapy in patients who suffered from PD [2]. LID symptoms can be rated in various ways by their topography (affected body regions) and their duration or consistency [2]. Thus, their detection and assessment during daily activities is of great interest. Current LID assessment mainly relies on clinical methods [2, 5] which lack of objectivity and they are not feasible for long-term assessment. To overcome these limitations several computer-based methods are developed using quantitative instrumental techniques such as: accelerometers and gyroscopes [5, 6], electromyography (surface) [7], force gauges [7], position transducers [8] and Doppler ultrasound systems [5, 7]. An important drawback of the aforementioned studies is that they employ a small number of motor tasks that have been performed in laboratory settings.

In this study we propose a three-stage methodology for the automated detection of FoG events and LID severity assessment using signals received from accelerometers/gyroscopes placed on different positions of the patient's body. In the first stage the pre-processing of the signals is performed, while a feature vector is extracted (for each second of the recorded signals) in the second stage. In the third stage this feature vector is used for FoG and LID assessment using Decision Tree (DT) and Random Forests (RF) algorithms.

2 Materials and Methods

In this study 16 subjects are enrolled with 24 recordings, 5 healthy subjects and 11 PD patients presenting all types of PD motor disabilities such as tremor, dyskinesia, FoG and LID (Table 1). The movements and postures are automatically measured using accelerometers/gyroscopes and a portable data recorder. Six sets of three orthogonal accelerometers are used, which are placed at: right and left wrist (RW, LW), right and left leg (RL, LL), chest (CH) and waist (WS). Additionally, two gyroscopes are used, that are placed in the chest and waist. All sensors transmit data using ZigBee protocol to a portable PC equipped with data acquisition hardware and software to collect and store the signals. Sampling rate is set to 62.5 Hz.

Table 1. Number of recordings and motor disabilities for PD patients

Patient Number	Number of recordings	Tremor	Bradykinesia	FOG	LID
1	4	√	√	√	
2	1			√	
3	1				
4	3	√	√	√	√
5	2				
6	2				√
7	2			√	√
8	1		√	√	
9	1				√
10	1				√
11	1				√

2.1 Methodology

In the first stage of the methodology, pre-processing of the signals is applied. The missing values, presented since there is loss of data in case of disconnection of a wireless sensor from the base station, are reconstructed using linear interpolation. Then, a finite impulse response (FIR) high-pass filter is used in order to remove the low frequency components of the raw signal.

The processed signals are used for feature extraction. A moving window with 2 second duration and 1 second overlapping is used and, for each window, the mean entropy is calculated as:

$$e_i(j) = \sum_{n=w(j)-fs}^{w(j)+fs}(p(x_i(n))logp(x_i(n)),\tag{1}$$

where $e_i(j)$ is the entropy of the j-th window for the i-th signal, fs is the sampling frequency, $w(j)$ is the time position of the j-th window, $x_i(n)$ is the n-th sample of the i-th signal and $p(x_i(n))$ is the probability of $x_i(n)$ (calculated using the histogram of x_i). Since eight sensors are used and each sensor records three signals, one for each axis (x,y and z axis), a total of 24 signals are collected and thus the feature vector characterizing each window contains 24 features (entropy for each axis for each sensor). However, several different experimental settings have been used, related to the selection of sensors which are employed. For each one of them, the number of features in the feature vector may vary based on the number of used sensors.

The feature vector is used for the assessment of each window of the signal related to FoG and LID. For this purpose, two classification techniques have been tested, decision trees (DT) and random forests (RF) [9]. A DT represents the acquired knowledge in the form of a tree. In order to construct the decision tree we use the C4.5 inductive algorithm [10]. This algorithm has the advantage of solving the overfitting problem by employing a post pruning technique which is based on the pessimistic error rate (sub-tree replacement). RF is a classifier consisting of a collection of tree-structured classifiers. Each classifier votes for one of the classes and an instance being classified is labeled with the winning class. For the construction of each tree of the forest a new subset of samples is selected from the dataset (bootstrap sample). The tree is built to the maximum size without pruning. In our study the RF consists of 10 trees.

3 Results and Discussion

Several different experimental settings (sensors selection) have been evaluated with two classification techniques (DT and RF) for FoG detection and LID severity assessment. For each one of the experimental settings, results are obtained in terms of classification accuracy, while the 10-fold stratified cross validation technique is used in all cases. The various combinations of signals used in each experimental setting and the obtained classification accuracy for DT and RF techniques, for both FoG detection and LID assessment are presented in Table 2.

Table 2. Experimental settings and classification accuracy results (%) using DT and RF classification techniques, for FoG detection and LID severity assessment

Sensors	Number of features	FoG Detection		LID assessment	
		DT	RF	DT	RF
LW,RW	6	-	-	89.01%	91.46%
LL,RL	6	93.74%	93.90%	89.99%	90.07%
CH	6	92.68%	93.11%	89.82%	90.81%
WS	6	93.13%	94.00%	90.29%	91.21%
LW,RW,LL,RL	12	94.83%	95.89%	90.54%	91.19%
CH,LW,RW,LL,RL	18	94.45%	96.05%	92.33%	92.81%
WS,LW,RW,LL,RL	18	94.57%	96.07%	92.23%	92.33%
CH,WS,LW,RW,LL,RL	24	95.08%	96.11%	92.58%	92.59%

The proposed methodology aims to automatically detect FoG events and LID assessment severity in patients with PD using features extracted from accelerometer and gyroscope sensors. The obtained results indicate high efficiency in distinguishing FoG and LID from other PD symptoms and in LID severity classification. Also, the methodology is able to deal with FoG detection and LID asessment under real-life conditions, since it has been developed using a dataset that reflects real-life conditions, since it includes all kinds of symptoms that a PD patient may suffer from and a variety of voluntary movements.

References

1. Braak, H., Ghebremedhin, E., Rub, U., Bratzke, H., Del Tredici, K.: Stages in the development of Parkinson's disease-related pathology. Cell. Tissue Res. 318, 121–134 (2004)
2. Jankovic, J.: Parkinson's disease: clinical features and diagnosis. J. Neurol. Neurosurg. Psychiatry. 79, 368–376 (2008)
3. Giladi, N., Treves, T.A., Simon, E.S., Shabtai, H., Orlov, Y., Kandinov, B., et al.: Freezing of gait in patients with advanced Parkinson's disease. J. Neural Transm. 108, 53–61 (2001)
4. Fahn, S.: The freezing phenomenon in Parkinson's disease. In: Fahn, S., Hallet, M., Luuders, H.O., Marsden, C.D. (eds.) Negative Motor Phenomena, pp. 53–63. Lippincott–Raven, Philadelphia (1995)
5. Keijsers, N.L., Horstink, M.W., Gielen, S.C.: Online Monitoring of Dyskinesia in Patients with Parkinson's disease. IEEE Eng. Med. Biol. Mag. 22, 96–103 (2003)
6. Burkhard, P.R., Shale, H., Langston, L.W., Tetrud, J.W.: Quantification of dyskinesia in Parkinson's disease: validation of a novel instrumental method. Mov. Disord. 14, 754–763 (1999)
7. Hoff, J.I., van Hilten, J.J., Roos, R.A.: A review of the assessment of dyskinesias. Mov. Disord. 14, 737–743 (2001)
8. Chelaru, M.I., Duval, C., Jog, M.: Levodopa-induced dyskinesias detection based on the complexity of involuntary movements. J. Neurosc. Meth. 186, 81–89 (2010)
9. Breiman, L.: Random Forests. Machine Learning 45, 5–32 (2001)
10. Quinlan, J.R.: C4.5. Morgan Kauffman, San Mateo (1993)

An Intelligent System for Classification of Patients Suffering from Chronic Diseases

Christos Bellos[1], Athanasios Papadopoulos[1],
Dimitrios I. Fotiadis[1], and Roberto Rosso[2]

[1] FORTH BRI Foundation for Research and Technology - Hellas, Biomedical Research,
Ioannina Greece
[2] TESAN Telematic & Biomedical Services S.p.A., Vicenza Italy
cbellos@cc.uoi.gr, thpapado@cc.uoi.gr, fotiadis@cs.uoi.gr,
rosso@tesan.it

Abstract. The CHRONIOUS system addresses a smart wearable platform, based on multi-parametric sensor data processing, for monitoring people suffering from chronic diseases in long-stay setting. An intelligent system, placed at a Smart Assistant Device, analyzes incoming data, facilitating data mining techniques and decides upon the severity of a probably pathological episode. Part of the intelligent system is the Mental Support Tool, which calculates a stress index and classifies the mental condition and stress levels of the patient. An additional component aiming at the personalization of the monitoring system is the Profiler which defines several patients' profiles and facilitates clustering techniques in order to associate each resulting cluster with one of the predefined profiles.

Keywords: Personalized treatment, Wearable Monitoring, Management of chronic disease.

1 Introduction

The CHRONIOUS system defines a European framework addressing people with chronic health conditions. In particular, it intervenes on the field of two chronic pathologies, chronic obstructive pulmonary disease (COPD) [1] and chronic kidney disease (CKD) [2], these being widespread and highly expensive pathologies in terms of social costs [3]. The CHRONIOUS goals achieved by developing a multidisciplinary, sophisticated, and adaptive chronic disease platform that integrates state of the art sensors and services in order to cover both patients and healthcare professional's needs [4], [5].

An open architecture design has been used to exploit the benefits of the final platform upon other chronic diseases, besides COPD and CKD. The system,as depicted in Fig. 1, consists of six primary functional blocks, which are the Sensors Framework, Data Handler (DH), Home Patient Monitor (HPM), Smart Assistant Device, CHRONIOUS Central System and Clinician Framework. Each block interacts to each other as well as with thetwo secondary functional blocks, which are the Communication Module to connect the primary blocks to each other and maintain interoperability

J. Lin and K.S. Nikita (Eds.): MobiHealth 2010, LNICST 55, pp. 39–46, 2011.
© Institute for Computer Sciences, Social Informatics and Telecommunications Engineering 2011

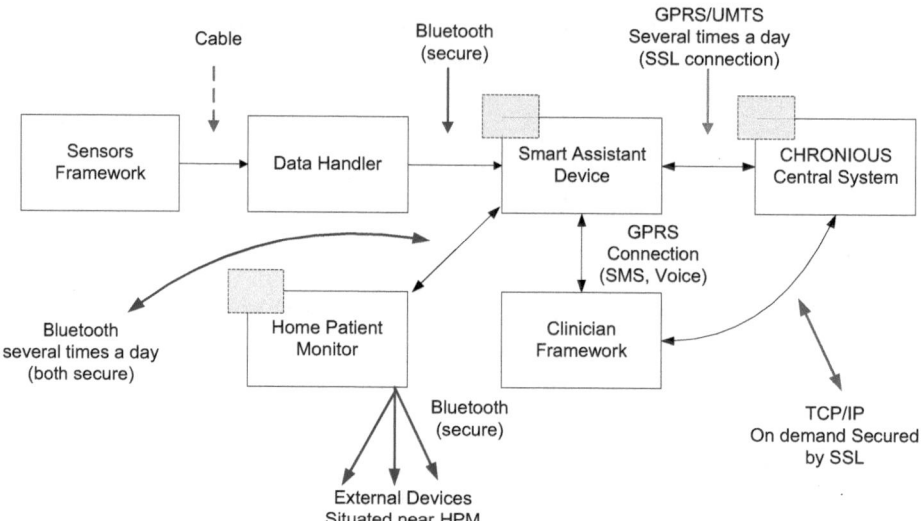

Fig. 1. The functional blocks of the CHRONIOUS system

and efficiency and the External Devices constituting by Body Weight Device, a Blood Pressure, a Blood Glucose Device and a Spyrometer device.

2 System Overview

The Sensors Framework is one of the most critical parts of the system. It consists of a tight-fitting and washable shirt which provides the support for the stabilization of the body sensor network. Several miniature sensor devices utilizing non-invasive methods are responsible for the recording of the characteristic signals and their further transmission for the analysis. The types of sensors which are utilized in this framework are: a 3-lead Electrocardiogram (ECG), a microphone as a context-audio sensor, a pulse oximeter, two respiration bands, an accelerometer and a sensor for measuring humidity as well as body and ambient temperature. Their position at the wearable jacket as well as their connectivity with the Data Handler device are shown in Fig. 2.

The data handler device is placed on the wearable part of the system at the lower part of the shirt. It has been designed and developed aiming at the collection of all the signals coming from the body sensor network. However, its role is the accurate collection and the transmission of the vital signals wirelessly – via a Bluetooth connection– to the Smart Assistant Device for their analysis.

The CHRONIOUS system facilitates several data mining techniques to extract knowledge and classify patient's health status with different levels of severity. These techniques are being nested in three different modules with various functionalities which interact to each other: The Patient Profiler placed in Central System; The Mental Support Tools and the Decision Support System formulating the CHRONIOUS Intelligence with emergency-direct feedback, which are placed in Smart Assistant Device.

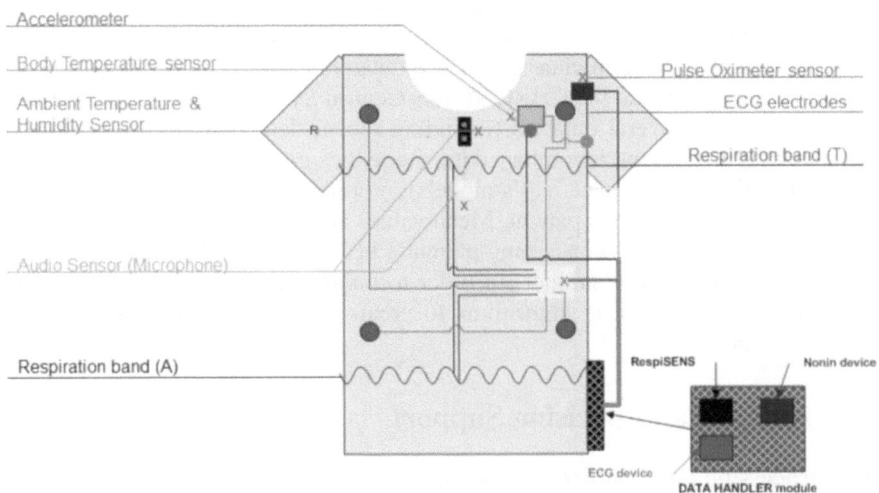

Fig. 2. The Sensors Framework integrated with the Data Handler device

The CHRONIOUS Intelligence constitutes of several sub-modules whose responsibility is to analyze the incoming data from the various sources, extract the useful features and retrieve knowledge using data mining techniques. In order to eliminate the energy consumption of the Sensors Framework and the Smart Assistant Device, a mechanism has been implemented as an add-on value to the integrated system. Several threshold values of the most critical signals are computed and stored in the Data Handler's (DH) memory. Each time these computations result to values outside the normal ranges, the Smart Assistant Device is restored from stand-by to normal mode.

The Decision Support System (DSS) is placed at CHRONIOUS intelligence core and constitutes one of the most important modules of the CHRONIOUS platform. Physically, it is installed and functions in the Smart Assistant Device. This module is an intelligent sub-system [6], combining an expert rule-based system and a supervised classification system, which may be an artificial neural network (aNN). The intelligent sub-system is responsible to categorize any abnormalities in the acquired data, evaluate the severity of the situation and provide an advice/recommendation and/or an alert to a caregiver/clinician regarding the health status of the patient. In case no abnormal situation has been tracked, the DSS takes no action and remains deactivated until the next pack of data are acquired. This triggering process takes part in the DH device when the values of the collected signal exceed the appropriate threshold for the specific patient. The normal ranges for each patient were extracted during the initial setup of the system(training phase), which is held several days before the real recording of patient's data.

Besides DSS, a patient's Mental Support Tool, located at CHRONIOUS Intelligence, is being implemented aiming in the control of patient's mental state and the parameters that affect it, in terms of detecting them on-time and providing the appropriate feedback to elevate patient's moral and strengthen his/her mental health. The purpose of this tool is to effectively detect and alert the patient for a stressful and possibly harmful condition in which he may be, by monitoring environmental parameters such as noise or air quality, physical parameters such as physical activity, heart rate variability (HRV), body temperature, blood pressure and all the parameters which are identified by the clinicians as stress indicators.

Patient Profiler, located at the CHRONIOUS Central System, aims at creating a patient model by using several datasets (including recent data acquired by sensors or inserted manually by patient, laboratory data, guidelines given by clinicians and clinical models including previous patient's models) in order to achieve personalization of the severity estimation for each patient. Mean values and variations of the most recent acquired data as well as data concerning patient's history, are input to the expert system (Patient Personal Model Trainer) in order to build a more dynamic profile. The Patient Profiler uses clustering algorithms to create a new, more personalized and accurate patient profile.

3 Data Analysis and Decision Support

3.1 Pre-processing and Feature Extraction

In CHRONIOUS platform, data acquired by sensors are being encapsulated in XML files by the Data Handler. The XML file that is being formed and transmitted contains the acquired data, error codes that might have occurred and threshold values indicated by the user.Several thresholds of the values of the wearable sensors as well as specific rules, specified and validated by clinicians, have been inserted in the kernel of the Data Handler to perform a preliminary validation of the patient's current health status. In case the system identifies an abnormal value, the Data Handler transmits a triggering signal, accompanied with the sensors' recent values, to the Smart Assistant Device for an advanced an analytical estimation of the current situation. Nevertheless, incoming data are complex enough to deter knowledge extraction and a pre-processing stage has been foreseen. The Feature Extraction Module applies XML de-encapsulation and reconstructs the acquired signal. In addition, de-noising and analysis methods are being applied specifically for the three continuous signals: ECG, audio and accelerometer signal.

The last phase of signal processing is the Feature Extraction which extracts the required features that have been indicated by clinicians or characterized as features with high diagnostic value by the evaluation process. These features constitute the attributes facilitated by the Intelligent System.There are several measures that can be obtained by the above mentioned signals, either in time or in frequency domain. The most important features, with a short description, are:

Heart rate variability (HRV). Is a physiological phenomenon where the time interval between heart beats varies. It is measured by the variation in the beat-to-beat interval. The HRV can be directly derived from the RR interval, using the formula:

$$HRV = \frac{60}{RR} \tag{1}$$

SDNN (msec). Standard deviation of all normal RR intervals in the entire ECG recording,

$$SDNN = \sqrt{\frac{1}{n}\sum_{i=1}^{n}(NN_i - m)^2}, \tag{2}$$

where NN_i is the duration of the i_{th} NN interval in the analyzed ECG, n is the number of all NN intervals, and m is their mean duration.

SDANN (msec). Standard deviation of the mean of the normal RR intervals for each 5 minutes period of the ECG recording.

SDNNIDX (msec). Mean of the standard deviations of all normal RR intervals for all 5 minutes segments of the ECG recording.

pNN50 (%). Percent of differences between adjacent normal RR intervals that are greater than 50 msec, computed over the entire ECG recording.

r-MSSD (msec). Square root of the mean of the sum of the squares of differences between adjacent normal RR intervals over the entire ECG recording

$$rMSSD = \sqrt{\frac{1}{n-1}\sum_{i=1}^{n-1}(NN_{i+1} - NN_i)^2}, \tag{3}$$

where NN_i is the duration of the i_{th} NN interval in the analyzed ECG and n is the number of all NN intervals.

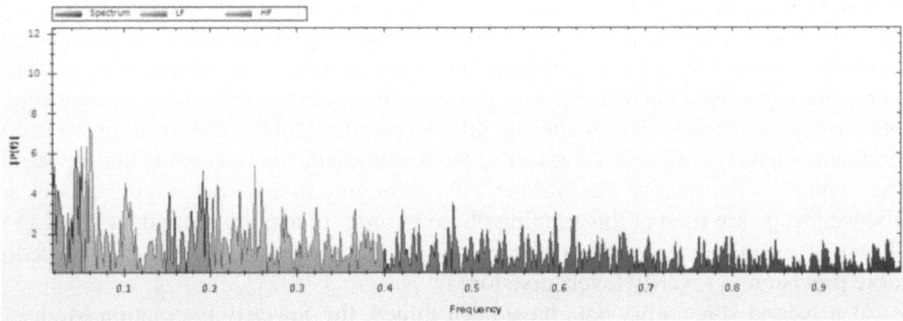

Fig. 3. The spectrum of HRV and the extracted Low–Frequency band (LF) and High–Frequency band (HF)

Regarding the frequency domain features, the main features involve sub-band powers. More specifically, the two bands that were utilized in the analysis are (Fig. 3):

The *Low–Frequency band* (LF), which includes frequencies in the area [0.03 – 0.15] Hz, the *High–Frequency band* (HF), which includes frequencies in the area [0.15 – 0.40] Hz and the ratio *LF/HF* is also utilized.

From the Respiration signal the more diagnostic features that have been extracted are:

Respiration Rate – The number of breaths per minute determined by the identification of the peaks of the respiration signal as displayed in Fig. 4.

Tidal Volume (VT). The normal volume of the air inhaled after an exhalation.

Vital capacity (VC). The volume of a full expiration. This metric depends on the size of the lungs, elasticity, integrity of the airways and other parameters.

Residual volume (VR). The volume that remains in the lungs following maximum exhalation.

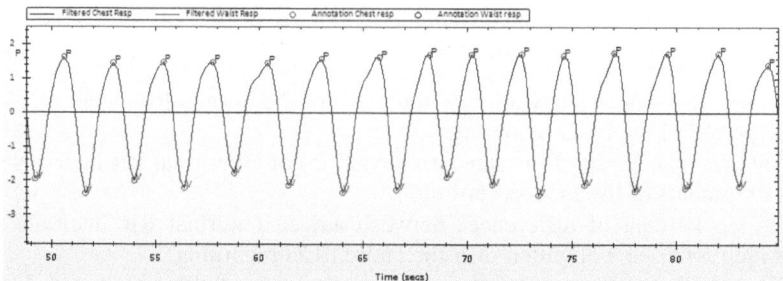

Fig. 4. Identification of the respiration signal peaks

3.2 Intelligent System

The DSS operates on demand, being triggered either by the Stand-by end mode Module, located at DH or by an internal clock a couple of times per day. Afterwards, the data are processed by an expert rule-based system and a supervised classification system running in parallel. The rule-based system is being used to make a first categorization of the nature of the severity of the episode and accompanies the output of the classifier in order to give an explanation of the severity assessment. On the other hand, the supervised classifier is being trained only during the training phase (once) and evaluates the severity of the identified episode. During this (training) session, clinicians identify different values of severity and mark the thresholds that divide the five layers of abnormality. Several patients, belonging to different staging classes and disease levels, are used at this training phase in order to acquire more data, track more abnormal events and improve the accuracy of categorization system by succeeding more precision in severity levels division.

At a second stage, after data have been mined, the Severity Estimation Module is being triggered, using simple if-then rules, in order to classify the decision of Decision Support Component and corresponding that with the respective action. These rules correlate the output of DSS with pre-specified thresholds, which have been indicated by clinicians and stored at CHRONIOUS repository.

An add-on value to CHRONIOUS Intelligence is the Mental Support Tool, where a stress index parameter is being calculated using a rule-based system. These rules have been formed after cooperation with clinicians in order to have clinical justification and physical meaning in real life scenarios. According to identified stress levels, there have been indicated four levels of stress: Normal, Mild, Moderate and Severe. In addition, the system provides to the patient the appropriate feedback (advice/alert) to assist him/her to overcome his/her stressful situation.

3.3 Applied Protocol and Classification Methods

Two healthy volunteers were recruited to the breath-down protocol based on the University of California, Institutional Review Board (UCSF-IRB) regulations [7]. Informed consent was obtained from volunteers prior to study commencement. The initial dataset is split to 11 instances with an applied time window and the 10 folds cross-validation method is used for testing.

Several algorithms have been utilized for the classification procedure. Mainly decision trees [8] have been explored since can classify both categorical and numerical data and are easy to understand which is crucial for the initial validation of the system. PARtial decision Trees [9]creates rules by repeatedly generating partial decision trees and builds a rule, while the J48 [8] algorithm generates a classification–decision tree for the given dataset by recursive partitioning of data. The Random tree [10] is a tree drawn at random from a set of possible trees and Naïve Bayes [11]is a simple probabilistic classifier.A multilayer perceptron (MLP) [12] is a feed-forward aNN model that consists of multiple layers of nodes in a directed graph. Due to the preliminary phase of the analysis and the small amount of collected data, the aNN has one hidden layer that isn't properly trained. Finally, Support Vector Machines (SVM) [13] have been developed and used for the classification system, but their proper training is still pending since the collected data aren't enough.

A preliminary implementation of the several supervised classifiers that are used for the initial analysis has been performed, but their performance isn't the same with the final that will conclude after the collection of more healthy and pathological data as well as after the annotation of the collected data by the clinicians. The mean absolute error will decrease drastically after the proper training of the classifiers and the readjustment of the attributes' weights.

4   Conclusions

The CHRONIOUS system exploits innovative IT solutions providing effective description of the health status of the patient as well as advanced messages and alerts about the severity estimation of the condition or possible critical health episodes. The Decision Support System exploits both a supervised classifier and a rule-based system in order to limit the error of the decision, increase the accuracy of the system and justify the identified events by providing the rule or the critical parameter to clinicians. A personalization of the decision is even more feasible with the CHRONIOUS system due to the fact that several profiles have been created, describing with accuracy the health status of the patient, and used as an input to the intelligent part of the System. In addition, the Mental Support Tool is an added-value to the final system, evaluating the stress level and contributing to disease monitoring by helping the patient to avoid or face stressful situations that may have implications to his health.

In order to increase the effectiveness and the accuracy of the CHRONIOUS system, healthy and pathological data will be collected as well as their clinical annotation resulting in the improvement of the accuracy of the system.

References

1. Viegi, G., Pistelli, F., Sherrill, D.L., Maio, S., Baldacci, S., Carrozzi, L.: Definition, epidemiology and natural history of COPD. Eur. Respir. J., 993–1013 (2007)
2. Tonelli, M., Wiebe, N., Culleton, B., House, A., Rabbat, C., Fok, M., McAlister, F., Garg, A.X.: Chronic Kidney Disease and Mortality Risk: A Systematic Review. J. Am. Soc. Nephrol. 17, 2034–2047 (2006)
3. http://www.aihw.gov.au/cdarf/diseases_pages/index.cfm

4. Lawo, M., Papadopoulos, A., Ciancitto, F., Dellaca, R.L., Munaro, G., Rosso, R.: An Open, Ubiquitous and Adaptive Chronic Disease Management Platform. In: Proc. pHEALTH Conf., Oslo, Sweden, p. 50 (2009)
5. Papadopoulos, A., Fotiadis, D.I., Lawo, M., Ciancitto, F., Podolak, C., Dellaca, R.L., Munaro, G., Rosso, R.: CHRONIOUS: A Wearable System for the Management of Chronic Disease. In: 9th International Conference on Information Technology & Applications in Biomedicine, Th.1.3.4, Larnaca, Cyprus (2009)
6. Tan, P., Steinbach, M., Kumar, V.: Introduction to Data Mining, ch. 8. Addison-Wesley, Reading (2006)
7. http://www.research.ucsf.edu/chr/Inst/chrInst_Cdc.asp
8. Quinlan, R.: C4.5. Morgan Kaufmann, CA (1993)
9. Frank, E., Witten, I.H.: Generating Accurate Rule Sets Without Global Optimization. In: Proceedings of the Fifteenth International Conference on Machine Learning, 24-27, pp. 144–151 (1998)
10. Cristianini, N., Shawe-Taylor, J.: An introduction to support vector machines and other kernel-based learning methods. Cambridge University Press, Cambridge (2000)
11. Friedman, N., Geiger, D., Goldszmidt, M.: Bayesian Network Classifiers. Machine Learning 29, 131–163 (1997)
12. Haykin, S.: Neural Networks: A Comprehensive Foundation. Prentice Hall, Englewood Cliffs (1998)

Session 3

Intelligent Home Monitoring

Autonomy, Motivation and Individual Self-management for COPD Patients, the Amica Project

Kostas Giokas, Ioannis Kouris, and Dimitris Koutsouris

National Technical University of Athens,
9, Heroon Polytechniou str., 15773 Zografou, Athens, Greece
{kgiokas,ikouris,dkoutsou}@biomed.ntua.gr

Abstract. AMICA Project targets to improve the quality of life of patients suffering from Chronic Obstructive Pulmonary Disease (COPD). Incorporating advanced signal analysis algorithms and custom designed monitoring devices with a Telemedical Platform (TP), an innovative system is under development to help elderly persons to reduce hospitalization time. After a brief analysis of COPD the sub modules that compose the TP will be described, along with the used technologies.

Keywords: e-Health, Telemedical Platform, COPD, monitoring device.

1 Introduction

COPD is also known as Chronic Obstructive Lung Disease (COLD) which is an umbrella term used to describe chronic lung diseases that are characterized by progressive obstruction of the airflow into and out of the lungs and increased shortness of breath [4]. COPD is an insidious disease, which is often diagnosed after some of the lung capacity is already lost. Other diseases related to COPD include emphysema and chronic bronchitis. Very little has been learned in past years about COPD, because the number of related studies is very limited. However, today, things are improving with some very encouraging studies, clinical trials and research for medications and treatments. COPD, though considered a chronic, debilitating and sometimes fatal disease, can be managed, controlled and slowed down [5].

Most significant COPD symptoms are coughing that produces large amounts of mucus, wheezing, shortness of breath and chest tightness. Smoking is one of the main causes of COPD. Most of the individuals diagnosed with COPD are active or old smokers. Long-term exposure to other lung irritants, such as air pollution, chemical fumes, or dust, also may contribute to COPD. The disease is usually diagnosed in middle-aged or older people. However, treatments and lifestyle changes can help the patient feel better, stay active and slow the development of the disease [11]. One of the main factors that contribute to a longer and healthier lifestyle include early detection of the problem, following of the medication treatment faithfully, acquiring of healthy eating habits, stop smoking, increase of personal exercise, education about each aspect of the disease and the related problems, and prevention of infections in order to limit exacerbations which can lead to additional lung damage.

J. Lin and K.S. Nikita (Eds.): MobiHealth 2010, LNICST 55, pp. 49–53, 2011.
© Institute for Computer Sciences, Social Informatics and Telecommunications Engineering 2011

2 Background

Related research targets to reproduce hospital environment at the patient's home, using sensors and medical devices that require medical protocols to be used properly and the presence of skilled health professionals. Other solutions are based on nursing outreach programs. In both cases, the dedicated systems are expensive and the patients' health conditions do not improve a lot [6].

The use of Information Computer Technologies (ICT) in routine practice is particularly limited in the field of respiratory medicine. Some researchers have focused on tele-consultation between professionals working at different levels of the health system. Other studies in respiratory telemedicine deal with the telemonitoring of lung transplant recipients and patients with chronic obstructive pulmonary disease, asthma, or cystic fibrosis [13, 14] With the exception of spirometry self-testing in the context of home telemonitoring, monitoring of physiological respiratory signs have been limited to a few preliminary studies on the application of new technologies in home mechanical ventilation. None of the applications have been incorporated into routine practice [10-12].

The AMICA Project targets to merge professional COPD supervision with patient self-management (PSM) in one complete, easy to use and cost effective TP. The use of advanced mobile devices for telemonitoring each individual's conditions targets to reduce hospitalization time of the patient. The complete platform will include a monitoring device, a base station, a communication module, a signal analysis module and a web platform for data exchange and surveillance [8-9].

3 Platform Analysis

AMICA TP is composed of distinct modules performing dedicated tasks. Each module has a dedicated role, although all of them communicate and exchange data through a common platform, developed for the purposes of the project.

3.1 Signal Acquisition

Spirometry is the golden standard in the management of COPD patients, but the patients' perception of the lung capacity does not always coincide with spirometry results. During the initial phase of clinical trials during fall 2009, a patented multifunctional sensor used for the signal acquisition [3]. The sensor was capable to capture tracheal sounds and accelerations. In order to capture the data, a housing of the sensor was especially designed in order the miniaturized sensor to fit and to be easily used by elder people. Captured signals were transmitted by wire to the base station (described below), although the final product will make use of wireless connectivity protocols, such as IEEE 802.11 and Bluetooth, to transmit the signal from the sensor to the base station.

The evaluation of the captured signals indicated that the information provided by the accelerometer did not significantly improve the accuracy of the recordings. In that sense, accelerometer data acquisition decided to be abandoned and more effort agreed to be dedicated to the signal analysis.

3.2 Base Station

Many research projects have worked towards telemedical platforms during the last years. User interfaces implicate many problems and are generally not well accepted in the "real-world" of medical applications. The HMI mechanisms of mobile devices that are not adapted to the needs and requirements of patients, especially for elderly people. The hardware used for the implementation of the Base Station (BS) of the AMICA Project is customized for the needs of the system and the design is modular in order to easy allow upgrades.

The portable device will be situated in the home of the patient. It will be used for signal acquisition, collection of the questionnaire answers and data transmission to the central server of the system (CSS). A prototype has been already designed and is equipped with a large touch sensitive display of 7" diagonal dimension. The hardware is customized to allow the reception of transmitted signals by the sensor, digitize them, using an ADC, and perform the communication with CSS via an installed GSM modem.

BS will include advanced software for the Human Machine Interaction (HMI). The software will provide instructions to the patient on how to use the sensor, in order to record tracheal sounds and will facilitate the patient to fill the medical questionnaire related to the disease progress. All data are saved locally and then are securely transmitted to the database of the system. Questionnaires have been defined and validated by the doctors that participate to the project. At the moment, the interaction between the end user and the Base Station is performed through the touch screen interface but a bi-directional voice interaction interface is under development.

3.3 Telemedical Platform Framework

Telemedical Platform Framework is used for secure data storage and transmission to the CSS. It is also used to execute the signal analysis. BS stores the data locally and then using secure connection transmits the data to the central system database, located in a secure place inside the hospital. Encryption is used, to guarantee the privacy of the data. Raw data from the sensor are analyzed by the signal analysis algorithm (performance and primary results are currently examined) and the results are stored into the system database [1-2]. Demographic data, medical history, medical exams, medication and medical scales are gathered to create the Patient Electronic Health Record (PEHR). PEHRs can be accessed by the authorized users, using an internet browser [7].

The users of the system are divided into three distinctive roles: Administrators, Physicians and Researchers. Administrators are responsible for the overall system security. Physicians are fully authorized to examine patients' data, register new patients, record medical exams and medication changes and access questionnaire results and signal analysis data. A Researcher may access the data but cannot identify the patient, as any identification information has been removed.

3.4 Signal Analysis

Signal analysis takes place in the CSS. The raw signals are recorded by the sensor and are transmitted to the CSS along with the answers to the questionnaires. Signal analysis is currently initiated by the researchers, but for the final product they will be automatically triggered upon the data arrival on CSS. The duration of sound recordings must be at least 10". A recording duration between 10 and 30 seconds seems to be enough for feature extraction. The algorithms are currently under evaluation. The features to be extracted will include ECG signals, lung sounds and heart rate. The results are compared to the physiological parameters and an estimation of disease progression is provided. Feature extraction aims to identify early signs of exacerbation and so to alert the physician to act and prevent patient hospitalization.

4 Future Work

Currently, BS station hardware is ready and software for HMI is under development. Sensor design is almost complete and ready to be manufactured. During the second phase of clinical trials feedback will be received by the end users and modifications will take place. Signal analysis algorithms results are under evaluation and will be reevaluated to optimize prognosis results. After the second phase of clinical trials, during fall 2010, the results will be collected and will be used to finalize AMICA TP development.

References

1. Anagnostaki, A.P., Pavlopoulos, S., Kyriakou, E., Koutsouris, D.: A novel codification scheme based on the "VITAL" and "DICOM" standards for telemedicine applications. IEEE Transactions on Biomedical Engineering 49, 1399–1411 (2002)
2. Choi, Y.B., Krause, J.S., Seo, H., Capitan, K.E., Chung, K.: Telemedicine in the USA: standardization through information management and technical applications. IEEE Communications Magazine 44, 41–48 (2006)
3. (Patent) Monitoring of the cardio-respiratory and snoring components received by an accelerometer (P200602453) (W070000254)
4. WHO World Health Organisation,
   http://www.who.int/respiratory/COPD/en/
5. National Collaborating Centre for Chronic Conditions, http://www.guideline.gov
6. Hailey, D., Roine, R., Ohinmaa, A.: Systematic Review of evidence for the benefits of telemedicine. Journal of Telemedicine and Telecare 8, 1–7 (2002)
7. Lin, J.C.: Applying telecommunication technology to health care delivery. IEEE Engineering in Medicine and Biology Magazine 4, 28–31 (1999)
8. Pattichis, C.S., Kyriacou, E., Voskarides, S., Pattichis, M.S., Istepanian, R., Schizas, C.N.: Wireless telemedicine systems: an overview. IEEE Antennas and Propagation Magazine (44), 143–153 (2002)
9. Pavlopoulos, S., Kyriacou, E., Berler, A., Dembeyiotis, S., Koutsouris, D.: A novel emergency telemedicine system based on wireless communication technology-AMBULANCE. IEEE Transactions on Information Technology in Biomedicine 4, 261–267 (1998)
10. Global Initiative for the Chronic Obstructive Lung Disease,
    http://www.goldcopd.com
11. Corral, J., Masa, J.F., Disdier, C., Riesco, J.A., Gomez-Esparrago, A., Barquilla, A., et al.: Respiratory teleconsultation: telespirometry, teleradiology and telemedical history between primary care clinics and pulmonary unit. Eur. Respir. J. 24, 280 (2004)

12. Koizumi, T., Takizawa, M., Nakai, K., Yamamoto, Y., Murase, S., Fujii, T., et al.: Trial of remote telemedicine support for patients with chronic respiratory failure at home through a multistation communication system. Telemed. J. E. Health 11, 481–486 (2005)
13. Wilkinson, O.M., Duncan-Skingle, F., Pryor, J.A., Hodson, M.E.: A feasibility study of home telemedicine for patients with cystic fibrosis awaiting transplantation. J. Telemed. Telecare 14, 182–185 (2008)
14. Adam, T.J., Finkelstein, S.M., Parente, S.T., Hertz, M.I.: Cost analysis of home monitoring in lung transplant recipients. Int. J. Technol. Assess Health Care 23, 216–222 (2007)

A Novel System for Hemodialysis Patients Home Monitoring

Eleni Sakka[1], Markela Psymarnoy[1], and Pantelis Angelidis[1,2]

[1] Mobihealth Research, 91 Aglandjia Avenue, Diogenes Incubator, 1678 Nicosia, Cyprus
[2] University of W. Macedonia, Kozani, 50100, Greece
research@mobi-health.eu

Abstract. Chronic renal patients and patients with end stage renal disease are a distinctive patient group with a serious, chronic and irreversible health condition, which is mainly treated at home. As such they are unique candidates for support via telehealth services. This paper introduces a novel monitoring system for hemodialysis patients. The leading aims of this system are the development of innovative biomedical signals management system and the implementation of integrated model medical signal projection and processing tools. The system is expected to contribute to the increase of the demand in the medical services field as well as to reduce the patient transfer abroad for recovery.

Keywords: home care telematics, renal telematics, telemonitoring, patient management.

1 Introduction

Hemodialysis has been a common medical treatment for the people with chronic renal failure. In Cyprus, every year 67 - 77 new incidents of final renal disease appear and though this number remains the same the last 10 - 15 years, the synthesis of patients has changed. The number of young persons with chronic renal disease has reduced, whereas the number of citizens over 60 years old and renal disease citizens due to diabetes has increased [1]. According to the statistics, 60 to 70 thousand people in Cyprus suffer from diabetes and it is anticipated that the number will increase. It has been noticed that the diabetic nephropathy is a complication of 30% of the diabetic patients.

The hemodialysis taking place in a hospital requires the transfer of the patient to the medical centre three times a week. It should be noted that between two visits for hemodialysis, the maintenance of the required quality of life as well as the restriction of side effects for the patient is a big challenge, depending on the ability of biosignal monitoring at home. These signals can be the weight of the patient, heart pulses, temperature and blood pressure and in some cases electrocardiogram and blood glucose (for patients with heart condition and diabetes respectively).

Identifying this problem, we have implemented a novel system for hemodialysis patients home monitoring. The basic scenario of system function is described below: the patient after being registered to the system during the scheduled visit in the Hemodialysis Centre, he/she is equipped with the portable and useful device. This

J. Lin and K.S. Nikita (Eds.): MobiHealth 2010, LNICST 55, pp. 54–60, 2011.
© Institute for Computer Sciences, Social Informatics and Telecommunications Engineering 2011

device communicates automatically with the, essential for the monitor of patient's health condition, digital medical devices, that record the biosignals. Measurements and other data concerning parameters of monitoring procedure can be added manually in the portable device, together with information regarding the general patient's situation. Data, that are collected either manually or automatically from the patient, are transmitted automatically to server during fixed time periods (at least once a day, depending on physicians directions). In the server the measurements are received and stored and are subjected to basic and advanced processing and analysis for the extraction of notifications/ alarms. The medical personnel during scheduled time periods e.g. daily, or after an alarm, reviews the patient's health condition, the patient's compliance to the physicians recommendations and the patient's response to the treatment. According to the processed data, the treatment plan can be revised and the physician is able to communicate with the patient in order to get more information, to refer the patient immediately to the closest medical centre or to modify the treatment.

2 Telemonitoring Service - Overview

The aim of this system is to monitor and manage renal disease patients that undergo hemodialysis. It is based on the recording of all essential biosignals for patient monitoring. The utilization of these signals optimizes the monitoring of these patients, whilst physicians can manage on time the possible complications between two hemodialysis sessions.

The system was based on the fact that patients undergoing hemodialysis every other day need to be monitored between the hospital visits. The system includes the functional units below:

- Patients' device for the collection of medical data that will be transferred telemetrically to the central hospital. The device, which is a PDA, is connected to the appropriate medical devices so as to wirelessly receive the patient medical data (i.e. vital signs), while it gives the option to the patient to add manually further information. The data are sent to the hospital unit via GPRS.
- Telemetry data collection unit, which receives the biosignals as well as all the information that are transferred from the patient unit. It manages them in order to provide basic and advanced services of processing, analyzing and file storing as well as giving the ability to the user to create notifications and alarms. The collection unit has been implemented with open interface so as to give the opportunity to third parties to integrate it with existing systems.
- Database with personal, medical and biomedical patients' data.
- Database with administrative data (user data, roles etc)
- Central system administrative unit (server) and basic communication centre between users (medical personnel, patients, administrators), which undertakes the medical data presentation to the medical personnel and supports the administration of system and of users (new patient registration, new medical personnel registration, roles management etc). The server is implemented with web services in order to facilitate the convenient and universal access, ensuring the essential security together with interoperability.

These basic functional units and their interconnection can be seen in Fig.1.

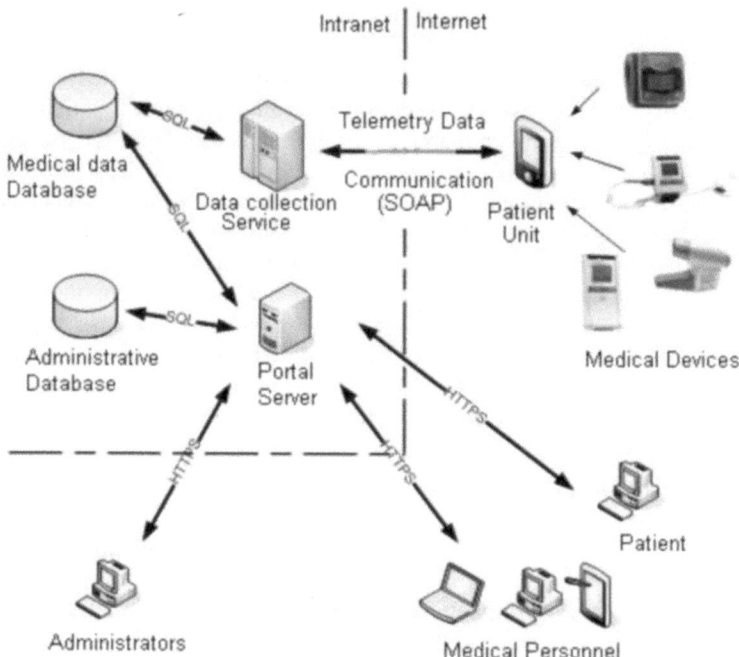

Fig. 1. Functional units of the system

2.1 Implementation

2.1.1 Patient Unit

The implementation of the patient unit was made on .NET Visual Studio 2008 [2] together with Windows Mobile 5.0 pocket pc SDK [3] and Microsoft SQL CE 3.5 [4] for the local storage of medical data and scheduled measurements program[1].

The patient after opening the application can choose to download the new plan of scheduled measurements, specified by his/her physician or to proceed in the perform-ance of a new emergency measurement in case he/she doesn't feel well. The patient unit communicates with the server and gets the configuration of the scheduled meas-urements as well as the monitoring plan that the attendant physician has defined. After that the unit displays the sequence of the scheduled measurement(s) that need to be taken by the patient. The appropriate medical devices (according to the scheduled measurement) are connected via Bluetooth and send the biosignals to the PDA. At the end of each session, the patient is asked whether to send the measurements to the server or not. Upon successful transfer, a confirmation message is shown to the pa-tient. Alternatively, the patient is notified in case of transfer failure, in order to re-send the data.

---

[1] The language of the user interface of the patient application is Greek.

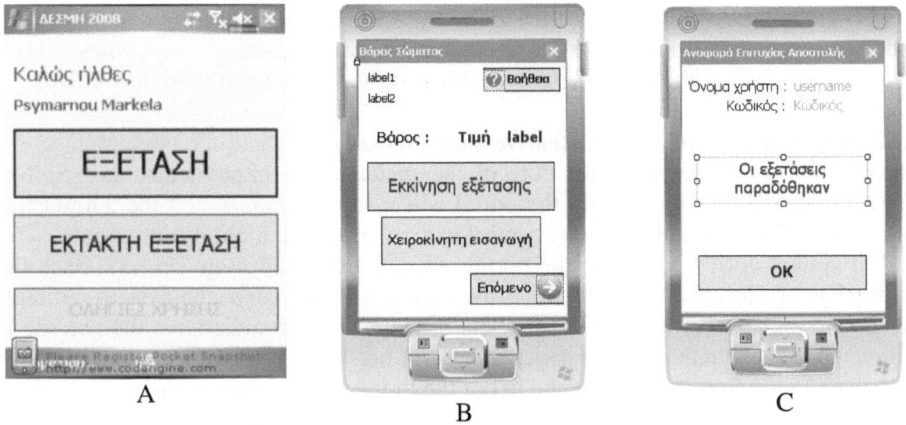

Fig. 2. Screenshots from patient unit. A) Welcome screen, b) Weight measurement insertion form and c) Successful data transmission message screen.

2.1.2 Telemetry Data Collection Service

The Telemetry data collection unit is basically an **XML** web service, developed in .Net Visual Studio 2008, using standard Internet based protocol SOAP. This gives the option to third party manufacturers to integrate their patient units to the system.

The web service enables the communication between the patient unit and the server. It encapsulates all the essential functions regarding the measurements configuration download, the programmed measurements download, the upload of the performed measurements as well as the upload of the errors that have potentially occurred during the execution of the patient application.

In the web service the check for the generation of notifications/alarms is performed. After the recording of the biosignals a control is performed whether the measurements, that were uploaded, where accomplished on time according to the schedule or not and in the latter case a notification is created to the attendant physician. Secondly a test is carried out whether the value of the measurement is between the physiological range of values. If it is above or below the normal values, and according to the criteria the physician has specified, either a notification or an alarm is created and the physician is informed. Finally the web service checks and creates the corresponding notification in case there are any measurements not performed (or sent) by the patient.

2.1.3 Personal and Medical Data Database and Administrative Database

Both databases are designed and implemented in MySQL server version 5.1 [5].

The personal and medical data database was implemented according to the system requirements for the regular function of the server. It includes all the necessary data tables for the patient management, the control of the measurements' plan, the administration of the necessary measurements required for the patient monitoring as well as the definition of the notifications/alarms.

The administrative database is generated by ASP.NET membership control system and it includes the fundamental data tables for the management of users, roles as well as information about the users' activity as long as they are logged in to the system.

2.1.4 Central System Administrative Unit (Server)

The central system server is the core of the system. It is implemented in ASP.Net Visual Studio 2008. It is mainly the portal where the physicians and the administrators of the system are able to view, control and process the patient information[2].

The system allows access to the portal only to authorized users (Fig 3). Once the credentials of the user are correct and the user is authenticated, the system redirects the user to the appropriate page. If the role of the user is administrative then he/she is redirected to the administrator's page, whereas if he/she is medical personnel he/she is redirected to the first page where the list of the monitored patients is shown (Fig 4).

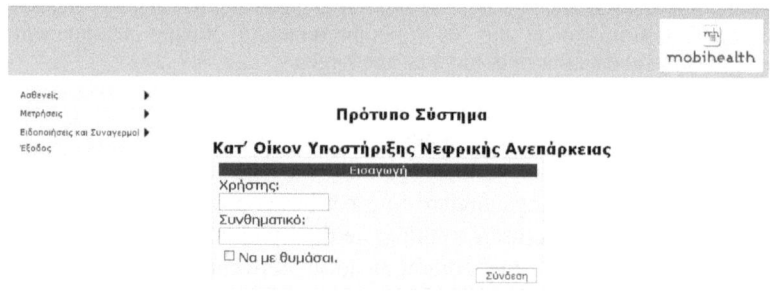

Fig. 3. Login page to the portal of the system

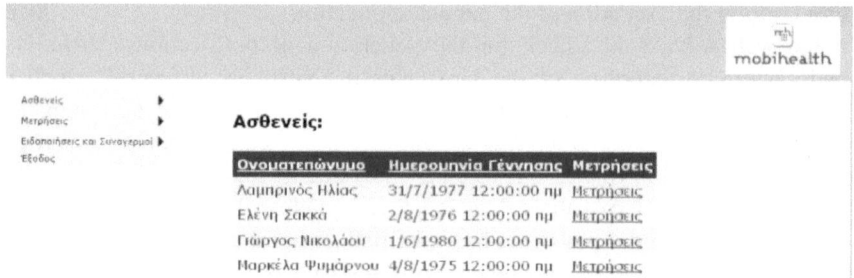

Fig. 4. Patients list for the logged in physician

The physician can view the scheduled measurements of his/hers patients, the measurement results of the patients, as well as the measurements that have not been carried out (Fig. 5). The system gives the ability to the physician to define special notifications that contribute to the patient monitoring and shows the alarms that were created according to these notifications' definitions. The physician can also add new patients to the system and he/she can define the program of measurements that patient needs to follow.

---

[2] The language of the user interface of the central system administrative unit is Greek.

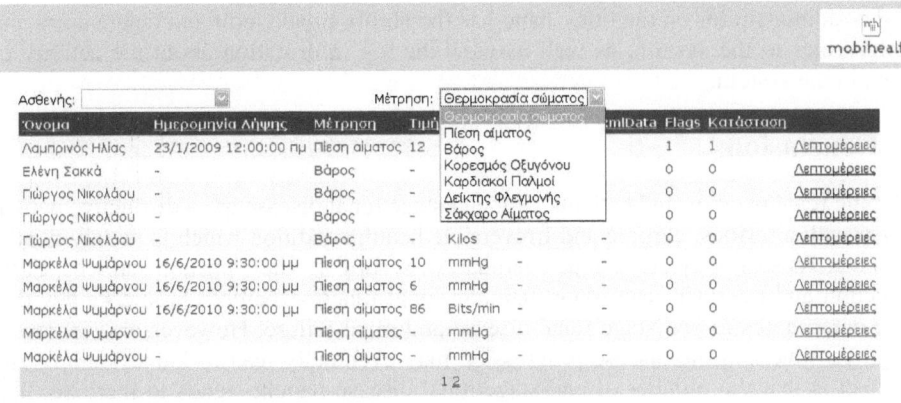

Fig. 5. Measurements list

Προσθαφαίρεση ρόλων
Προσθαφαίρεση χρηστών σε ρόλους
Εισαγωγή νέων χρηστών
Εμφάνιση στοιχείων χρήστη
Log out

Δημιουργήστε νέο χρήστη

User ID: username

Password:

Email: myemail@foo.org

Ερώτηση για το   Ποιο είναι το γένος της μητέρας σας
Password:

Απάντηση:

            Δημιουργία χρήστη

Fig. 6. Add new user to the system

Προσθαφαίρεση ρόλων
Προσθαφαίρεση χρηστών σε ρόλους
Εισαγωγή νέων χρηστών
Εμφάνιση στοιχείων χρήστη
Log out

Εισάγετε το νέο ρόλο:

            Δημιουργία

Η λίστα των διαθέσιμων ρόλων φαίνεται παρακάτω.

User Name	
Administrator	Remove Role
Doctor	Remove Role
Patient	Remove Role

Επιλέξτε εδώ για τη διαχείριση των ρόλων των χρηστών.

Fig. 7. Create new role to the system

The administrator on the other hand has the ability to add, edit and delete users and assign roles to the system, as well as view the log information about the activity of users in the system.

3 Conclusion

Chronic renal patients and patients with end stage renal disease are a distinctive patient group with a serious, chronic and irreversible health condition which is mainly treated at home. As such they are unique candidates for support via telehealth services. Early detection and treatment can often maintain renal function before chronic kidney disease deteriorates to end stage renal disease and renal failure. However, this is not always possible and the disease progression may eventually lead to kidney failure and the fact is that the number of end-stage renal disease patients tends to increase. It is therefore becoming all the more imperative to take measures for the prevention and the better management of end stage renal disease. Close monitoring may prove a good measure for early diagnosis, treatment adjustment and rehabilitation.

The above described system has been implemented in order to help the aforementioned problem. Aim of this system is to contribute to the increase of the demand in the medical services field as well as to reduce the patient unnecessary transfer. It is a novel system for hemodialysis patients home monitoring, where medical personnel is able to monitor renal patients at home between hemodialysis session which take place in to the hospital.

Patient's satisfaction and self-esteem increases as a result of not being forced to visit hospital daily and therefore enjoys a better quality of life. From physician's point of view, the described system gives the opportunity for a better patient management, integrated support and increased prestige duo to the fact that he/she is able to put into practice novel and pioneer methods in everyday patients' treatment. Finally, concerning the healthcare system, the aforementioned solution not only ameliorates the quality of provided services but also reduces the cost of the hemodialysis services provided, and helps for the optimal resources usage (human, technical, and financial).

Acknowledgments. The system was developed under the National Framework Program for Research and Technological Development 2008 of Research Promotion Foundation in Cyprus.

References

1. Renal problems Week, Nicosia, Cyprus, November 13 (1998),
   http://www.hri.org/news/cyprus/kypegr/1998/
   98-11-13.kypegr.html
2. Microsoft .NET Visual Studio (2008),
   http://msdn.microsoft.com/en-us/vstudio/default.aspx
3. Windows Mobile 5.0 SDK for Pocket PC,
   http://www.microsoft.com/downloads
4. Microsoft SQL Server Compact 3.5,
   http://www.microsoft.com/sqlserver/2005/en/us/Compact.aspx
5. MySQL Enterprise Server 5.1,
   http://www.mysql.com/products/enterprise/server.html

Post Cardiac Surgery Home-Monitoring System

Efthyvoulos Kyriacou[1,2], Panayiota Chimonidou[1], Constantinos Pattichis[1],
Ekaterini Lambrinou[3], Vassilis I. Barberis[4], and George P. Georghiou[4,5]

[1] University of Cyprus
[2] Frederick University Cyprus
[3] Cyprus University of Technology
[4] American Heart Institute Cyprus
[5] Tel. Aviv. University Israel
e.kyriacou@frederick.ac.cy, pattichi@cs.ucy.ac.cy

Abstract. One of the major factors limiting but also causing the application of modern technology in medicine is the response time to patients, should they need specialized medical care. In this work we propose a solution that is aiming to help and improve the patients' life after a cardiac surgery. This is a group of patients that have to be monitored for a short period after the operation. The aim of this project is to give the opportunity to these patients to be monitored at home after their operation so as to keep their rehabilitation period as smooth as possible and avoid unnecessary visits to the hospital or prevent adverse events. This is going to be achieved by creating an integrated web- based system which can regularly monitor several biosignals like ECG, blood pressure, arterial SpO2 and parameters like body weight and provide the tools to identify any unusual events.

Keywords: Cardiac surgery patients, home monitoring, biosignals monitoring, web based telemedicine systems.

1 Introduction

Cardiovascular disease (CVD) is the leading cause of death and adult disability in the industrial world. Despite advances in the diagnosis and treatment of coronary heart disease (CHD), it remains the single most frequent cause of death in Americans older than 65 years old [1]. International statistics parallel those of the USA with an increasing epidemiology of CHD occurring worldwide [2]. A recent study by the World Health Organization revealed that by 2015 almost 20 million people will die from CVD, mainly from CHD and stroke [3]. Coronary artery bypass graft (CABG) surgery is the most frequently performed major surgery for CHD in the United States [2].

As the prevalence of CVD is increasing, new strategies need to be developed in order to reduce the cost of health care services and at the same time to improve patients' quality of life. As a result, there is an increasing interest in care delivery models that incorporate information-communication technology, with the transfer of physiological data [such as blood pressure, weight, electrocardiogram (ECG), oxygen saturation], via the internet, the mobile phones, the wireless communications from home to health care providers.

J. Lin and K.S. Nikita (Eds.): MobiHealth 2010, LNICST 55, pp. 61–68, 2011.
© Institute for Computer Sciences, Social Informatics and Telecommunications Engineering 2011

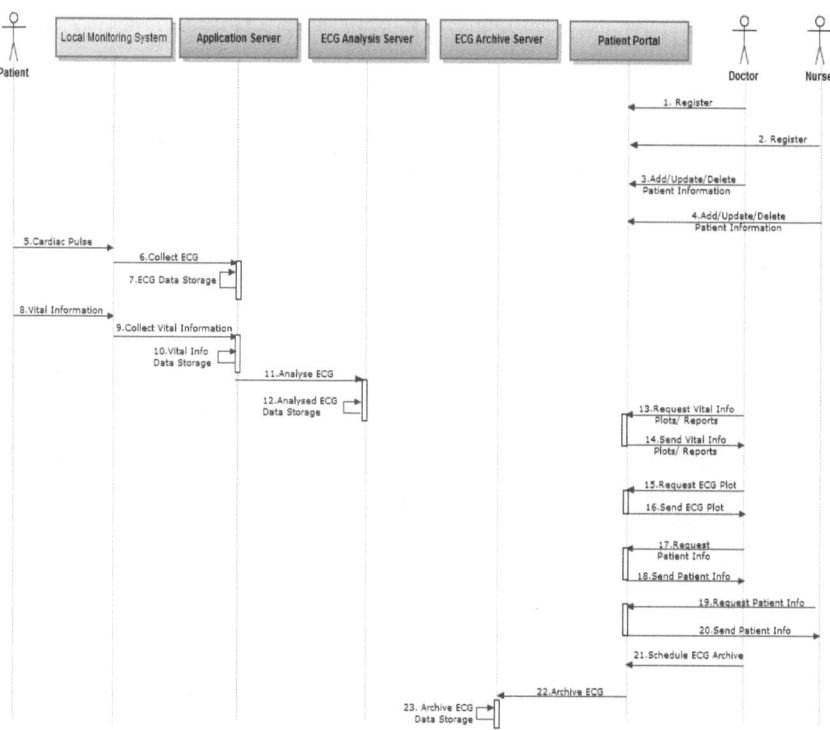

Fig. 1. Portal Sequence Diagram

The production of revolutionary medical monitoring systems we are proposing includes a system that will enable physicians to monitor patients undergoing cardiac surgery after hospital discharge.

A considerable proportion of patients experience adverse events or are readmitted within a few weeks after discharge, leading to worse outcomes and/or increased costs. These problems are likely to increase over the next few decades as the longevity of the population increases [4- 6]. The impact of structured telephone support on the risk of readmissions and rehospitalization after cardiac surgery have been proved in several studies. These systems proved to be useful from the actual monitoring point of view as well as the psychological point of view. They also give the opportunity for significant savings in the health care system, improvements to patient's care and at the same time, to patients' health related quality of life [7-11].

Like every web-based application, in order to achieve a respectable level of status, the system must offer substantial services. Some typical facilities that our system includes are: doctor registration and collaboration, patient's ECG monitoring and automatic analysis in order to extract useful information for the physicians. This method of management of patients after discharge for cardiac surgery can be very beneficial in combating episodes of exacerbation and preventing rehospitalizations, urgent care visits, and emergency room visits.

The other important objective of this system is to help patients. With the use of this system a patient will not have to visit the hospital almost every day just for some minutes or whenever thinking that something is wrong. The impact of the system support on the risk of readmissions can be attributed in part to the triage of patients at the first sign of clinical deterioration by the specialist nurse, and the consequent immediate intervention of a primary care physician. Alternatively with the help of specialized sensors and other equipment, involving daily transmission of vital signs (eg ECG, blood pressure, and oxygen saturation), symptoms and weight lead to earlier detection and management of clinical deterioration by both the patient and/or the health care professional.

The current project was build upon and further past research [12], incorporating multiple, disparate technologies in one cohesive system, focusing on the reasoning and inferencing components of the system via the application of innovative machine learning techniques, transferring this into a viable home based product that can handle this complex domain and meet the needs of patients at need.

2 Methodology

2.1 System's Purpose and System Functions

The system will gather all the necessary information concerning patients, such as weight, blood pressure, oxygen saturation and ECG. The ECG signal is automatically analyzed by the system in order to identify possible arrhythmias and facilitate extra and helpful information to the doctor. Each doctor can see his patients' information; on the other hand, he must have the ability to give or remove access to other doctors, in order to enable collaboration between them and help each other to get some decisions.

The web portal provides site functionality such as historical information storage and maintenance. Medical background information, patient hospitalization information, and patients' symptoms data. Questionnaires completed before and after the treatment in order to calculate Physical, Emotional, Global and Sum Score, finally patient's calls and follow up information.

Furthermore the system is used to store, analyze and archive patients' information. The system is able to facilitate and provide all the necessary functionality to the doctors and the nurses. An overall sequence diagram showing the sequence of actions being done from the users (Patient, Doctors, and Nurses) can be seen in fig. 1.

2.2 Basic System Operations and Functions

In general the System facilitates the following operations and functions:

- Doctor registration
- Patient Registration which can be done by the doctor or the nurse
- Doctors have the ability to give access to another doctor as contributor or just as a viewer.
- Before and after patient's treatment several scores are measured based on predefined questionnaires.
- Historical information relating to previous diseases, medical background and symptoms are handled.

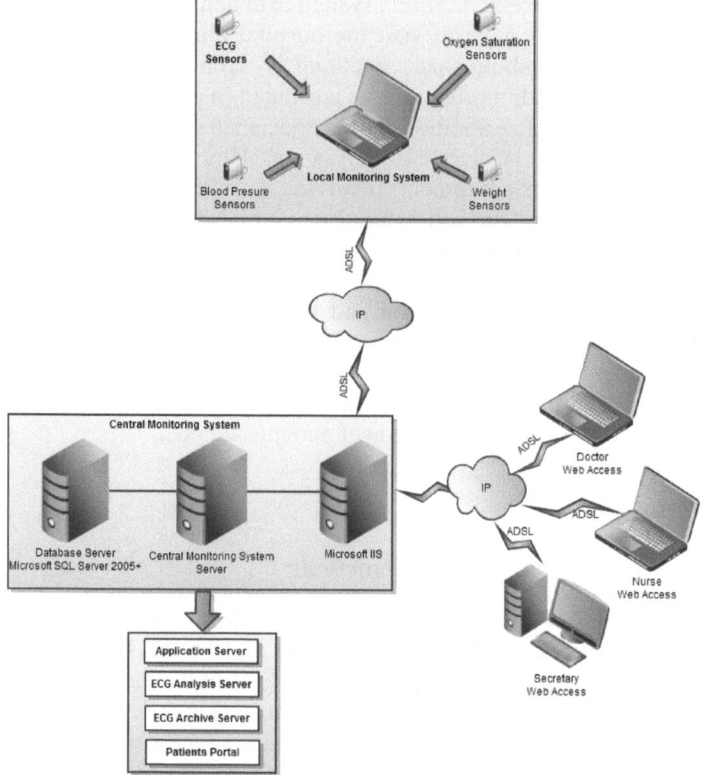

Fig. 2. Overall System Architecture

- Patient calls and follow-up information are handled by the system.
- Several statistics about biosignals and overall graphs of other parameters can be provided to the doctor. These refer to:
  - ○ ECG
  - ○ Weight
  - ○ Blood pressure
  - ○ Oxygen saturation
  - ○ Score statistics
- Automatic analysis of ECG signals for possible arrhythmia detection. The analysis is being done based on an open source arrhythmia detection algorithm provided by E.P Limited [14]
- The doctor has the ability to schedule an archive process for the patient's ECG.

2.3 System Architecture

The overall architecture of the system can be seen in fig.2. It's actually a web based application and mainly consists of the central web server and the local monitoring systems. The communication between the two systems is being done using a dedicated web service and predefined XML message over the IP network.

The Local Monitoring System consists of a dedicated PC with the appropriate software, ECG sensors, Blood pressure, Oxygen Saturation sensors and a digital weight scale. This unit is responsible for collecting and uploading all vital information from the patient. Currently we are using a Dyna-Vision© (DVM-010S) ECG and SpO$_2$ acquisition device [13] (connected with the pc using Bluetooth or USB) and CONTEC08A (CONTEC© Medical Systems) for Non Invasive Blood Pressure.

The Central Monitoring Web Server collects the vital information from the Local Monitoring Systems. It includes four major processes. The first one is the Application Server which is the central process that is used to collect and store vital information and side information. The second one is the ECG Analysis Server which is used to analyze (detection of possible cardiac arrhythmias) and store the ECG. The third major process is the ECG Archive Server which is used to archive the ECG that was scheduled by the doctor. Finally, the most important process is the Patients Portal, which is used to collect and display the patients' information and their vital information. The portal is accessible through a web interface. Doctors, nurses, secretaries and patients can apply their user name and password and in this way they are able to maintain and view the patients' information. Security of the system was developed using different access levels for each group. It is being done by using a Microsoft Membership provider from ASP.NET© [16]. Password code of each user is Hashed using a one-way hashing algorithm and a randomly generated "salt" value.

A snapshot of the initial screen of the system can be seen in fig. 3 where on this screen a user doctor can see all recent uploads from his patients' and select any subsection to see either past medical information, follow up, vital info etc related to any of his patients.

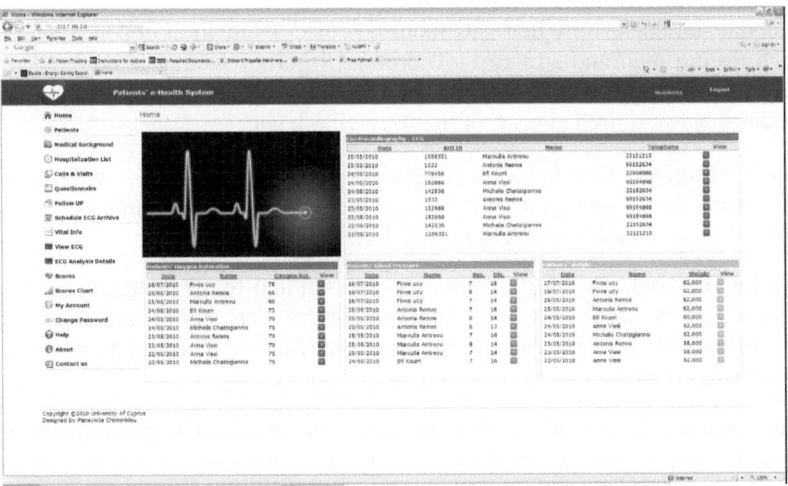

Fig. 3. Initial system screen displaying patients that have recently uploaded information and links to several screens of the system

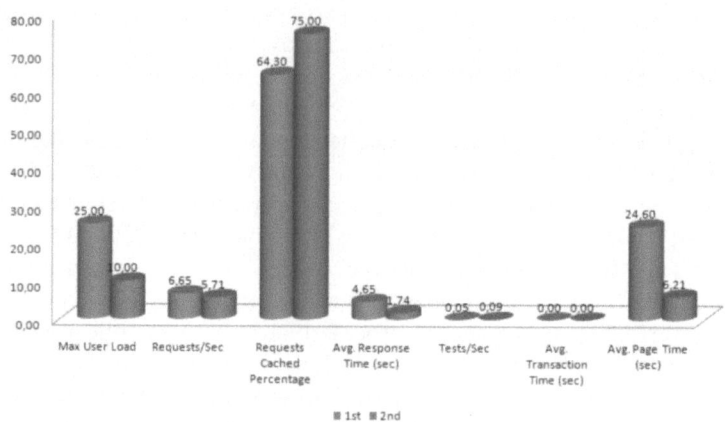

Fig. 4. Overall testing results

2.4 Tools Used for System Implementation

For the implementation of the system we had used the Microsoft Visual Studio 2008 with ASP.NET and Visual Basic.NET [15-16], as the main programming tool. Microsoft SQL Server 2008 was used as the database management system. Furthermore, Ajax Toolkit 3.5 was used for several enhancements on the user interface. Finally for the ECG graphs over the web, the National Instruments Measurements Studio was used [17].

3 Results

Professional statistics show that satisfactory project evaluation depends heavily on a thorough testing plan and strategy. Therefore, rigorous testing is demanded for the effective evaluation of the finished end-product. Successful testing of the system's performance was required at each of the following levels:

Module Testing. For this type of testing, each individual module was tested to determine whether all the system's modules are logically and functionally correct. If an error occurred, a suitable debugging procedure was followed.

Integration Testing. This form of testing was applied to all interfaces among modules to ensure that transfer of both data and control were performed correctly. This testing method included the run-time evaluation of all variables that are passed from one module to another.

Function Testing. The results and outcomes of the program were evaluated after the execution of the program in which every functional menu selection had been activated systematically in turn.

Final System Testing. The objective of this type of testing was the full test of the entire system on the completion of the system development period. In order to achieve this several testing tools e.g. the load test, the unit test that the visual studio 2008 offers helped us with testing in order to discover programming errors and potential problems. The system was tested with simulations for data input, retrieval and ECG automatic analysis. The results for 25 and 10 users running for 10 minutes gave a warm-up duration of 30 and 60 seconds respectively. Tests were applied to the pages that have the most significant processing functions like ECG Preview and VitalInfo.

The graphical representation of overall results can be viewed in fig. 4. Blue bars display the first case that the scenario was simulating 25 simultaneous accesses to the Patients Portal and the red bars indicate the scenario with 10 users. As expected the results of the second case are much better than the first case. Request cached, Average Response Time and the Average Page time are better in the case that we have 10 users accessing the patient portal. The "average page time" from 24.60 seconds it is decreased to 6.21 seconds. In any case the results depend on the server lines and hardware used.

4 Conclusions

These are the initial steps followed in order to create a system that will be used for monitoring patients after cardiac surgery. The system has been completed and the next step will be the actual system and acceptance testing before moving into the final use of the system in real cases. The system will be tested with real data, with the patients' and doctors' help. The goal is to use this system to the minimum number of 50 patients initially, in order to ensure that everything is working correctly and it satisfies all requirements.

References

1. American Heart Association, Heart disease and stroke statistics-2008, update, Dallas, Texas (2007), http://www.americanheart.org/presenter.jhtml
2. Kleinpell, R.M., Boaz, A.: Integrating telehealth as a strategy for patient management after discharged for cardiac surgery. Results of a pilot study. Journal of Cardiovascular Nursing 22(1) (2007)
3. World Health Organisation, Fact sheet No 317 (February 2007), http://www.who.int
4. Giordano, A., Scalvini, S., Zanelli, E., Corrà, U., Longobardi, G.L., Ricci, V.A., Baiardi, P., Glisenti, F.: Multicenter randomised trial on home-based telemanagement to prevent hospital readmission of patients with chronic heart failure. International Journal of Cardiology 131(2), 192–199 (2009)
5. Schwarz, K.A., Mion, L.C., Hudock, D., Litman, G.: Telemonitoring of heart failure patients and their caregivers: a pilot randomized controlled trial. Progress in Cardiovascular Nursing 23(1), 18–26 (2008)
6. Wakefield, B.J., Ward, M.M., Holman, J.E., Ray, A., Scherubel, M., Burns, T.L., Kienzle, M.G., Rosenthal, G.E.: Evaluation of home telehealth following hospitalization for heart failure: a randomized trial. Telemedicine Journal and E Health 14(8), 753–761 (2000)
7. Rodrνguez, J., Dranca, L., Goρi, A., Illarramendi, A.: A Web Access to Data in a Mobile ECG Monitoring System. Stud. Health Technol. Inform. 105, 100–111 (2004)

8. Ryan, A., McCann, S., McKenna, H.: Impact of community care in enabling older people with complex needs to remain at home. International Journal of Older People Nursing 4(1), 22–32 (2009)

9. Glascock, A., Kutzik, D.: The Impact of Behavioral Monitoring Technology on the Provision of Health Care in the Home. Journal of Universal Computer Science 12(1), 59–79 (2006)

10. Sixsmith, A.: An evaluation of an intelligent home monitoring system. Journal of Telemedicine and Telecare 6(2), 63–72 (2000)

11. Drennan, V., Levenson, R., Goodman, C., Evans, C.: The workforce in health and social care services to older people: developing an education and training strategy. Nurse Education Today 24, 402–408 (2004)

12. Kyriacou, E., Pattichis, C., Hoplaros, D., Kounoudes, A., Milis, M., Jossif, A.: A System for Monitoring Children with Suspected Cardiac Arrhythmias Technical Optimizations and Evaluation. In: XII Mediterranean Conference on Medical and Biological Engineering and Computing, MEDICON 2010, Chalkidiki, Greece (2010)

13. RS TechMedic BV, ECG monitors,
    `http://www.dyna-vision.com/products.html`

14. Hamilton, P.S.: Open Source Arrhythmia detection Software DOI,
    `http://www.eplimited.com`

15. MSDN website, `http://msdn.microsoft.com/`

16. The Official Microsoft ASP.NET Site, `http://www.asp.net`

17. National Instruments, `http://www.ni.com`

INDEPENDENT: Technology Supported Autonomous Living

Pantelis Angelidis and Eleftheria Vellidou

Vidavo S.A., 9th Klm Thessalonikis Thermis Av.,
57001, Thessaloniki, Greece
{projects,pantelis}@vidavo.gr

Abstract. ICT enabled Service Integration for Independent Living (INDE-PENDENT) is an ICT – PSP project funded under objective 1.3 ICT for ageing well / independent living. Work has started as early as February 2010 and expected to finish after 3 years. INDIPENDENT will address current limitations of telehealth and telecare platforms to serve needs for support and delivery of support to the elderly which is not limited to a single sector (healthcare or social care) but spans the two sectors and empowers informal carers and the third sector to participate in delivery of support. This paper will discuss the Greek experience when drafting pilot scenarios that fit into the project's goals.

Keywords: elderly, social care, health care, autonomous living, third sector, integrated platform of communication, informal carer.

1 Introduction

Large demographic changes are underway in the EU which will lead to significant increases in old age dependency ratios. Ageing and health care along with long-term care expenditures appear to be highly related. Ageing populations pose major economic, budgetary and social challenges. By 2060, projections agreed within the Member States set the increase in age-related expenditure at an average of 4¾ percentage points (pp) of GDP inside the EU. At the same period Europe will move from having four people of working age for every person aged over 65 to a ratio of 2 to 1. Ageing will already start affecting most EU economies in the coming decade. According to Eurostat, Europe is an ageing continent. Statistics say that [1]:

- The size of the EU population will fall from 376 million in 2000 to 364 million in 2050. Big declines will take place in Italy, Spain and Germany whereas increases are projected in France, Ireland, Luxembourg and the UK;
- The number of young persons (aged between 0 and 14) will fall from 69 million in 2000 to 58 million in 2050
- The working-age population (aged between 15 and 64) will fall by some 20%, from 246 million in 2000 to 203 million in 2050
- The numbers of elderly persons (aged 65 and over) will rise significantly from 61 million in 2000 to 103 million in 2050.
- Within the 60+ age group, there will also be a significant growth in the number of "very old", i.e. people aged 80 years and over. Whereas the very old

J. Lin and K.S. Nikita (Eds.): MobiHealth 2010, LNICST 55, pp. 69–76, 2011.

constitute 3% of the European population today, 11 of the former EU-15 Member States will have at least 10% of their population aged 80 or over by 2050.

Eurostat also predicts that by 2060 almost a third of the population of the present EU countries will be aged over 65. The current proportion is one in six. The population aged above 65 as percentage of the population aged 15 to 64 is shown in Figure 1:

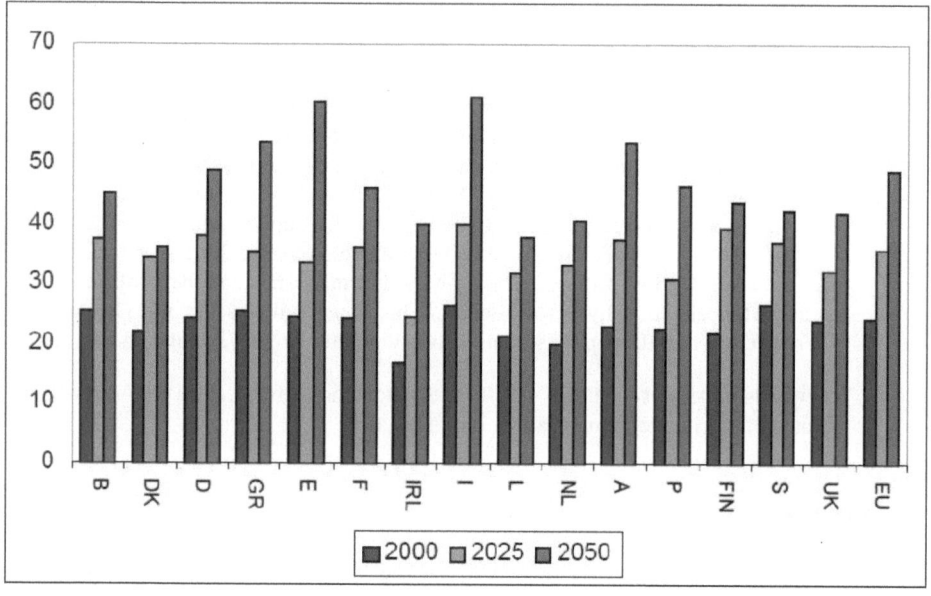

Fig. 1. Old Age Dependency Ratio in EU member states 2000, 2050[2]

The main reasons behind the trend are:

- Increased life expectancy
- Low birth rate
- "Modernization" of lifestyles
- The growing ability of medicine to intervene and keep alive people who previously would have died
- Much higher proportion of the population living with chronic conditions and, in many cases, multiple conditions.

In Europe, all national care systems are faced with three major challenges, as the population of Europe is ageing, health care is increasingly effective but also becoming more expensive, and patients, having become true consumers, are also more demanding. Expenditures in the global market for telemedicine are expected to grow at an annual rate of 19% till 2012, from 4.7 Billion in 2007 to 11.2 Billion in 2012[3].

2   A Criticism on Support Mechanisms

As Europe's population ages, the way we support older people will have to change. The National Health Systems as well as the individuals cannot afford to have the elderly being looked after in institutional care as it is widely done today, nor even our older people want to lose their independence in this way. Healthcare and social care to older people at home is growing in importance, and care service provision is empowered and improved by ICT-enabled solutions, by modern telecare and telehealth systems. However, for a number of reasons these systems are not adapted to the needs of the elderly and consequently to our needs as we grow older.

So far we have designed ICT-enabled forms of support as an embedded integral part of healthcare and social care organisational "silos" hence living unexploited the great potential of solutions such as telecare and telehealth. Up until quite recently, national welfare and health systems and regional/local support practices were developed in a highly specialized way and boundaries between them were well defined preventing them from cooperation [4].

However, when it comes to supporting older people living in the community, today's reality is still characterised by fragmentation and bureaucracy in current provision systems resulting in disjointed and patchy support services. Recently the dangers of closed silo service provision have been widely recognised at the policy level and steps taken to spread responsibility more widely and introduce cooperative structures, including third sector and citizens groups. Many governments are now beginning to seek to improve collaborative support of older people living in the community. Evidence points into the direction that "models of integrated health and social care for the elderly can result in improved outcomes, client satisfaction and/or cost savings"[5]. ICT suppliers have not yet properly responded to this trend.

The design of today's components for telehealth and telecare reflects their customers' specialisation in separate sectoral "silos" respectively for healthcare provision and social care provision. This has restrained them from the wide scope cooperative approach now increasingly seen as essential, and restricted them in particular to integration of responsibilities and tasks performed by family or volunteers usually called the third sector. Current platforms for vital signs monitoring provided by healthcare organisations are generally not accessible for care personnel outside the directly responsible health institution. While first generation systems provided only capture and transmission of vital signs, the current generation of such platforms is beginning to support interaction with the cared for individual, but typically communication is restricted to those having access to the vital signs server in the clinic. Apart from this, state-of-the-art platforms for chronic disease management are currently designed for use only within the healthcare sector, though the care tasks including training and measurement or quality triage can better (more cost-effectively) be provided outside the periphery of the formal health care sector.

ICT platform for social care, primarily social alarm or more generally telecare, are somewhat more open to the transfer of information from the cared-for person to the family and other informal or voluntary carers. Currently, this openness is mainly limited to sending alerts and messages outside the system. These home platforms, in the inward direction, are exclusively accessible from professionals working in the sector though outward communication from the home is available to some extent.

Platforms provided for social alarms by community alarm providers are not in any way fully accessible to care personnel outside the alarm centre directly responsible.

Existing and additional functionality – messaging, reminders, questionnaires etc. - could be used more effectively if controlled and secure access were given to informal carers and other authorised support givers outside the specific service provider organisation operating the platform.

In addition to opening up current telehealth and telecare solutions and providing functionality on unspecialized platforms, the organisations and individuals, supporting the elderly need tools to effectively cooperate with eachother. Back office inter-organisational services in support of collaboration have also largely remained yet unrealised.

Some progress has been made to removing an emerging telehealth island within healthcare, e.g. Philips has implemented the Continua xHR standard to connect telehealth systems with existing electronic health record (EHR) systems. Shared usage of ICT infrastructures across established domain boundaries to support cross-sectoral collaboration, e.g. by medical and social professionals, though intra-sector integration is being tackled in this way, is nowhere near reality in neither Europe nor elsewhere [5].

Together all these factors contribute to the fact that the vast potential that innovative ICT solutions do generally hold for supporting older people in living independently in the community has yet remained largely unexploited, with negative impacts on the quality of life of those whose independence is threatened by social and other circumstances that tend to appear when growing older. Additionally, this situation has negative impact on the economic sustainability of welfare and health systems. It is widely recognised that models of formal support provisioning to the elderly need to change, to reflect the budgetary pressure and the demographic changes, including different ways of accessing formal carers and co-ordination of informal care. This creates obvious needs for integrated means of communication and for the supporting technology. It also highlights the potential for familiar user and home technology performing a role within the supporting network.

3   Mission and Objectives of the INDEPENDENT Project

Therefore,

- given that in the ageing societies of Europe and elsewhere the pressure is increasing to improve and extend support to independent living of older people, and
- given that a purely sectoral professional approach in healthcare and social care will fail to deliver and it is recognised that working collaboration and task sharing must be established between professional healthcare and social care services, informal and family support and voluntary sector organisations, and
- given that extension and interoperable opening of today's sectoral ICT solutions and replication of functions and interoperability onto low cost consumer devices provides an opportunity to make this collaborative cross-sector load sharing affordable and bearable;

The mission of the INDEPENDENT project is to define, deliver and pilot a multiplatform digital infrastructure supporting coordinated cross-sector delivery of sufficient and timely support, thereby effectively preventing or at least slowing the way many older people today inexorably slip towards the edges of safe independent living.

In line with this mission the project will pursue a dedicated programme of service process innovation complemented by adaptation of technology. Digital support infrastructure and related services will be set up and piloted:

- using appropriate existing technology to provide as many older people as possible with digital access to the support services they need and enabling them to be reached appropriately by digital techniques by those who can support them and
- augmenting and opening sectoral platforms to enable coordinated cross-sector support delivery,
- developing of care coordination applications to run on informal care platforms, such as scheduling, automatic messaging, voice and video telephony support,
- adopting a clearly demand-driven, choice-giving approach and avoiding all technology 'push'.

4   Mature Starting Points in Trikala, Implemented by Vidavo S.A.

In services currently used by 298 users, elderly people are equipped with light-weight handheld devices and record their vital signs which are then transferred (via the telecare center) to the municipality hospital over PSTN or GPRS for review and feedback by the experts. This combines the components of self-care health service, professional health service, and vital signs remote monitoring. Teams of nurses and physicians visit the older people at home. The nurse records their vital signs and forwards them to the hospital (via the telecare center) for review and feedback by the experts. This combines the components of professional health service, and vital signs monitoring.

The solution complies with a variety of standards as well as promotes and safeguards present and future interoperability with other systems. For this reason:

- The development of the platform was based on open source technologies, and only where required utilisation of proprietary systems took place
- For the interconnection amongst systems, and for future interconnection with HIS, the HL7 protocol is utilised
- For the wireless transmission of the various data, established protocols and technologies are utilised such as the Bluetooth technology for the short range communication between devices.
- The eHealth Interoperability Standards mandate (M403) is followed closely.

A schematic representation of the platform is shown in Figure 2:

The health status monitoring offered is based on the electronic health record (EHR) of the elderly who participate in the scheme. The existing EHR consists mainly of medical components such as latest diagnostics, prescriptions, ECGs, etc. with no reference to the individual's mental health status. Some demographic data are also

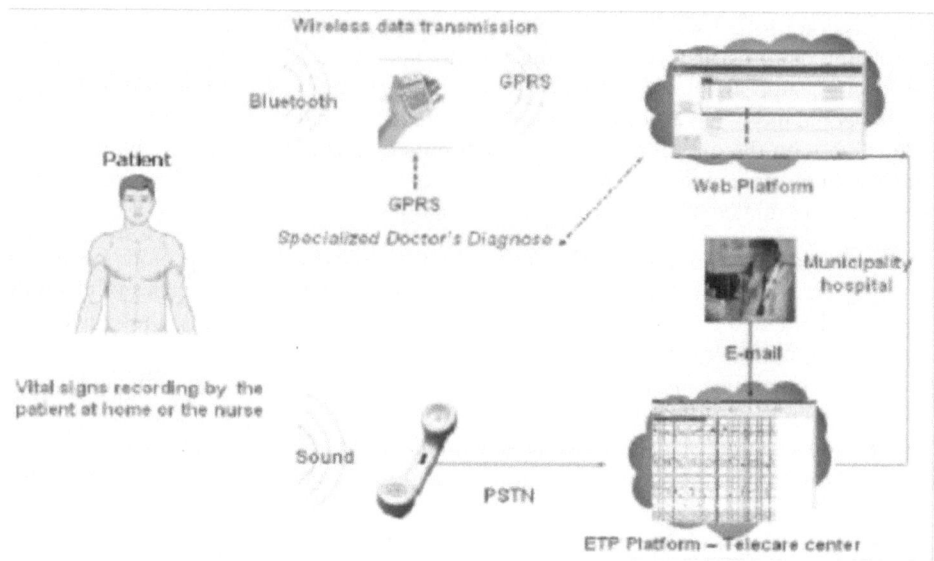

Fig. 2. Trikala's already installed platform

included for facilitating the EHR administration. So far access to the EHR is only allowed to physicians from both the General Hospital of Trikala as well as from Sotiria Hospital in Athens acting as the centre of excellence for the chronic syndromes from which the majority of the elderly suffers. Communication between the health care practitioners (regardless of specialty) and the social services of the Trikala Municipality has retained its traditional paper or oral format.

5 The Solution Envisaged for Trikala in the Context of INDEPENDENT

The Municipality of Trikala, with the aid of VIDAVO S.A. through INDEPENDENT project plans to develop:

- An integrated platform, for common use from the care and health services, with the use of ICT, based on an extended health and care multilevel records and enables cross-sectoral access in particular to augment support to users of remote health monitoring systems.
- study and make the necessary organisational re-formulation of the existing care and health services, on the basis of the integrated platform of INDE-PENDENT
- tele-videoconference for psychological support
- Create a single point entry for the elderly to the health and care services of the Municipality that will cut across organizational boundaries of the various present service models.
- provide efficient integrated care to provide communication and exchange of data between the social and health services by sharing common information

resources and by providing to them new tools to support the process of care of the elderly at home.

- Increase the users or the care and telehealh services by reducing complexity, overlaps of care provision and repetition which decrease efficiency.

In order to better combat depression as a medical cum social condition there is a need for enhancing the monitoring of the individual's status by including psychometric characteristics. The same principle applies to EHRs, they should also be upgraded to incorporate psychiatric diagnostics, prescriptions, free text from consultation, treating practitioners comments etc. The enhanced EHR should not be limited to the medical practitioners; social workers who play a very important role in the community should also interact with this ICT tool. Their shared locus of operation is the elderly and the new tools provide the means for uninterrupted and efficient communication between the two categories of professionals thus allowing for continuity of the overall health care. Informal carers or the elderly could also have access to the EHR in an effort to create awareness for specific conditions and in some cases to reassure someone on his/her actual health status.

In terms of procedure an alarm system could be generated that every time there is a new insertion from either group (social or medical) the others will receive an e-mail prompting them to access the file so they can be updated on the newest developments on the elderly monitoring. This change in process will impose the principal of non repudiation for the practitioners and it will also ensure through the historic data stored in the EHR that even professionals who have never worked with the individuals before, they will have access to all the necessary information for continuing offering their services in the most efficient way.

The services will also strengthen the daily interaction with their social sphere - partners and caregivers, giving them the feeling of safety and preventing their social isolation.

This set of services will be integrated in the scope of the project, evaluated and tested in realistic conditions with real users. The integration will be performed on already existing hardware facilities providing thus the end-product service for the users involved.

This necessitates the holistic approach that will be followed in the project and that will involve the broad expertise and role of the participating partners, and the continuous convergence of the individual components to the service on the integrated platform.

6 Conclusions

The difficult changes that many elderly individuals face—such as the death of a spouse or medical problems—can lead to mental ailments such as depression, especially in those without a strong support system. Left alone, it does not only prevent older adults from enjoying life like they could be, it also takes a heavy toll on health. Although depression in the elderly is a common problem, only a small percentage gets the help they need because the condition is so often overlooked. The consequences of this oversight are high. Untreated depression poses serious risks for older adults, including illness, alcohol and prescription drug abuse, a higher mortality rate, and even suicide. For the condition's treatment the close cooperation between social services, informal carers and mental health professionals is considered mandatory.

In the context of the INTEPENDENT project, the Municipality of Trikala along with VIDAVO S.A. as technology provider will attempt through an ICT empowered solution to integrate health and social care services into one powerful platform that will allow its elderly users to prolong their autonomous living in their familiar surroundings.

References

1. Economic Policy Committee: Budgetary challenges posed by elderly populations, Executive Summary, EPC/ECFIN/630-EN final, October 24 (2001),
   `http://europa.eu/epc/pdf/summary_en.pdf`
2. European Commission, Economic and Financial Affairs: 2009 Ageing Report,
   `http://ec.europa.eu/economy_finance/publications/`
   `publication14992_en.pdf`
3. Telemedicine; Opportunities For Medical and Electronic Providers. BCC Research
4. Kelly, D.: Touching People's Lives with Technology. Presentation at the Silver Economy in Europe Conference, Bonn, Germany, February 16-17 (2005)
5. MacAdam, M.: Frameworks of Integrated Care for the Elderly: A Systematic Review (2008)

Session 4

Interoperability in e-Health

Towards Interoperability for Telemedicine Systems

Lamprini Kolovou, Evy Karavatselou, and Dimitrios Lymberopoulos

Electrical and Computer Engineering Department, University of Patras
University Campus, 265 04 Rio Patras, Greece
lamprinik@wcl.ee.upatras.gr, karavats@upatras.gr,
dlympero@wcl.ee.upatras.gr

Abstract. The analysis, the modeling and the implementation of an intermediate system for facing the syntactic interoperability problem within an e-health domain for telemedicine applications and related medical information systems is the target of this work. The proposed architecture provides a unique service for interoperability utilizing distributed functional entities and specially structured messages. It facilitates different medical information systems and telemedicine application to visibly handle real world events and information, without any interference in the basic structure of these systems. The performance of the proposed system has been tested using special mechanisms and the evaluation was also performed. The extracted statistics validated the high degree of system's effectiveness and efficiency.

Keywords: telemedicine, interoperability, messaging, medical information systems.

1 Introduction

In recent years telemedicine applications have proved their necessity in the provision of qualitative healthcare. The evolution of telemedicine services is its expansion to cover the various areas for remote provision of health care.

In a physically integrated e-health domain, telemedicine applications are not autonomous as far as their interoperability is concerned [1]. Cooperation with other departments within a medical unit and therefore communication with other medical information systems, such as Radiology Information Systems (RIS), Laboratory Information Systems (LIS), Health Electronic Record (HER), is required [3].

The main aim and the next step towards interoperability is the integration of all systems and applications, thus allowing them to operate as a single entity, facilitating their communication and efficiency in transferring and exchange of administrative and medical data. The purpose of this is two-fold: a) the creation of updated and consistent medical files and b) the support of the necessary mobility both for patients and medical personnel. A basic requirement is that the medical files information is immediately available and manageable from all systems, when this is required by the workflow for the provision of medical care within and outside a medical unit. To achieve the necessary integration and as a result of the above requirements, interoperability among telemedicine and the other medical information systems must be ensured.

J. Lin and K.S. Nikita (Eds.): MobiHealth 2010, LNICST 55, pp. 79–86, 2011.

From its general definition, interoperability for telemedicine systems is considered as the ability of different functional entities (applications and data stores) of related systems to (a) exchange information (functional), (b) exchange information that is processible (syntactic) (c) exchange information that is comprehensible (semantic) [2].

For the functional layer, interoperability solutions are provided by the telecommunication networks. In the syntactic and semantic layers there exist gaps due to the existence of many different standards used from the various medical information systems and the freedom in the development and their use [5].

This paper proposes an architecture for syntactic interoperability among telemedicine and other medical information systems, which can be extended to the semantic layer, *provided that the application entities employed will include the necessary translation mechanisms*. Firstly, design considerations and modeling of the proposed architecture are presented, then the implementation and the valuation issues follow.

2 Basic Design Considerations

For providing interoperability service efficiently, a model for the system's architecture was designed taking into account the conditions of the environment described as: (a) telemedicine systems are totally distributed systems, (b) different types of networks are utilized in order to connect two distant points and various means might be interposed, (c) communicating systems and networks should respond and transfer data the faster possible, (d) the communication between a telemedicine system and other information systems within the healthcare enterprise is frequently local, but distant communication is also required for providing its special healthcare services.

The above requirements were taken into account for specifying the basic design considerations of the proposed architecture meeting the special conditions that arise from the environment where telemedicine applications are applied:

- The proposed system follows the distribution of telemedicine systems in various domains and shares its functionality to different sites that participate in communication and exchange of information.
- The proposed systems described not only the functional aspects of the designed architecture but also the syntax of the application messages that are transferred. These messages that have a special structure are able to be adopted from different networks and transfer valid information.
- The proposed architecture and the distribution of functionality keep response times in a qualitative level as the added information that supports the functionality of the system is the less possible and it is not accessed from all functional system's elements.
- The service of structuring and transferring these messages is available to any application and data store that is related to telemedicine application without interfering to their implementation. The provided services elements are locally and distantly provided by special functional entities, properly designed and implemented in each site.

To cover these requirements the proposed system was analyzed and designed distinguishing two basic perspectives: (a) functional features of the system that are linked to the technical specifications of the implemented infrastructure and (b) the provided interoperability service.

3 Modeling Interoperability Service and the System Architecture

3.1 The Functional Aspect

From its functional perspective the proposed system is fully defined by the following aspects.

As users of this system are considered the applications and the data stores of tele-medicine and other related medical information systems that are to exchange informa-tion, independently of the messaging protocol that they use. The specification of users' profile, the administration of sessions and the application of information secu-rity policies are supported by diverse information classes and by their conceptual relations.

The general architecture of the proposed system consists of an intermediate transfer system (TS) and dedicated interfacing entities for the users. The TS is the core unit of the system serving messages created by all users and supporting translating functions as well. The collection of all functional entities and its users, in common with their appropriate operational settings, constitutes a management domain.

During the session, the end-to-end user communication process is organized by a special service, named '*interoperability service (int service)*' that is following de-scribed. At any time instance, each user may be the originator or the recipient of a message. According to the needs of the session, any user may alternate its role.

The common structure of the exchanged messages is defined as well. These mes-sages consist of two parts (Fig. 1): (a) the envelope part that constitutes four segments of fields; (b) the content part that includes the initial user's message. The envelope part is used to provide the *int-service* consistently and its structure is dependent on the telecommunication protocol that the user applies in the application layer.

```
<message>
    <envelope>
        <originator></originator>
        <recipient></recipient>
        <conditions>
            <protocol></protocol>
            <coding></coding>
            <message_type></message_type>
            <content_type></content_type>
            <priority_level></priority_level>
        </conditions>
        <identifiers>
            <session_ID></session_ID>
            <message_ID></message_ID>
        </identifiers>
    </envelope>
    <content>application message</content>
</message>
```

Fig. 1. XML structure of message

3.2 Int-service Design

Service of interoperability is designed as an end-to-end user communication service. The specification of service considers that:

- During any session, the *int-service* utilizes the functional entities of intermediate system in order to establish the appropriate communication path between users (originator and recipient).
- The operation of the *int-service* is accomplished through submission, transfer and delivery interactions. An interaction is considered as the 'means' by which the HT-messages are transferred between users' domains and TS.
- The creation of the communication paths and the performance of all interactions are achieved through the use of a complete set of service elements.

Interactions. The proposed specification of int-service allows submission, transfer and delivery interactions.

Submission interaction is the means by which an originating user's interfacing entities submit the message to TS. The envelope fields of the submitted HT-message (submission envelope) contain information that leads TS to select and apply the appropriate service elements. This information represents identification data of the originator and recipient, as well as special identifiers and formatting conditions for the application data that are included in the content part.

Transfer interaction is the means by which user's interfacing entities transfer the message to TS. During transfer interaction, TS reformats the content of messages, if the originator and recipient use different messaging standards.

Delivery interaction is the means by which TS delivers the message to a recipient's site. The envelope of the HT-message (delivery envelope) contains the delivery information of the HT-message. This information is similar to that of the submission envelope.

Service Elements. The features of the above interactions are implemented by sixteen (16) basic service elements, provided by the functional entities. The total service elements constitute the int-service and are organized in:

The *Message Transferring service elements* (10) are responsible for the transferring of the messages and handling the message addressing, identification and conversion as well as user capabilities negotiation.

The *Message Storing service elements* (4) handle the transmission and receipt conditions of HT-messages from or to the message storing entities.

The *Resource Verification service elements* (2) are responsible for the verification and maintenance of the connection between user interfacing entities and the TS.

4 Implementing the System

4.1 System's Architecture

The presented system has the structure that is depicted in Fig 2. The entities of the proposed architecture are of three types: (a) agents that are used for message processing

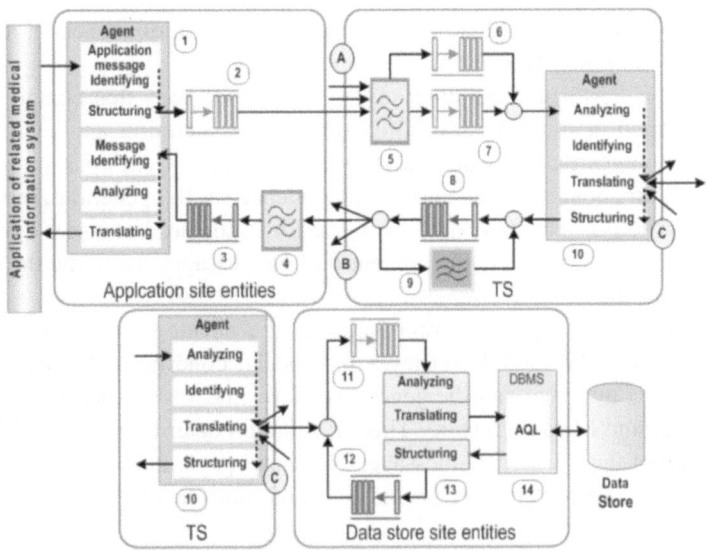

Fig. 2. The proposed architecture implements the various functional entities and supports the provided service

and include proper modules, (b) message stores that are used for message queuing and (c) filters that are used for error checking and message recover functions.

TS performs storing, transferring and reformatting processes of HT-messages using four entities; an agent (10), three message stores: (6) for application-to-application sessions, (7) for application-to-data store session, and a message store for outbound messages (8). Additionally, TS includes two message filters, (5) for inbound messages and (9) for outbound HT-messages.

The users access TS through individual and dedicated interfaces. Application's interfacing is performed by an agent (1), two temporarily data storage entities for the inbound and the outbound messages (3) and (2) and a message filter (4). Data store's interfacing is performed by another agent (13), two message data stores −(11) for inbound messages and (12) for outbound messages- and a special entity called Access Query Library (AQL) (14). AQL provides extra security mechanism protecting data store's hosted information and controlling the access to this information, with predefined queries that specify all the possible and allowed interactions that the parent data store might perform.

4.2 Special Mechanism Modules

Translation: Translation is one of the core functions of the proposed system. The entities of each sender's domain use the content part (payload) of the messages as carrier of their initially originated messages. If two users communicate applying the same messaging standard, there is no affect on the messages payload, in the transmission process. If users communicate applying incompatible standards, TS translates accordingly the messages payload from the standard format of the sender to this of the recipient, activating its "Translating" module.

Translation is performed utilizing: (a) *"Users' Catalogue"* that contains -in users' profiles- information about the special conditions that each user applies for the structure of the messages that they send and receive; (b) the *"Meta-data store"* that contains information about relations and correspondence for the general rules of message coding and structure that the different messaging standards of users apply; (c) the *"Translator"* that re-constructs the content part of messages using the information of the two previous units.

Translation depends upon the information in the envelope of the message. In the case of translation, the module retrieves the special conditions that the users apply from the Users' Catalogue and the general rules for message structures of messaging standards, from the Meta-data store. This information determines the 'final' structure of the payload of the transferred message. The 'new' payload is then forwarded to the next module, in order to construct the message and transfer it to its recipient.

Error handling: This mechanism operates at the application level of the utilized telecommunication infrastructure and includes: (a) supervision of the sessions' performance with the use of special fields of the messages' envelope; (b) check of system resources before starting every session from the users' interfacing entities; (c) administration of queues in message stores with priority in that messages that are signaled with special flags in their envelope; (d) use of filters for: correct routing of the messages, feedback in the case of failed forwarding and temporary storage of messages until the sessions regular termination. In special cases of system's failures, the system recovers its last normal operational status. Messages that arrive simultaneously in message stores are retrieved with priority. First are these that "belong" to sessions in progress and then the initially originated messages. If the messages are of the same case, these are retrieved with a random order. In any case of failure, TS sends special notifications to the originators.

Auditing: This mechanism is in function continuously and produces log files including tracing information of the sequential processes that are recorded. For each process the exact time details (timestamps) are marked so the extraction of the desired results is possible.

The auditing information that is recorded to the log files is divided in three main categories. The first includes the details of the connections between the different entities of the system and between the various computational systems. In the second category the details of sending a message are transcribed. The fields of this section of the log file describe the start and end of messages' transfer, the success or failure notifications, the re-sending procedure's details, filtering results and the identification data of message/session. The third category audits contain the receive process of messages including start and termination time points, filtering results, types of notifications and identification data of message/session.

5   Development Issues

The above described technical features of the system are basically developed as executable modules. These of the intermediate system are installed in an autonomous computational system. These of users' interfacing are embedded as autonomous software modules to the application programs and installed in the users' terminals.

The Users' Catalogue and the Meta-data Store have been implemented as independent relational databases that are hosted to the same database server.

For the development of users' interfacing and TS's modules Java language were utilized. HL7 messaging procedures were developed by means of the NeoTool Library. Databases were hosted by means of Oracle10g RDBMS and for access to the AQLs the ADO technology and SQL DML language were applied. DICOM services and message definitions were implemented using the CTN open source software (Washington University of Saint Louis).

6   Evaluation

The developed system was tested and evaluated using two medical information systems that are usually related with telemedicine applications in every day workflow. These are Laboratory Information System (LIS) and Picture Archiving and Communication System (PACS), administering medical exams, laboratory and imaging in respective. During the test, the telemedicine application was requesting the retrieval of the proper laboratory and imaging examinations of a patient, related to the same medical incident with the intention to create a unique record for this patient.

To measure the performance of the system the Auditing mechanism was used and the produced recorded information was properly processed in order to estimate the following quality factors: functionality, reliability, efficiency, maintainability and portability (according to the ISO 9126 model [6]).

Functionality, reliability and efficiency were estimated using the evaluation parameters recorded to the log files and the rest of the quality factors were studied based on the features of the designed and developed system. The first three factors were measured at the levels of 99,2 to 99.7 % verifying that the designed system meets the initially stated requirements at a very satisfactory level.

Maintainability and portability are measures of the difficulty in adjusting the system under new operational requirements. These two factors are answered by the methods and standards that were used to develop and evaluate the system. For maintainability, the evaluation mechanism enables the surveillance of the processes that occur and any fault can be easily diagnosed. For portability, the tools and the standards that were used for the implementation allow the easy installation of TS to different environments and compatibility with already used software solutions. A basic issue that is put forward concerns the technical features of the used hardware as messages' processing requires high computational power.

7 Conclusions

Nowadays, the healthcare information domain is oriented to distributed systems manipulating, with a uniform and unbounded manner, information created by medical applications with different specialties and capabilities. In this domain telemedicine applications keep a significant role and interoperability within this domain is a main issue. The presented system is an effort to overcome this problem, focusing on the syntactic interoperability. While most solutions face interoperability from the technical point of view, the current system contributes to the standardization approach, applying the specifications of a model for structuring a distributed system that shares its service to the different participating sites. This approach can lead to more viable solutions, while no constraint regarding the used messaging standards or technologies is set. Better administration, maintenance and surveillance of the provided *int-service* is achieved.

References

1. Vargas, B., Pradeep, R.: Interoperability of hospital information systems: a case study. In: Proceedings of 5th International Workshop on Enterprise Networking and Computing in Healthcare Industry, June 6-7, pp. 79–85 (2003)
2. CEN/ISSS e-Health Standardization Focus Group: Current and future standardization issues in the e-Health domain: Achieving interoperability. In: CEN 2005 (2005)
3. Mantzaris, D., Anastassopoulos, G., Adamopoulos, A., Gardikis, S.: A non-Symbolic Implementation of Abdominal Pain Estimation in Childhood. Information Sciences 178(20), 3860–3866 (2008)
4. Berler, A., Pavlopoulos, S., Koutsouris, D.: Design of an interoperability framework in a regional healthcare system. In: 26th Annual International Conference of the ISSS, EMBS, San Francisco, CA, USA, September 2004, pp. 3093–3096 (2004)
5. Bicer, V., Laleci, G.B., Dogac, A., Kabak, Y.: Artemis message exchange framework: Semantic interoperability of exchanged message in the healthcare domain. SIGMOD Record 34 (September 2005), http://www.srdc.metu.edu.tr/
6. ISO/IEC 9126, International Standard, Information Technology – Software Product Evaluation – Quality characteristics and guidelines for their use (1991),
   http://www.usabilitynet.org/tools/r_international.htm

Personal Health Systems for Patient Self-management: Integration in Pervasive Monitoring Environments

Andreas K. Triantafyllidis, Vassilis G. Koutkias, Ioanna Chouvarda,
Georgios D. Giaglis, and Nicos Maglaveras

Lab. of Medical Informatics, Faculty of Medicine, Aristotle University of Thessaloniki,
P.O. Box 323, 54124, Thessaloniki, Greece
{atriant,bikout,ioanna,giaglis,nicmag}@med.auth.gr

Abstract. Various personal health systems have been applied in pervasive health monitoring, in which the need for patient involvement and self-management support with appropriate health information management tools has been highlighted. This paper presents a novel approach towards constructing a personalized mobile system, introduced as add-on to existing remote monitoring systems, for the management of health information by the patient himself/herself, with a Personal Health Record (PHR) constituting the system backbone. Particular emphasis is given to interconnection aspects with the monitoring system, so as to enable enhanced customization and management of monitoring-driven information provided to the patients according to their requirements/preferences. Communication issues between the monitoring and the proposed system are handled by using well-defined Web service interfaces for data exchange. Our prototype implementation, along with an application scenario presented, illustrate the applicability and virtue of the current work.

Keywords: Health Information Management; Self-management; Personal Health Records; Pervasive Health Monitoring; Service-oriented architecture.

1 Introduction

Several health monitoring systems enabled by pervasive computing technologies have been introduced for healthcare services delivery [1]. Moreover, various approaches have been proposed targeting on the generation and management of health information by the user/patient [2]. The patients' central role in the management of their health is indicated by a number of educational programmes aiming to provide them with skills and knowledge in order to cope with their diseases on a daily basis [3]. It is expected that patients' participation in self-management activities can be beneficial in terms of enhancing their communication with their doctor, helping them to focus on the treatment plan and be adherent, growing their level of self-confidence, and better managing their well-being [4].

Although various personal health systems have been applied in pervasive health monitoring, patient's participation in the involved procedures has not been systematically elaborated, while the need for better tools for self-managed care has been

J. Lin and K.S. Nikita (Eds.): MobiHealth 2010, LNICST 55, pp. 87–94, 2011.
© Institute for Computer Sciences, Social Informatics and Telecommunications Engineering 2011

highlighted [5]. Considering in particular personal health information management by the patient, this typically involves user-to-system interactions which are rather limited, tight to the monitoring plan, and dedicated to the monitoring system functionality, all of which reduce actual patient involvement with respect to customization and filtering of information [6]. Moreover, in continuous health monitoring, supported by sensor-enhanced wearable/mobile systems and appropriate medical procedures initiated by healthcare professionals, the monitoring system may not generate appropriate feedback to the patient (e.g., in terms of false alerts in regard with the health status observed), due to a number of reasons associated with the variable context related to the patient (e.g., time, location, activity, situation, etc.) [7].

In the current work, we present a mobile, personal health management system (PHMS) targeted at chronic patients, who are using remote monitoring systems (RMS), are highly aware of their disease, and may wish to play a more active role in their disease management. The system relies on the Personal Health Record (PHR) notion [8] for self-reporting and is interoperable with typical RMSs [9]. This interoperation involves configurations related to patient decisions on the value of the monitoring output, as well as presentation preferences, which may increase system usability and acceptance. A mobile base unit (MBU) is used as the patient's personal terminal for health information display and management, and the communication hub for data exchange between the two systems. The basis of PHMS is a set of appropriately defined communication structures following the service-oriented architecture (SOA) paradigm [10], whereas terminology services are used for medical concept resolution and system interoperability. Thus, the PHMS and the RMS constitute two autonomous, yet interacting systems. The PHMS can be used as an add-on to monitoring systems capable of providing a suitable layer of Web service clients to their back-end infrastructure for chronic patients' self-management.

2 Functionality Overview

The functionality of the proposed PHMS is partially distributed between the MBU, residing in the patient site and aimed at recording patient-provided health information, and the system's server side, for the persistence of information recorded by the patient, as well as the provision of communication interfaces to the RMS and external services/applications. In the current implementation, the particular focus is on recording various conditions or symptoms. The afore-mentioned information constitutes the *Patient-driven Information* (PDI), i.e., information which is recorded manually by the patient himself/herself, as extensively analysed in [8].

In a pervasive health monitoring setting, the feedback provided to the patient via clinical-site initiated procedures is usually related to condition-specific content, i.e., various kinds of event-driven recommendations/alerts (e.g., a prompt message with exercise recommendations upon weight increase), periodic reports (e.g., sets of alerts/recommendations within a time-period), and questionnaires for the identification of subjective symptoms. We refer to this type of feedback as *Monitoring-driven Information* (MDI). In the current work, this information provided to the patient is considered as input to the PHMS, enabling the patient to process and filter it according to his/her needs, aiming to generate a personalized output.

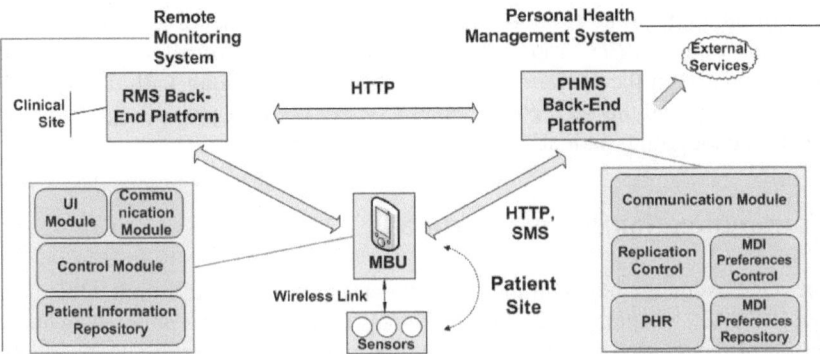

Fig. 1. Overall system architecture

In our current system realization, the patient is supported with advanced options to manage the provided MDI. Thus, the PHMS interacts with the RMS and the patient is able to configure the MDI insertion by providing the decision on whether and when the specified MDI is allowed to be inserted in the PHR. The above-mentioned patient's management operations are independent from the RMS, so as not to intervene with the medical personnel's initiated monitoring procedures. Finally, explicit system adaptations related to the terminology used, the level of MDI detail, and information access rights are provided, as these constitute personalized options, that may have impact on the patient's adoption of the system and long-term commitment. In this context, the patient is provided with a holistic view of personal health information integrating both his/her observations and reports as well as those generated by the RMS as encapsulated in PDI and MDI, respectively.

3   System Architecture

The primary objective of the proposed system architecture is to decouple the monitoring procedures from the PHMS functionality to the extent possible. Thus, the PHMS is conceived as an add-on to existing monitoring systems, allowing easy interconnection and avoiding complex configurations and communication mechanisms. This requirement is addressed via the definition of appropriate interfaces on a service layer upon HTTP, as well as a request/response model.

Figure 1 depicts the overall system architecture, comprising of the MBU in the patient site for patient's management of health information, the PHMS back-end used both as the surrogate host and communication gateway of the PHMS, and the monitoring back-end typically established in the clinical site. The MBU consists of four layered components: a) The *Patient Information Repository* constituting the record management system for persisting information about PDI, MDI and patient's preferences; b) the *Control module*, encapsulating the application logic; c) the *UI module*, responsible for UI adaptations as these apply according to certain patient preferences, and d) the *Communication module*, handling communication with the PHMS back-end. Requested data from the latter may be persisted in the Patient Information Repository or/and delivered to the UI module. Likewise, the PHMS back-end platform consists of an appropriate *Communication module* for connection with the MBU and the RMS, as well as a *PHR* repository and a *Replication Control module* for replicating data persisted in the *Patient Information Repository*, along with the *MDI Preferences Repository* and the *MDI Preferences Control* used for persisting and controlling information concerning patient's preferences, respectively.

4 Communication Infrastructure

For message exchange between the communicating parties, the Simple Object Access Protocol (SOAP) (http://www.w3.org/TR/soap/) encodings are adopted, whereas the definition of the service interfaces is provided via the Web Service Description Language (WSDL) (http://www.w3.org/TR/wsdl/). SOAP and WSDL provide the necessary communication infrastructure, so that the MBU and the PHMS back-end can communicate in an interoperable manner according to the SOA paradigm, offering also loose coupling and extensibility in the proposed approach [10].

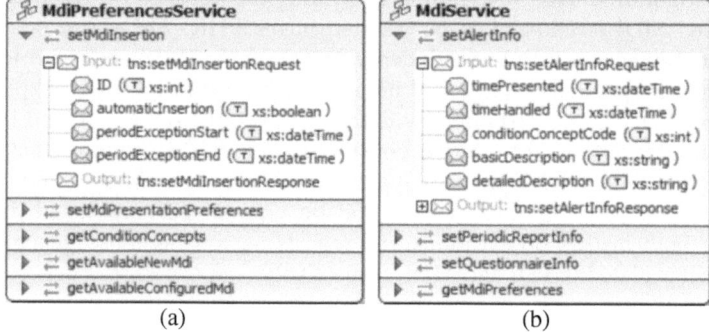

Fig. 2. Example Web service operations for: (a) patient MDI preferences and (b) MDI control

Two distinct service interfaces are offered: a) The *PHMS back-end – MBU interface* (Fig. 2 (a)) that is required for the transmission of user's MDI preferences to the system's back-end, as well as for the replication of data persisted in the MBU to the server side. b) The *PHMS back-end – RMS interface* (Fig. 2 (b)) that allows the RMS to set the MDI and transmit it to the PHMS back-end. Especially for the communication between the PHMS and the RMS, it is important to address interoperability issues in regard with the content semantics embodied in MDI. Although the support of a clinical standard-based format, e.g., HL7/CDA [11] could be applicable, this would introduce an additional layer of information de-serialization, as well as an unnecessary overhead in the transmission of document-based services. Thus, enabling access to widely adopted, medical terminology services was preferred for medical concept resolution. The PHMS back-end can then interpret the relevant concept identifier, e.g., for a condition/symptom, in a dynamic fashion by initiating appropriate connections to the defined terminology services e.g., by using the UMLSKS (Unified Medical Language System Knowledge Source Server) service interface (http://umlsks.nlm.nih.gov/).

5   MDI Insertion and Presentation Preferences

The MDI insertion into the PHR according to patient's preferences and needs is a fundamental element in enabling health information management by the patient in pervasive health monitoring. Thus, the patient can be provided with options to configure the insertion of the MDI to his/her PHR, e.g., with "Yes", "No", or a "Send me a notification to decide" options. A sequence diagram illustrating the afore-mentioned feature is depicted in Fig. 3 (corresponding to the operations of services (a) and (b) depicted in Fig. 2). Additionally, sophisticated preferences are supported, so as to enhance the manipulation of MDI by the patient. For example, these include the configuration of a context dimension, such as time. Thus, the patient may control which MDI can be logged into the PHR by defining e.g., temporal exceptions.

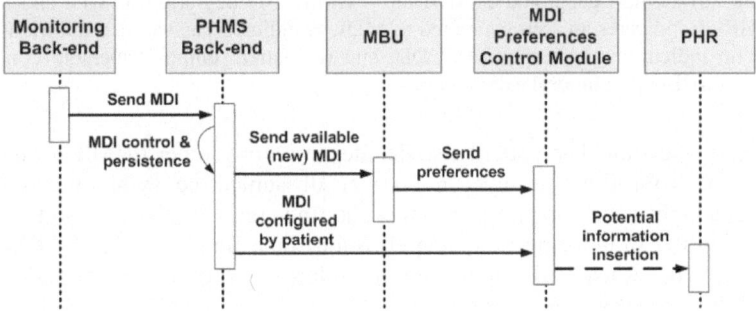

Fig. 3. Sequence diagram illustrating the potential MDI insertion into the patient's PHR

Three are the main dimensions according to which patient preferences are provided: a) the *level of MDI detail* that includes beyond basic information about an observed alert/condition, details, such as the conditions which lead to the MDI generation, description of correlated events, etc.; b) the *medical vocabulary used*, as according to user's configuration, the medical information presented to the patient may contain either user-defined terms possibly used in everyday natural language communication, or formal medical concepts as defined in medical terminologies, and c) *information access rights*, which are associated with the user's permission to view, edit, or delete an MDI instance. Such configuration capabilities can help the patient to focus only on system interactions of personal interest.

6   Application Scenario and Prototype Implementation

Jane, a 53-year old school teacher, is newly diagnosed with a heart condition and is prescribed with the appropriate medication. She is also provided with a wearable RMS to track her condition, and it is suggested to her to use the PHMS for personal health information management. According to her health status, it is decided by her doctor that a number of parameters will be monitored via the RMS, including blood pressure (BP), with the use of a specific sensor, depression, with the use of a short, standardized test, administered every other week, and dyspnoea, with the use of a

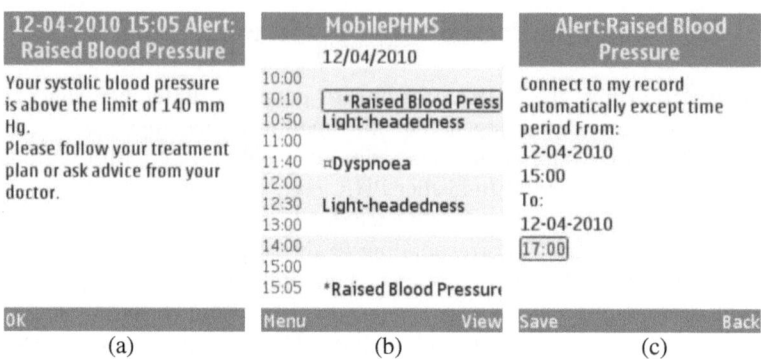

Fig. 4. Screenshots from the mobile PHMS application deployed in a Nokia N95 smartphone illustrating: (a) an alert generated as MDI into PHMS, (b) integration of MDI and PDI in patient's PHR (*: indicates an alert generated as MDI, ¤: indicates answer to a question generated as MDI, no indications correspond to PDI), and (c) patient empowerment to configure the insertion of MDI with temporal exceptions.

simple daily question. The patient also decides to record in her PHMS her medication intakes and, from time to time, a number of subjective symptoms (e.g., light-headedness, night-time coughing, etc.) that she finds relevant to her condition.

Accessing her monitoring system/application, Jane finds out that the RMS has issued a couple of "Raised BP" alerts and that it has incorporated in her periodic report almost daily increases of BP during afternoons. Jane realizes that these high BP bouts coincide with her visits to her local fitness-training center. Soon afterwards, she opens her mobile PHMS application (Fig. 4 (a), (b)) and realizes also that the same bouts have been logged into her personal record, since the default PHMS functionality is associated with the automatic insertion of all kinds of MDI into the PHR. In a next step (Fig. 4 (c)), Jane formulates a rule that no "Raised BP" alerts should be recorded in her PHR during the times and days she is training (while the monitoring procedures remain unaffected). From a technical perspective, the rule activation forces the PHMS back-end to check via the *MDI Preferences Control* module, whether the alert generation time is within the user-defined time period, whenever an alert of this type is received. This includes the resolution of the "Raised BP" concept using UMLS (in this case, "Raised Blood Pressure" with concept identifier 271647008). Following the approach of this hypothetical scenario, Jane is able to view health-related information on her PHR, combining personal observations (i.e., PDI) and objective information (i.e., MDI), filtered according to her personal preferences.

Aiming to explore the technical feasibility of such scenarios, in our prototype implementation, a sensor-enhanced RMS with an MBU, namely the Citizen Health System (CHS), was deployed [12]. CHS particularly targets at patients suffering from diabetes or heart failure, and provides the necessary communication infrastructure, such as mobile communication components, Component Object Model (COM) technology, etc., for information exchange between the patient and the clinical site. The most dominant type of system-generated feedback provided to the patient is the so-called "Tip" in the form of a recommendation, e.g., "Reduce your salt-intake" included in event-driven (e.g., raised blood pressure) educational sessions.

A testing service client layer for Web service consumption was implemented on the CHS back-end infrastructure with which information concerning event-driven educational sessions could be delivered to the PHMS. In the PHMS back-end infrastructure, the Apache Tomcat Server was used as Web application container, Apache Axis2 as the underlying SOAP engine for the Web services enablement, while UMLSKS Web service clients were constructed for dynamic medical concepts resolution. Although this deployment was performed using CHS, any RMS capable of supporting a Web service layer interface with the PHMS could be used.

A Nokia N95 smartphone was used acting as the MBU device, while Java Micro Edition (JavaME) was the chosen development environment to implement a prototype mobile application realized as the front-end of the described PHMS. In regard with the SOAP/WSDL approach, the communication with the PHMS back-end was achieved via JSR (Java Specification Requests) 172 Web Services API that utilizes the generation of appropriate client structures according to the specified WSDL documents. An open source SMS gateway (http://smstools.meinemullemaus.de/) was used for implementing the push operations of back-end requests via SMS, whenever the PHMS back-end initiates communication with the MBU, e.g., in case of sending a notification whether to insert or not MDI into the PHR.

For privacy and security reasons, all data held in MBU memory were encrypted via a 128-bit key based AES algorithm [13]. The key is generated upon the initial user registration in the mobile application via username and password credentials. The above mentioned functionality was implemented via the Bouncy Castle Crypto API for Java (http://www.bouncycastle.org/). Moreover, an authentication Web service was implemented requesting as input the same credentials and returning as response a session key for communication between the MBU and the PHMS back-end.

After the conduction of several communication tests, Web service invocations initiated by the MBU were found to last on average about 1.5 seconds (till reception of response), while service invocations from the CHS back-end lasted on average about 0.5 seconds. Thus, concerning performance, the proposed PHMS was found to provide fast enough request/response times for SOAP messages exchange.

7 Conclusion and Future Work

Although the importance of patient self-management towards effective healthcare has been stressed [4], this aspect has not been systematically elaborated in pervasive health monitoring environments. The current work introduces a novel approach towards building a personalized mobile system as add-on to RMSs for the management of health information by the patient himself/herself. In this regard, interoperability issues with RMSs have been elaborated, so as to enable the provision of customizable, advanced and personalized feedback to the patient.

Our prototype implementation constituted a technical proof-of-concept effort, in the direction of enabling the interaction between PHMSs and RMSs for supporting patient self-management. Such an interaction resulted in an integrated mobile system for patient health information management, aiming to contribute in continuity of care, independent living, and well-being.

The proposed system targets at patients willing to actively engage in their health management processes for the potential gain of self-management benefits [5]. This approach is in line with the notion of collaborative healthcare, where the patient's role is further enhanced in healthcare delivery. It is evident, though, that the presented system has to be evaluated in terms of usability, patient acceptance and medical procedures in appropriate clinical field studies.

The current work constitutes a basic step towards personalized and patient-targeted monitoring adaptations in pervasive health. In this regard, our future work involves the development of a generic methodology introducing patient's observations and personal preferences on the received monitoring feedback, handling of contextual parameters such as time and location, behavioral monitoring, and appropriate clinical decision support methods.

References

1. Varshney, U.: Pervasive healthcare and wireless health monitoring. Mob. Netw. Appl. 12(2-3), 113–127 (2007)
2. Mattila, E., et al.: Empowering citizens for wellbeing and chronic disease management with Wellness Diary. IEEE Trans. Inf. Technol. Biomed. 14(2), 456–463 (2010)
3. Warsi, A., Wang, P., LaValley, M., Avorn, J., Solomon, D.H.: Self-management education programs in chronic disease: a systematic review and methodological critique of the literature. Arch. Intern. Med. 164(15), 1641–1649 (2004)
4. Lorig, K.R., Sobel, D.S., Ritter, P.L., Laurent, D., Hobbs, M.: Effect of a self-management program on patients with chronic disease. Eff. Clin. Pract. 4(6), 256–262 (2001)
5. Demiris, G., et al.: Patient-centred applications: use of information technology to promote disease management and wellness. J. Am. Med. Inform. Assoc. 15(8), 121–126 (2008)
6. Koch, S.: Home telehealth – current state and future trends. Int. J. of Med. Inf. 75(8), 565–576 (2006)
7. Zheng, J.W., Zhang, Z.B., Wu, T.H., Zhang, Y.: A wearable mobihealth care system supporting real-time diagnosis and alarm. Med. Bio. Eng. Comput. 45, 877–885 (2007)
8. Tang, P.C., et al.: Personal Health Records: definitions, benefits, and strategies for overcoming barriers to adoption. J. Am. Med. Inform. Assoc. 13(2), 121–126 (2006)
9. Hermens, H.J., Vollenbroek-Hutten, M.M.R.: Towards remote monitoring and remotely supervised training. J. Electromyogr. Kinesiol. 18, 908–919 (2008)
10. Singh, M.P., Huhns, M.N.: Service-Oriented Computing: Semantics, Processes, Agents. J. Wiley and Sons, Chichester (2005)
11. Dolin, R.H., et al.: HL7 Clinical Document Architecture, Release 2. J. Am. Med. Inform. Assoc. 13(1), 30–39 (2006)
12. Maglaveras, N., et al.: The Citizen Health System (CHS): A modular medical contact center providing quality telemedicine services. IEEE Trans. Inf. Technol. Biomed. 9(3), 353–362 (2005)
13. Daemen, J., Rijmen, V.: The Design of Rijndael: AES - The Advanced Encryption Standard. Springer, Heidelberg (2002)

A Portal for Ubiquitous Access to Personal Health Records on the Cloud

Vassiliki Koufi, Flora Malamateniou, and George Vassilacopoulos

Department of Digital Systems, University of Piraeus,
Karaoli & Dimitriou St. 80, 18534 Piraeus, Greece
{vassok,flora,gvass}@unipi.gr

Abstract. Recently, there has been a remarkable upsurge in activity surrounding the adoption of Personal Health Records (PHRs) whose architectures are based on the fundamental assumptions that the complete records are centrally stored and that each patient retains authority over access to any portion of his/her record. Although the consumer/patient is the primary beneficiary and user of PHRs, healthcare professionals stand to benefit from their use as well. In particular, the integration of leading-edge networking technologies, such as cloud-based services and mobile communications, with PHRs has the potential to improve delivery of healthcare by rendering PHRs ubiquitously accessible. This paper presents a portal application which provides access to PHRs on the cloud. Cloud-based services can prove important in healthcare provision, but the inherent nature of medical records underscores the need for clouds to be private to ensure data security is better maintained. Thus, the proposed portal application comes with a suitable security mechanism, in order to ensure secure access to healthcare information.

Keywords: Personal Health Records, cloud computing, web services, ubiquitous access, access control, portal.

1 Introduction

Throughout their lives individuals may receive care by various providers and under various circumstances, resulting in patient data being scattered around disparate and geographically dispersed information systems hosted by different healthcare providers [1][2]. The lack of interoperability among these systems, as is often the case, impedes optimal care since it leads to unavailability of important information regarding a patient health status when this is mostly needed (e.g. in case of an emergency).

Recently, there has been a remarkable upsurge in activity surrounding the adoption of Personal Health Record (PHR) systems [2] as both patients and healthcare providers have realized that their use may entail a number of benefits, such as better access to information, increased patient satisfaction and continuity of care [2][3]. A PHR is a consumer-centric approach to making comprehensive electronic health records (EHRs) available at any point of care while fully protecting patient privacy [4][5]. In particular, a PHR can be defined as a set of tools that allow patients to access and coordinate their lifelong health information and make appropriate parts of it available

J. Lin and K.S. Nikita (Eds.): MobiHealth 2010, LNICST 55, pp. 95–101, 2011.

to those who need it. PHR data can come from EHRs or directly from the patient – including non-clinical information (e.g. exercise habits, diet, etc) [6]. The key difference between PHRs and EHRs is that, unlike traditional EHRs that are based on the "fetch and show" model, PHRs' architectures are based on the fundamental assumptions that the complete records are held on a central repository and that each patient retains authority over access to any portion of his/her record [3] [4]. Thus, an entire class of interoperability is eliminated since the system of storing and retrieving essential patient data is no longer fragmented.

Although the consumer/patient is the primary beneficiary and user of PHRs, healthcare professionals stand to benefit from their use as well [7]. In particular, healthcare professionals, due to the high level of mobility they experience, require ubiquitous access to relevant and timely patient data in order to make critical care decisions [8]. The integration of leading-edge networking technologies, such as cloud-based services and mobile communications, with PHRs can meet this requirement since it can enable easy and immediate retrieval of PHRs from anywhere, via almost any device. Hence, healthcare providers are increasingly considering migrating to cloud computing in an attempt to increase flexibility and agility of patient data access, processing and storage and enhance quality and safety of patient care [9-10]. In this context, protection and confidentiality of personal data must be ensured owing to the inherent nature of medical records.

Along these lines, a prototype web portal is presented, namely NefeliPortal, which provides a web interface to workflow-based healthcare processes. In particular, NefeliPortal provides pervasive and ubiquitous access to healthcare processes which are modeled as flows of cloud-based web services that provide access to PHR data, residing within a cloud infrastructure. The aforementioned processes may involve access to medical data by authorized users or triggering a new healthcare process, such as the e- prescribing process.

2   Motivating Scenario

The basic motivation for this research stems from our intervention in a recent project concerned with designing and implementing a PHR system in the context of a prototype e-prescription system developed for the needs of the Greek Health and Social Security System. Essentially, the system assumes that an effective drug prescription mechanism should be based on providing a rich picture of the patient's heath record so that quality of care improvement and cost containment are both met concurrently.

Suppose a healthcare delivery situation where an individual is transferred to the emergency department (ED) of a hospital. Upon arrival to the ED, the patient registration procedure is performed by specifying the patient's identity somehow and by undergoing through triage to determine the nature and severity of his/her case. Upon completion of emergency case management, which may have involved drug prescription and/or administration, the patient is either admitted to the same hospital (e.g., to a clinical department, the Intensive Care Unit - ICU) or transferred to a more specialized hospital or even discharged. As ED visits are unplanned and urgent, there is a need to ensure that information regarding patient's health status (e.g. health problems, allergies, medication history, recent diagnostic and therapeutic procedures) is

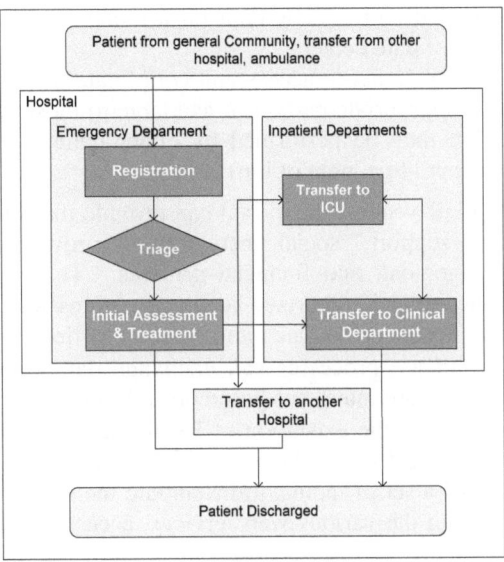

Fig. 1. Emergency Patient Flow

automatically made available to ED physicians. Thus, care inefficiencies, in the form of redundant testing, care delays, and less-effective treatments prescribed are eliminated and quality of care is enhanced [11-20].

Figure 1 shows an indicative high-level view of the patient flow from the time of arrival to a hospital's ED to the time of leaving the ED. Two of the roles participating in the emergency patient's care are the roles of the ED physician and specialized ED nurse.

3 System Architecture

Figure 2 shows a high-level view of the cloud PHR architecture that underlies Nefeli-Portal, where patient data are accessed via web services deployed through Business Process Execution Language (BPEL). It is essentially a cloud-based system architecture that coordinates reliable, secure and high-performance deployment of NefeliPortal services and comprises software elements on the mobile device (i.e. a Personal Digital Assistant - PDA) and on the cloud.

The PDA client is running an HTTP(S)-based client, which is the PDA's web browser and provides user interaction with the system. The cloud, which essentially constitutes the NefeliPortal's environment, consists of the following software components:

- **PHR platform:** it is a platform used for the implementation of the PHR system. The platform comprises:

i. *a data repository* - it stores PHR data on a cloud data storage system which relies on a number of data centers.

ii. *a portal* - it allows patients to access and coordinate their lifelong health information and make appropriate parts of it available to those who need it. Authorization propagation may be performed by either patients themselves or by an assigned "gatekeeper" (e.g. next of kin) [21].

Depending on the PHR vendor, this portal can provide the following categories of services: decision support, social networking, provider-patient interaction, disease/health management, and financial services. Thus, patients can actively manage their own health and authorized healthcare professionals (e.g. general practitioners) can timely access up-to-date patient data (e.g. drug prescription data).

- **Web Services:** healthcare processes can exchange data with the PHR platform through a series of software interfaces based on web services standards.
- **BPEL Engine:** it handles the execution of BPEL-based healthcare processes provided in the healthcare settings. The role of the BPEL engine is, given a BPEL process definition and a set of inputs, to instantiate the healthcare process, executing the tasks by calling the various web services, accessing PHR data and routing the data between them.
- **Web Portal:** it provides a web-based front end to healthcare processes and, in turn, to PHR data accessed through the execution of these processes. It consists of a JSR-168 [22] compliant portlet container that hosts and manages the main portlet of NefeliPortal, namely NefeliPortal BPEL portlet, as well as the portlets of the workflow (BPEL) applications. A portlet is a java web component that generates dynamic content in response to processed requests [23]. NefeliPortal BPEL portlet provides the Web browser-based portal user interface to the BPEL Engine where all healthcare processes are deployed. Thus interaction with the corresponding workflows is enabled. This interaction is performed through certain portlets developed to facilitate the physicians' interaction with the relevant tasks of the workflows.
- **Web/Application Server:** it provides the hosting environment to the aforementioned components.

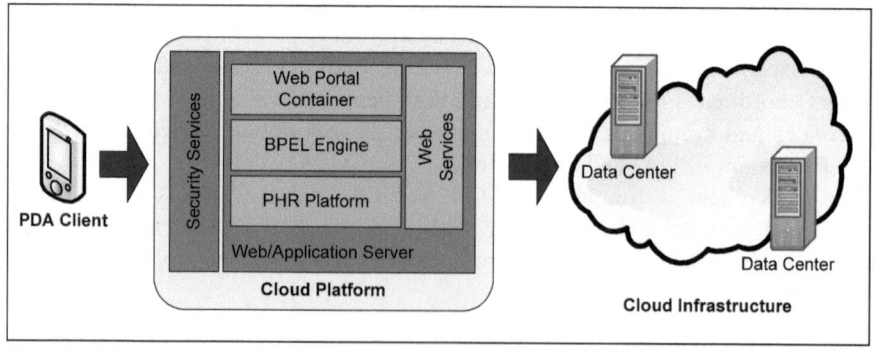

Fig. 2. System Architecture

4   Implementation Issues

The prototype implementation of the proposed portal application has been developed on a laboratory cloud computing infrastructure. The system has been developed as a web application using the Apache/Tomcat as Web/Application Server. The BPEL engine used for the execution of BPEL healthcare processes is ActiveBPEL [24], an open source BPEL Engine [24]. NefeliPortal that provides access to this engine is based upon IBM WebSphere portal framework [25], a JSR-168 compliant portal [22]. The platform used for the generation of sample patient records is Care2X Integrated Healthcare Environment [26]. Although Care2X is not a PHR platform but an open source Web based hospital information system, it has been considered sufficient for the purpose of our research. As illustrated in Figure 2, PHR data are stored on multiple data centers on the cloud. To this end, the cloud storage model is used. Essentially, cloud storage is a model of networked online storage where data is stored on multiple, virtual servers, generally hosted by geographically dispersed third parties, rather than being hosted on dedicated servers [27]. In our prototype, these servers lie behind a firewall (i.e. the cloud is private) and serve as large data centers that are exposed as storage pools, which healthcare providers can use to store PHR data objects.

Access to data stored in Care2X repository is achieved by means of web services which make use of the Care2X Application Programming Interface (API) and are deployed on the cloud computing infrastructure. One of the web services developed is the PHR access enabler (PHRE) which encompasses the tasks that are concerned with ED physician accesses to patient record data.

Development of cloud computing applications that provide readily access to integrated healthcare information at the point of care introduces security risks especially with regard to authorization and access control. To this end, a suitable security mechanism is embedded into the proposed cloud portal application, which ensures authorized data access through the invocation of relevant web services. Authorization decisions are made subject to the constraints imposed by the execution context.

When on duty, an ED physician needs to gain access to the PHRs of the patients he is treating. To this end, each time the ED physician needs to view the PHR of a patient he attempts to invoke PHRE. Thus, a request for the invocation of this web service is issued which is identified by the authorization and access control mechanism incorporated in NefeliPortal. At the same time, the collection of relevant context information (e.g. physician id, patient id, time of attempted access, location of attempted access) is initiated and the acquired values are passed to the security mechanism, which, in turn, evaluates the relevant contextual constraints and decides whether access to the PHRE should be permitted or denied.

Due to lack of space, more details regarding the implementation of NefeliPortal and the security mechanism incorporated in it are presented elsewhere.

5   Concluding Remarks

Healthcare organizations are faced with the challenge to improve healthcare quality, preventing medical errors, reducing healthcare costs, improving administrative efficiencies, reducing paper work and increasing access to affordable healthcare. A Personal Health Record (PHR) is a way for patients to have control of their own health data, while providing an interoperable platform for sharing relevant clinical data between providers. Moreover, if deployed on a cloud computing infrastructure, PHRs can provide readily access to integrated healthcare information at the point of care. To this end, suitable cloud computing applications need to be developed which will streamline and automate healthcare processes and will provide timely access to the relevant PHRs. This paper presents a cloud portal application, NefeliPortal, which renders medical information immediately available to people who need it via remotely accessible, secure and highly usable PHRs. NefeliPortal is portlet-based and accessible via any portable device (e.g Personal Digital Assistant - PDA).

The evaluation of the proposed architecture requires its application in a wider spectrum of healthcare processes in order to reveal its potential strengths and weaknesses. This is a task to be undertaken in the near future.

References

1. Tang, P.C., Ash, J.S., Bates, D.W., Overhage, J.M., Sands, D.Z.: Personal health records: definitions, benefits, and strategies for overcoming barriers to adoption. J. Am. Med. Inform. Assn. 13(2), 121–126 (2006)
2. Wiljer, D., Urowitz, S., Apatu, E., DeLenardo, C., Eysenbach, G., Harth, T., Pai, H., Leonard, K.J.: Patient accessible electronic health records: exploring recommendations for successful implementation strategies. J. Med. Internet Res. 10(4) (2008)
3. Lauer, G.: Health Record Banks Gaining Traction in Regional Projects, http://www.ihealthbeat.org/features/2009/health-record-banks-gaining-traction-in-regional-projects.aspx
4. Yasnoff, W.A.: Electronic Records are Key to Health-care Reform, BusinessWeek (2008)
5. Win, K.T., Susilo, W., Mu, Y.: Personal Health Record Systems and Their Security Protection. J. Med. Syst. 30, 309–315 (2006)
6. Alberta Health Services: Engaging the patient in healthcare: An overview of Personal Health Record Systems and Implications for Alberta, White Paper (2009)
7. U.S. Department of Health and Human Services: Personal Health Records and Personal Health Record Systems, A Report and Recommendations from the National Committee on Vital and Health Statistics (2006)
8. Tentori, M., Favela, J., Rodriguez, M.D.: Privacy-Aware Autonomous Agents for Pervasive Healthcare. IEEE Intell. Syst. 21(6), 55–62 (2006)
9. Shimrat, O.: Cloud Computing and Healthcare, San Diego Physician.org (2009)
10. van der Burg, S., Dolstra, E.: Software Development in a Dynamic Cloud: From Device to Service Orientation in a Hospital. Environment. In: 2009 ICSE Workshop on Software Engineering Challenges of Cloud Computing, Vancouver, Canada (2009)
11. Schiff, G.D., Rucker, T.D.: Computerized Prescribing: Building the Electronic Infrastructure for Better Medication Usage. J. Amer. Med. Assoc. 279(13), 1024–1029 (1998)
12. Evans, R.S., Pestotnik, S.L., Classen, D.C., Clemmer, T.P., Weaver, L.K., Orme Jr., J.F., Lloyd, J.F., Burke, J.P.: A Computer-Assisted Management Program for Antibiotics and Other Antiinfective Agents. New Engl. J. Med. 338(4), 232–238 (1998)
13. Ash, J.S., Berg, M., Coiera, E.: Some Unintended Consequences of Information Technology in Health Care: The Nature of Patient Care Information System Related Errors. J. Am. Med. Inform. Assn. 11(2), 104–112 (2004)

14. Bates, D.W., Leape, L.L., Cullen, D.J., Laird, N., Petersen, L.A., Teich, J.M., Burdick, E., Hickey, M., Kleefield, S., Shea, B., Vander Vliet, M., Seger, D.L.: Effect of Computerized Physician Order Entry and a Team Intervention on Prevention of Serious Medication Errors. J. Amer. Med. Assoc. 280(15), 1311–1316 (1998)
15. Bates, D.W., Teich, J.M., Lee, J., Seger, D., Kuperman, G.J., Ma'Luf, N., Boyle, D., Leape, L.: The Impact of Computerized Physician Order Entry on Medication Error Prevention. J. Am. Med. Inform. Assn. 6(4), 313–321 (1999)
16. Gandhi, T.K., Weingart, S.N., Borus, J., Seger, A.C., Peterson, J., Burdick, E., Seger, D.L., Shu, K., Federico, F., Leape, L.L., Bates, D.W.: Adverse Drug Events in Ambulatory Care. New Engl. J. Med. 348(16), 1556–1564 (2003)
17. Teich, J.M., Merchia, P.R., Schmiz, J.L., Kuperman, G.J., Spurr, C.D., Bates, D.W.: Effects of Computerized Physician Order Entry on Prescribing Practices. Arch. Intern. Med. 160(18), 2741–2747 (2000)
18. Bell, D.S., Cretin, S., Marken, R.S., Landman, A.B.: A Conceptual Framework for Evaluating Outpatient Electronic Prescribing Systems Based on Their Functional Capabilities. Am. Med. Inform. Assn. 11(1), 60–70 (2004)
19. Higashi, T., Shekelle, P.G., Solomon, D.H., Knight, E.L., Roth, C., Chang, J.T., Kamberg, C.J., MacLean, C.H., Young, R.T., Adams, J., Reuben, D.B., Avorn, J., Wenger, N.S.: The Quality of Pharmacologic Care for Vulnerable Older Patients. Ann. Intern. Med. 140(9), 714–720 (2004)
20. Doolan, D.F., Bates, D.W.: Computerized Physician Order Entry Systems in Hospitals: Mandates and Incentives. Health Affair 21(4), 180–188 (2002)
21. Power, K.: Global Mobile Healthcare An Electronic Framework for Portability of Health Records. Medical Tourism Magazine (2009)
22. JSR-168 Portlet Specification,
    http://www.jcp.org/aboutJava/communityprocess/final/jsr168/
23. Del Vecchio, D., Hazlewood, V., Humphrey, M.: Evaluating Grid portal security, Supercomputing, Tampa, FL (2006)
24. Active Endpoints, ActiveBPEL Open Source Engine Project,
    http://www.activebpel.org/
25. IBM, IBM Websphere, http://www.ibm.com/websphere
26. Care2X Integrated Healthcare Environment, http://www.care2x.org/
27. IBM Cloud computing White paper, IBM Point of View: Security and Cloud Computing (2009),
    ftp://public.dhe.ibm.com/common/ssi/sa/wh/n/tiw14045usen/
    TIW14045USEN_HR.PDF

Session 5

Signal Processing Techniques for Monitoring Services

Early Diagnosis of Alzheimer's Type Dementia Using Continuous Speech Recognition

Vassilis Baldas[1], Charalampos Lampiris[2],
Christos Capsalis[2], and Dimitrios Koutsouris[1]

[1] Biomedical Engineering Laboratory, National Technical University of Athens,
Greece
[2] Wireless Communication Lab, National Technical University of Athens,
Greece
baldas@biomed.ntua.gr, clamp@mail.ntua.gr, ccaps@central.ntua.gr,
dkoutsou@biomed.ntua.gr

Abstract. One of the most important social problems that many of
the developed countries face is the constant rise of the percentage of the
elderly population values. A major health issue affecting this part of the
population is the appearance of dementia of the Alzheimers type (AD)
which is the most common case of dementia, affecting around 50 million
people worldwide. In addition, the frequency of the AD related cases is
expected to grow three times over the next 50 years.

The proposed AD status monitoring system (ADSMS) is processing
a person's speech habits to train itself and extracts specific statistic parameters. After that necessary training process, it constantly monitors
and analyzes new spontaneous speech data, in order to classify them. In
this way, it is possible for the ADSMS to predict possible signs of AD
that need further investigation with the common methods of diagnosis
by a physician.

Keywords: Dementia, Alzheimer, Continuous Speech Recognition,
Speech Analysis.

1 Introduction

One of the most important social problems that many of the developed countries
face, is population aging. Demographics show that there is a constant rise in
the percentage of the elderly population values. One of the main health issue
affecting this part of the population is the appearance of dementia [1]. The
dementia of Alzheimer s type (AD) is the most common case of dementia and
affects around 50 million people worldwide and the frequency of the AD related
cases is expected to grow three times over the next 50 years [2].

Alzheimer's and other dementias are also a great social and fiscal burden for
the nations, therefore an early detection will be of significant importance for
both the patients and the health and social care system. Early diagnosis leads to
early access to pharmacological treatment, access to information and education

J. Lin and K.S. Nikita (Eds.): MobiHealth 2010, LNICST 55, pp. 105–110, 2011.
© Institute for Computer Sciences, Social Informatics and Telecommunications Engineering 2011

for everyone involved, organization of the counseling and community support, cognitive training and even lifestyle advice. The benefits of early institutionalization and improved physical and mental health will also result in better public health and potentially lower costs [3].

Some work has been done on the field of early detection of AD using electroencephalographic (EEG) recordings and classifiers [4], and also by analyzing the MRI volumes in search of volumetric atrophy of the gray matter (GM) in areas of neocortex of AD patients. Most of these techniques use machine learning methods to classify brain images (MRI or fMRI) in order to short and discriminate the characteristics of normal vs neuropathological subjects [5]. In general, most of the previous work on early detection of AD is based on analysis of medical signals and images, and on gene information extraction [6].

Some researchers though, managed to extract information about a person's cognitive status from analyzing his written or spoken language [7] [8]. The described solution uses these methods as the basic theory behind the AD detection system.

1.1   The Proposed Method for Early Detection of AD

Nowadays, personal computers along with various multimedia and communication systems are present in every home. This fact can be used to design a pervasive long-term AD status monitoring system, based on continuous speech recognition and analysis. The person whose mental and cognitive level we are interested on tracking, is hereinafter called *subject*.

The AD status monitoring system (ADSMS) extracts specific statistical measurements using data from the subject's speech analysis, to train itself. After the training process is complete it constantly analyzes new data that are entered to the system in order to classify them. Thus, it is possible for the ADSMS to predict possible signs of AD that need further investigation with the common methods of diagnosis by the subject's physician.

2   Description of the Proposed System

The overall architecture of the proposed system and the main modules that contribute to the final result, are shown on Fig 1.

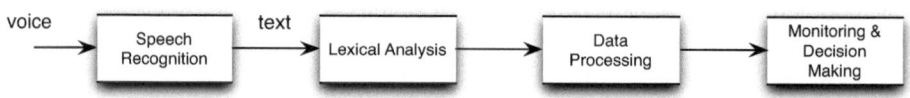

Fig. 1. The basic functions of the proposed system

ADSMS consists of three primary modules and each of them is composed of further subsystems. These parts are presented below.

2.1   Speech Recognition

The first part of ADSMS is the speech recognition module. This is the subsystem that is responsible for collecting the voice samples from the subject via a microphone or a network of multiple microphones, and transforming them to raw text that is later going to be further analyzed. Many methods in bibliography have been presented on accurate and fast speech recognition [9]. Two of the most used technologies on the field are hidden Markov modeling (HMM) and dynamic programming search techniques for large-scale networks [10]. Some of these works manage to succeed in translating speech to text even on noisy environments, and even with mobile devices as the processing platform.

For ADSMS, we propose a voice recognition system like the one described on [9], that uses multiple microphones in a room to collect the samples of the subject's voice and then convert them to text. The speech recognition subsystem of ADSMS is considered to be the most trivial part, as the research that has been done on this area is impressive and the results are satisfying.

2.2   Lexical Analysis

We begin by defining the concept of *Speech Matrix*, that will be used further on. Assuming we have a total of n words in the speech recognizer (SR) database, we map each of those words to a respective place in a speech vector of size $1 \times n$. Assuming also that the SR runs constantly each day, at the end of each day the respective speech vector for the i-th day will be of this form: $W_i = (t_{i,1} \ t_{i,2} \ \cdots \ t_{i,n})$ where $t_{i,j}$ is the number of times the j-th word is spoken on the i-th day.

For k days, we can represent the total speech body of the subject by the speech matrix:

$$W_k = \begin{pmatrix} t_{1,1} \ t_{1,2} \ \cdots \ t_{1,n} \\ \vdots \qquad\qquad \vdots \\ t_{k,1} \ t_{k,2} \ \cdots \ t_{k,n} \end{pmatrix}$$

At the same time, all the sentences are analyzed for *part-of-speech-tagging* (POST) that is required on later stages for the analysis. Words are classified based on eight parts of speech: verb (V), noun (N), pronoun (PN), adjective (AJ), adverb (ADV), preposition (PP), conjunction (CJ), and interjection (IJ). Using the algorithm described on [11] we compute for the i-th day a POST vector $POST_i = (V_i \ N_i \ PN_i \ AJ_i \ ADV_i \ PP_i \ CJ_i \ IJ_i)$ where χ_i is the number of words that were identified as belonging to the χ part-of-speech. Following the same rules as with the speech matrix, we can build a POST matrix for k days ($POST_k$).

Using the data from the W_k and the $POST_k$ matrices, we can extract important statistic values that provide information about the subject's cognitive status.

2.3   Interpretation of Results

Some previous work has been done on correlating spontaneous speech statistical patterns with AD [7] [8]. The authors use lexical analysis of the patient's words to get results of the severity of the AD. The stylometric measures that can be used to analyze the subject's W_k and $POST_k$ matrices are borrowed from the linguistics, and the ones that will be used by ADSMS are shown on Table 1.

Table 1. The stylometric measures that can be used to distinguish AD patients from healthy subjects

Symbol	Definition
Total Words (N)	Number of words spoken
Vocabulary Size(Voc)	Number of different words
Noun rate (N_{rate})	$\frac{nouns}{N}$
Pronoun rate (P_{rate})	$\frac{pronouns}{N}$
Adjective rate (A_{rate})	$\frac{adjectives}{N}$
Verb rate (V_{rate})	$\frac{verbs}{N}$
Type-Token Ratio (TTR)	$\frac{Voc}{N}$
Brunét's index (W)	$N^{Voc^{-0.615}}$
Single Vocabulary (Voc^{single})	Number of different words spoken once
Honorés Statistic (R)	$\frac{100 \log N}{1 - \frac{Voc^{single}}{Voc}}$

Bucks et al. [8], found that AD patient's have different speech patterns than normal subjects. These findings, along with findings from [7] are summed up on Table 2.

Each of the metrics can be easily computed from the subject's W_k and $POST_k$ matrices by manipulating and combining the rows.

2.4   Training of the ADSMS for Each Subject and Implementation Notes

Different subjects present different metric values, so it is important to train the ADSMS per person in order to obtain the best results. The training process must be done while the subject is in good cognitive condition so that the system is able to have the normal condition's results, which are the control values. Constant periodical comparison between these normal values and the new data will make it possible to monitor the subject's cognitive status and provide possible alerts for further investigation by his physician.

Table 2. Stylometric results. AD vs. healthy groups.

Metric	Result
Noun rate (N_{rate})	$N_{rate}^{AD} \leq N_{rate}^{normal}$
Pronoun rate (P_{rate})	$P_{rate}^{AD} \geq P_{rate}^{normal}$
Adjective rate (A_{rate})	$A_{rate}^{AD} \geq A_{rate}^{normal}$
Verb rate (V_{rate})	$V_{rate}^{AD} \geq V_{rate}^{normal}$
Type-Token Ratio (TTR)	$TTR^{AD} \leq TTR^{normal}$
Brunét's index (W)	$W^{AD} \leq W^{normal}$
Honorés Statistic (R)	$R^{AD} \leq R^{normal}$

Aging of the subjects is also expected to bring changes to some metrics [7] [8], so it is clear that the control (normal) values have to be updated when this change affects the results.

The speech recognition and data collecting module of the ADSMS has to work constantly in order to capture the data. The heavy work of data processing, analysis, monitoring and decision making can be done on a personal computer during the idle time as a background process.

3   Conclusions and Future Work

We have presented a method for constant monitoring of a subject's speech that can analyze the lexical data and decide on whether or not his cognitive status may be deteriorating due to AD. The described system can be installed on every space, and it's technological requirements are trivial.

Future additions and improvements may include the integration of the whole system into one wearable device that is constantly on the subject's body, and the extension of this research into constant monitoring of other health conditions to investigate if they present similar patterns.

References

1. De Castro, A.K.A., Pinheiro, P.R., Pinheiro, M.C.D.: Applying a decision making model in the early diagnosis of alzheimer's disease. In: Yao, J., Lingras, P., Wu, W.-Z., Szczuka, M.S., Cercone, N.J., Ślęzak, D. (eds.) RSKT 2007. LNCS (LNAI), vol. 4481, pp. 149–156. Springer, Heidelberg (2007)
2. Ramrez, J., Grriz, J., Salas-Gonzalez, D., Romero, A., Lpez, M. lvarez, I., Gmez-Ro, M.: Computer-aided diagnosis of alzheimer's type dementia combining support vector machines and discriminant set of features. In: Information Sciences (2009)
3. Todd, S., Passmore, P.: Alzheimers disease, the importance of early detection. European Neurological Review (2009)

4. Cichocki, A., Shishkin, S.L., Musha, T., Leonowicz, Z., Asada, T., Kurachi, T.: Eeg filtering based on blind source separation (bss) for early detection of alzheimer's disease (ENY-ARTICLE-2009-243. AZ I07/2005/I-022) (Sie 2004). 9p Clinical Neurophysiology 116(3), 729–737 (2005)

5. Savio, A., García-Sebastián, M., Hernández, C., Graña, M., Villanúa, J.: Classification results of artificial neural networks for alzheimer's disease detection. In: Corchado, E., Yin, H. (eds.) IDEAL 2009. LNCS, vol. 5788, pp. 641–648. Springer, Heidelberg (2009)

6. Schenk, D., Barbour, R., Dunn, W., et al.: Immunization with amyloid-beta attenuates alzheimer-disease-like pathology in the pdapp mouse. Nature 400, 173–177 (1999)

7. Thomas, C., Cercone, N.: Automatic detection and rating of dementia of alzheimer type through lexical analysis of spontaneous speech. In: Proc. of IEEE ICMA (2005)

8. Bucks, R., Singh, S., Cuerden, J.M., Wilcock, G.K.: Analysis of spontaneous, conversational speech in dementia of alzheimer type: Evaluation of an objective technique for analysing lexical performance (2000)

9. Yamamoto, K., Masatoshi, T., Nakagawa, S.: Privacy protection for speech signals. Procedia - Social and Behavioral Sciences 2(1), 153–160 (2010); The 1st International Conference on Security Camera Network, Privacy Protection and Community Safety (2009)

10. Jiang, H.: Confidence measures for speech recognition: A survey. Speech Communication 45(4), 455–470 (2005)

11. Schmid, H.: Probabilistic part-of-speech tagging using decision trees. In: Proceedings of the International Conference on New Methods in Language Processing, Manchester, UK (1994)

An Investigation of Acoustical and Signal Processing Techniques for Classification, Diagnosis and Monitoring of Breathing Abnormalities in Sleep

Sandra Morales Cervera, Dragana Nikolić, and Robert Allen

Institute of Sound and Vibration Research, University of Southampton
University Road, Highfield, Southampton SO17 1BJ, United Kingdom
{d.nikolic,r.allen}@soton.ac.uk

Abstract. Snoring is the often earliest symptom of Obstructive Sleep Apnoea (OSA) and other respiratory problems. A successful medical outcome depends on an accurate preoperative diagnosis of the anatomical reason for snoring. The perception of snoring is highly subjective; therefore, there is a need for an objective measurement of snoring for an accurate patient assessment and the evaluation of treatment effects. The main objective of this study was to distinguish between two types of snoring: palatal and non-palatal snoring considering the acoustic characteristics of the snoring signal. A key innovation is that the snoring signals are not analyzed only subjectively by a medical specialist but also objectively by analyzing recorded snoring signals. The patient's snoring has been recorded non-invasively during sleeping and processed in both time and frequency domains to determine the origin of the snore and to identify the key features useful to the medical specialist.

Keywords: Respiratory/breathing problems, Sleep apnoea, Obstructive Sleep Apnoea (OSA), Palatal snoring.

1 Introduction

Snoring can be defined as a respiratory noise generated during sleep when breathing is obstructed by a collapse in the upper airway. The sound of snoring consists of a series of impulses caused by the rapid obstruction and reopening of the upper airway. Several factors can cause snoring, including the sleep positioning, diet, drugs and allergies. It is more common in males than in females and in overweight people of both genders [1]. Some years ago it was firmly believed that snoring is nothing but a social nuisance, without any adverse health consequences to the snorer. But when the sleep apnoea syndrome (when a person stops breathing for short periods while asleep) began to be studied deeply, snoring achieved a totally different new status, being elevated from a social nuisance to an important clinical symptom. Indeed, current epidemiological data indicate that the sleep apnoea syndrome is second to asthma in the prevalence league table of chronic respiratory disorders.

Obstructive Sleep Apnoea (OSA) is a breathing disorder which occurs during sleep and is caused by the transient closure of the upper airways. At first, OSA is not

J. Lin and K.S. Nikita (Eds.): MobiHealth 2010, LNICST 55, pp. 111–116, 2011.
© Institute for Computer Sciences, Social Informatics and Telecommunications Engineering 2011

harmful. However, irregular breathing during the night usually wakes up the patient and leads to an excess of sleepiness and overall fatigue during the day and, if not treated, it can result in serious health problems.

The severity of OSA is often established using the apnoea/hypopnoea index (AHI), which is the number of apnoeic and hypopnoeic periods per hour of sleep. A hypopnoea is a medical term for a disorder which involves episodes of overly shallow breathing or an abnormally low respiratory rate. This differs from apnoea in that there remains some flow of air. Hypopnoea events may happen while asleep or while awake. This disruption in breathing cause a drop in blood oxygen level which may disrupt the different stages of sleep. Thus, AHI gives an overall severity of sleep apnoea including sleep disruptions and desaturations (a low blood oxygen level).

For patients seeking treatment, some options available to help them sleep better and to have less breathing problems during sleep range from losing weight and moderating alcohol intake, to the use of passive devices to modify the nasal or oral airway during sleep, nasal Continuous Positive Airway Pressure (CPAP), and ultimately to surgical re-modelling of the structures involved where this is feasible. A successful surgical outcome is dependent on an accurate preoperative diagnosis of the anatomical site of snoring and the identification of the airway structures involved in producing the noise, as palatal surgery only works if palatal flutter is present. Thus, an objective measurement of snoring is required for an accurate patient assessment and the evaluation of treatment effects.

There are different methods to classify the snoring sound based on the snoring region origin, depending on the acoustic properties or according to the type of snore generation. These categories are non-exclusive as some types of snoring sounds may be described by the use of two or more of them. Endoscopic appraisal of the pharyngeal structures during snoring has revealed that the complex-waveforms are linked with palatal snoring and the simple-waveforms with tongue-based snoring [2].

The main objective of this study was to employ acoustical signal processing techniques to distinguish between palatal and non-palatal snoring from overnight audio recordings of a snorer. The patterns of snores have been recorded and examined in order to determine the snore origin and to identify the key features useful to the medical specialist.

2 Method

Direct recordings from mobile phones have been taken and studied for four different subjects. Between three to five minutes of recording have been made by a patient's relative or friend with a mobile phone placed close to the mouth and nose of the snorer. Each sound record is converted into a ".wav" format with a sampling frequency of 16 kHz and further processed using Matlab software. In order to extract snore-related parameters, the snore recordings have been analyzed in the frequency domain to determine the site where the snore is produced, and in the time domain to distinguish between simple- and complex-waveform snoring. Furthermore, the snoring signals have been analyzed regarding the periodicity of breaths and the duration of the silences between them to determine apnoea episodes. Since such a recording method could not be standardized due to different recording characteristics of each mobile phone as well as varying positions (distances and angles) of the phones from the patient's mouth and nose, it is not possible to determine the perception of loudness of the snoring signal. Initially, the aim was to record snoring signals by making a call to the hospital, but the telephone line has a bandwidth from 400 Hz to 3400 Hz while the main frequencies of all the types of snoring are in the low frequency spectrum (except for the tongue-based snoring). For instance, palatal snoring is between 105 Hz and 190 Hz, and tonsillar snores are about 170 Hz [3]. Thus, in spite of capturing all the frequencies of interest with the phone microphone, the telephone line can reduce information important for snoring analysis.

Taking the recordings directly from the mobile phone as an audio file also has limitations – most of the mobile phones use an ".amr" file format for storing speech audio filtered to 200-3400 Hz with the sampling frequency of 8 kHz and 13-bit resolution using AMR (Adaptive Multi-Rate) codec. It is also important to take into consideration that every subject has been recorded with a different device, in a different position regarding the mouth and nose, at a different distance from the sound source, during different times of the snorer's sleep, and during different lengths. All these create significant difficulty in determining a sound level reference and these pilot measurements demonstrate how different recordings can be obtained from the patients, since the method of recording cannot be standardized.

To reduce ambient noise, the recorded signals are bandpass filtered between 5 Hz and 3000 Hz. The amplitudes of recorded signals are normalized to the range [−1,1] to allow a comparison of different signals and distinguishing between breathing and snoring. The sound signal from breathing exhibits a pattern that repeats itself over subsequent breathing cycles. However, some variation in the intensity and envelope can be seen not only between different individuals but also between breathing cycles from the same individual [4].

3 Experimental Results

Relevant information about four subjects participated in this experiment is given in Table 1 and the experimental results are shown in Fig. 1. Since medical diagnoses of the subjects were not available, the investigation is based on prior research and is given as a comparison of the time and frequency domain analysis of the recorded snoring signals with the results obtained in previous investigations.

For subjects 1 and 4, the interval between frequency peaks is equal to the rate of appearance of sound structures in the snores. The first peak represents the frequency of oscillations, and it coincides approximately with the interval between frequency peaks in the spectrum and with the value calculated from the time waveform. Thus, the frequency of oscillation is around 82-86 Hz for subject 1 and 96-100 Hz for subject 4. Snoring of subject 2 is completely different from those of subjects 1 and 4, having only three main frequency peaks separated by 80 Hz and the frequency of oscillation around 400 Hz which coincides with the highest peak in the spectrum. Therefore, the interval between the frequency peaks is neither the oscillation frequency nor a main frequency in the spectrum in this case.

Table 1. Relevant information about the subjects in this experiment

Subject	Gender	Age	Height [cm]	Weight [kg]	Smoker	BMI [kg/m²]	Weight category
1	Male	57	172	95	No	32.11	Obese (C1)
2	Female	34	164	73	Yes	27.14	Overweight
3	Female	55	170	100	No	34.6	Obese (C1)
4	Female	50	160	68	Yes	26.56	Overweight

Table 2. Types of waveform and two main frequencies of the snoring signals recorded in this experiment compared to the one obtained from the literature [5]

Waveform type	Subject	Frequency f_1 [Hz]	Frequency f_2 [Hz]
Complex	Beck et al. [5]	600	450
	Subject 1	250	164
	Subject 4	391	297
Sinusoidal simple	Beck et al. [5]	110	-
	Subject 2	407	-
Asymmetric simple	Beck et al. [5]	160	320
	Subject 3	226	461

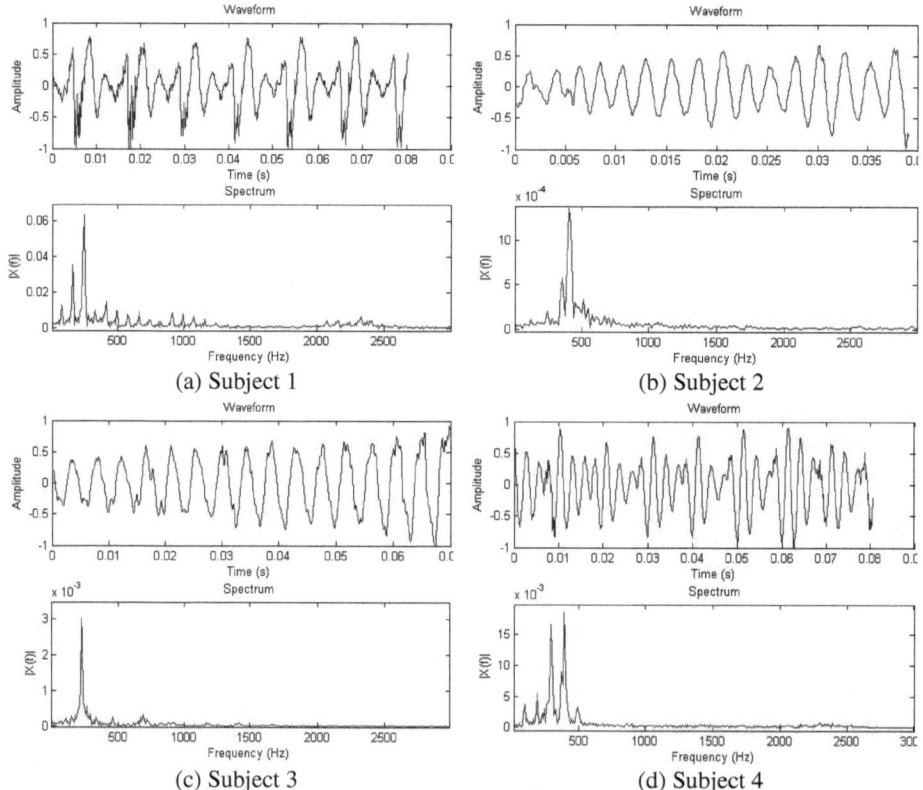

(a) Subject 1   (b) Subject 2

(c) Subject 3   (d) Subject 4

Fig. 1. Time segments (top) and frequency spectra (bottom) of the recorded snoring signals for each of four subjects

Snoring of subject 3, which is an asymmetric simple-waveform snoring, has a spectrum similar to the subject 1's one but with the energy located in low frequencies below 1000 Hz. The frequency of oscillation is 226.6 Hz, and the two next peaks are located at 461.4 Hz and 696 Hz. A separation between the peaks of 234 Hz is very close to the main frequency of 226.6 Hz, and this difference probably can be explained with a low frequency resolution.

4 Discussion

According to Osborne et al. [6], the audible rattle of palatal snoring is around 20 Hz and represents the movement of the palate itself. Since the low frequency content is omitted from the experimental results in this study due to the AMR codec, regular explosive peaks of sound at very low frequencies characteristic for a palatal snoring cannot be identified. However, as noted by Quinn et al. [2], a complex-waveform is associated with palatal snoring and a simple-waveform with tongue-based snoring. Consequently, two complex-waveform and two simple-waveform snorers are identified in this pilot experiment. Thus, the diagnoses given by medical specialist for all 4 subjects are required for an adequate evaluation of the experimental results obtained.

In prior studies, the mean frequency of tongue-based snores has been found to be over 400 Hz (Herzog et al. [7]) or around 1243 Hz (Agrawal et al. [3]). For subjects 1 and 3, some energy is located between 400 Hz and 1200 Hz meaning that those patients have some signs of tongue-based snoring. On the other hand, for three of the subjects, there is some energy in quite high frequencies comparing with prior studies – subjects 1 and 4 have a low energy activity around 2300 Hz, and subject 2 around 2500 Hz. These could be caused by the airflow through the nose or mouth (open mouth or nasal congestion). Moreover, a relation between the ends of the fall of the sound traces and the waveform of the snores could be drawn – subjects 1 and 4 show an abrupt ending of the sound trace, while subjects 2 and 3 show a smooth fall at the end of the event. Conversely, subjects 1 and 4 show an abrupt beginning whereas subjects 2 and 3 show a soft increasing of the amplitude at the beginning. The logical explanation of this is, in the second case, because the airflow is increasing gradually until the speed of the air makes the palate vibrate and it occludes the airway producing a higher amplitude snore. For subjects 1 and 4, the explanation is probably that the occlusion is already there before starting to breath, so it could be any of the non-palatal snores.

Unfortunately, none of the hypothesis described before is currently demonstrable owing to the fact that the previous scientific research is contradictory and there is not a medical diagnosis to compare the results with.

5 Conclusions

The initial idea in this study was to analyze snoring sounds for diagnosis of the underlying pathology, by making a phone call and leaving 4-5 minutes of the snoring sound as a message in a voice mail database for further processing. Although this would be an inexpensive and noninvasive method, it is not yet recommended for clinical implementation as the recorded signal would be filtered below 400 Hz by mobile phone codec or by the telephone line and this appears to be where most of the important characteristics of the snore are located.

In this investigation, the snoring recordings were obtained from the file created by a mobile phone recording, and, as a result, low frequency characteristics were not available. Moreover, the method of recording (i.e. distance, position, and device) is not standardized and therefore no information can be extracted from the amplitude of the signals.

From the available set of four recordings, two complex-waveform and two simple-waveform snorers were identified. The waveform characteristics are similar to the ones described by Beck et al. [5], however, the frequencies do not align. Therefore, there are some differences between previous studies: it has been assumed that complex-waveform is associated with palatal snoring and simple-waveform with tongue-based snoring, but the frequencies do not coincide. In our study, it was not possible to confirm the types of snoring for each patient because medical diagnosis has not been available. Also, due to the loss of low frequency information in the recordings, it was not possible to classify the types of snoring with high certainty.

Although there are some aspects which could not be determined in the present work due to low numbers of subjects in the pilot investigations, together with the number and quality of the recorded signals and due to the lack of a medical diagnosis of the available data, there are several opportunities to improve this investigation in the future. The analysis of the acoustical properties of snores may prove to be a non-invasive and reliable alternative to current diagnostic methods for breathing disorders in sleep. It is believed that this type of data analysis could lead to important conclusions if the results could be compared to a specialist's medical diagnosis.

References

1. Lugaresi, E., Cirignotta, F., Coccagna, G., Piana, C.: Some epidemiological data on snoring and cardiocirculatory disturbances. Sleep. 3, 221–224 (1980)
2. Quinn, S.J., Huang, L., Ellis, P.M.D.: The differentiation of snoring mechanisms using sound analysis. Clin. Otolaryngol. 20, 360–364 (1995)
3. Agrawal, S., Stone, P., McGuinness, K., Morris, J., Camilleri, A.E.: Sound frequency analysis and the site of snoring in natural and induced sleep. Clin. Otolaryngol. 27, 162–166 (2002)
4. Hult, P., Wranne, B., Ask, P.: A bioacustic method for timing of the different phases of the breathing cycle and monitoring of breathing frequency. Medical Engineering and Physics 22, 425–433 (2000)
5. Beck, R., Odeh, M., Oliven, A., Gavriely, N.: The acoustic properties of snores (1995)
6. Osborne, J.E., Osman, E.Z., Hill, P.D., Lee, B.V., Sparkes, C.: A new acoustic method of differentiating palatal from non-palatal snoring (1999)
7. Herzog, M., Schieb, E., Bremert, T., Herzog, B., Hosemann, W., Kaftan, H., Kühnel, T.: Frequency analysis of snoring sounds during simulated and nocturnal snoring. Eur. Arch. Otorhinolaryngol. 256, 1553–1562 (2008)

Performance Investigation of Empirical Mode Decomposition in Biomedical Signals

Alexandros Karagiannis and Philip Constantinou

Mobile RadioCommunications Lab, National Technical University of Athens
Iroon Polytechneiou 9, Athens, Greece
{akarag,fkonst}@mobile.ntua.gr

Abstract. In this paper, the performance of Empirical Mode Decomposition (EMD) applied in biomedical signals is investigated and especially it is considered the case of electrocardiogram (ECG). Synthetic ECG signals corrupted with White Gaussian Noise (WGN) as well as real ECG records are employed and a variety of time series lengths is processed with EMD in order to extract the Intrinsic Mode Functions (IMF). Computation time is measured upon the completion of the process in simulation campaign stage and real records stage and the results are compared in both cases. Spectral characteristics of the time series as well as the tendency to exhibit extrema are the key factors with significant impact on both computation time as well as the total number of IMFs produced.

Keywords: Empirical Mode Decomposition, ECG, Intrinsic Mode Functions, extrema, time of computation.

1 Introduction

Extraction of meaningful information derived from signals corrupted by noise is accomplished with the utilization of data analysis methods. Many traditional methods for processing are employed under the assumption of stationarity of the sampled signal and the linearity of the physical process that produces these signals.

Fourier transform is a widely used technique, albeit ineffective in processing nonstationary data and signals originating from nonlinear systems, because of the properties of the basis functions that are incapable of following spectral changes in time. Wavelet analysis [1,2] and the Wigner-Ville distribution [3] are designed for nonstationary data extracted out of linear systems with intrinsic limitations in characterizing in a detailed fashion the time-frequency composition of signals from nonlinear processes.

A joint function in both time and frequency domains is considered to be an efficient approach towards overcoming the limitations of the traditional techniques [4]. However, Short-time Fourier transform [5], a characteristic tool for time-frequency representation, has fixed time and frequency resolution in order to follow signals with bursts and quasi-stationary components. Research on the field of time-frequency representations is ongoing and fruitful in terms of number of different methods that

J. Lin and K.S. Nikita (Eds.): MobiHealth 2010, LNICST 55, pp. 117–124, 2011.
© Institute for Computer Sciences, Social Informatics and Telecommunications Engineering 2011

tackle with certain limitations. Still most of the existing nonlinear time series analysis methods refer to stationary signals [6] and a necessary condition for the processing of nonlinear and nonstationary data, namely the adaptive basis, is often underestimated.

Most of the biosignals are related to the dynamic biological systems ruled by nonlinear equations and they are considered to be nonlinear and nonstationary. Dealing with nonlinearity and nonstationarity requires an adaptive nature of the processing method. A priori defined sophisticated basis functions face difficulties in meeting the requirement of adaptation which a data driven basis function implies.

A recently proposed method, the Hilbert-Huang Transform (HHT) [7], satisfies the condition of adaptation employed in processing of nonlinear and nonstationary data. The HHT consists of EMD and Hilbert Spectral Analysis (HSA) [8]. The lack of mathematical foundation and analytical expressions poses a problem for the theoretical study of the method. Nevertheless there has been an exhaustive validation in an empirical fashion especially in the time-frequency representations [9].

The core of the method is Empirical Mode Decomposition which resolves a signal into its components adaptively without using an a priori basis. The decomposition is based on the local time scale of data. The adaptive nature of the process successfully decomposes time series from nonlinear processes and nonstationary signals in the time domain. Each component extracted from the original signal through an iterative and sifting process is required to satisfy certain conditions in order to be characterized as IMF.

Application of EMD in time series data results in the production of a set of IMFs and a residual signal. The notion behind this procedure is that a subset of the IMFs is directly related to the underlying physical process. The decomposition is based on the assumption that data consists of different simple intrinsic modes of oscillations and after the production of the IMF set, well-behaved Hilbert transforms compute physically meaningful instantaneous frequencies, thus constructing the Hilbert spectrum.

Unlike wavelet processing, Hilbert-Huang transform decomposes a signal by direct extraction of the local energy associated with the time scales of the signal. This feature reveals the applicability of HHT in both nonstationary and nonlinear signals.

Literature references' variety reveals the extensive range of EMD applications in several areas of the biomedical engineering field. Particularly there are publications concerning the application of EMD in the study of Heart Rate Variability (HRV) [10], analysis of respiratory mechanomyographic signals [11], ECG enhancement artifact and baseline wander correction [12], R-peak detection [13], Crackle sound analysis in lung sounds [14] and enhancement of cardiotocograph signals [15]. The method is employed for filtering electromyographic (EMG) signals in order to perform attenuation of the incorporated background activity [16]. Numerous research papers have been published concerning applications of EMD in biomedical signals and especially towards the direction of optimizing traditional techniques of acquisition and processing of signals such as Doppler ultrasound for the removal of artifacts [17], the analysis of complex time series such as human heartbeat interval [18], the identification of noise components in ECG time series [19] and the denoising of respiratory signals [20].

The contribution of this work is twofold. First, it proposes a mixed scheme based on EMD with an additional pre-processing stage, prior to the EMD application, to be defined according to signal's special characteristics. In this paper, both simulated and experimental ECG time series are employed and some types of filters are used as a filtering stage. Number of IMFs is measured for both filtered and non filtered cases in order to comparatively evaluate the introduction of the pre-processing stage in terms of number of extracted IMFs. Secondly, this work investigates the role of basic parameters such as time series length and signal to noise ratio (SNR) involved at the determination of the total computation time.

2   Synthetic and Experimental ECG Time Series

Synthetic electrocardiogram time series (Fig. 1) are produced artificially by a (software) generating function. The amplitude is expressed in normalized voltage values, taking into account the magnitude scales of the various complexes from experimental time series. For comparison purposes MIT-BIH ECG signals [21] are used as reference signals.

Simulated ECG time series are corrupted by White Gaussian Noise in order to produce noisy ones in multiple SNR levels from 0dB to 35dB. Data length varies from 500 to 8000 samples in numerical experiments where simulated noisy ECG time series are incorporated.

Two series of tests are conducted targeting to measure the total number of IMFs as a function of time series length and SNR in simulated ECG time series and the total computation time after the application of EMD until the completion of the whole process. A small sample incremental step is chosen for simulations targeted to evaluate the impact of time series length on the number of extracted IMFs. On the other hand, the maximum number of samples for the process of estimating the computation time in respect to time series length and SNR is 8000 and the step is 1000.

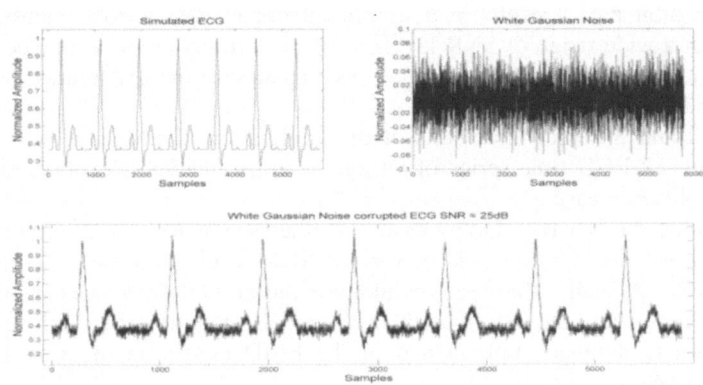

Fig. 1. Simulated ECG and addition of white Gaussian noise in 25dB SNR

In the case of real MIT-BIH ECG time series, the SNR as independent variable is not considered since these recordings already contain noisy components which are generally uncontrollable and unknown. However, time series lengths are selected without any restrictions sharing a common range with the simulated ones.

3   Results

3.1   Number of IMFs as a Function of Time Series Length and SNR

The study for the effect of time series length on the total number of IMFs is carried out comparatively by employing two widely used ECG filters. The variable of SNR as the second independent variable is determined by the process of noise addition to the simulated ECG time series and the production of the White Gaussian noisy simulated ECG time series. The composite impact study of time series length and SNR into the total number of IMFs reveal the indirect relation of noise level with the outcome of EMD method through the determination of the extrema and the distribution of them at the time series. An intrinsic mode function set is considered to be related at least for a subset with the underlying physical process that produces the biomedical signal. Application of Hilbert Transform on the IMFs set delineates the instantaneous frequencies and forms a time-frequency distribution of the signal for each IMF. The number of the IMF set is critical in the sense that any procedure applied on the time series may distort the signal characteristics resulting in a different IMF set. Currently, there is no robust methodology (optimum algorithm thresholds or filter's characteristics) in order to produce the optimum IMF set in terms of richest physical meaning or undistorted instantaneuous frequencies.

In the first case, a Savitzky Golay filter is incorporated due to the well known behavior in the preservation of the time series extrema. Various synthetic ECG time series of multiple lengths are processed with EMD and the total number of IMFs is monitored. Secondly, a low pass filter with frequency cutoff equal to 40Hz [22] is employed which tends to affect high frequency content of the time series and the extracted IMFs exhibit attenuated power in higher frequencies, resulting in a degraded peaky nature compared to the unfiltered one. Distortion in the tendency of the time series to exhibit peaks results in a significant impact on the total number of IMFs produced at a wide range of SNR levels. Low pass filters are used in electro cardiology to limit artifact for routine cardiac rhythm monitoring and reduce 50 or 60 Hz power line noise.

Figure 2 and 3 depict the results of the application of EMD on White Gaussian noisy simulated ECG time series of various lengths and SNR levels compared with the non application case.

Concerning the Savitzky-Golay case, the filter seems to have minimum effect on the filtered and non filtered case in various SNR levels in terms of number of extracted IMFs. Actually, these curves indicate the good performance of this filtering method in preserving the extremas in ECG signals and stress the high sensitivity of interpolation techniques implemented in the EMD algorithm in terms of accurate detection of peaky values.

3.2   Computation Time

The computation time for the EMD processing of simulated and real records ECG time series is related to the nature of the processed signal and the tendency to exhibit extremas. Apart from the number of extremas, another significant parameter is considered to be the distribution of the peaks in the whole range of time series length and inside the various ECG complexes.

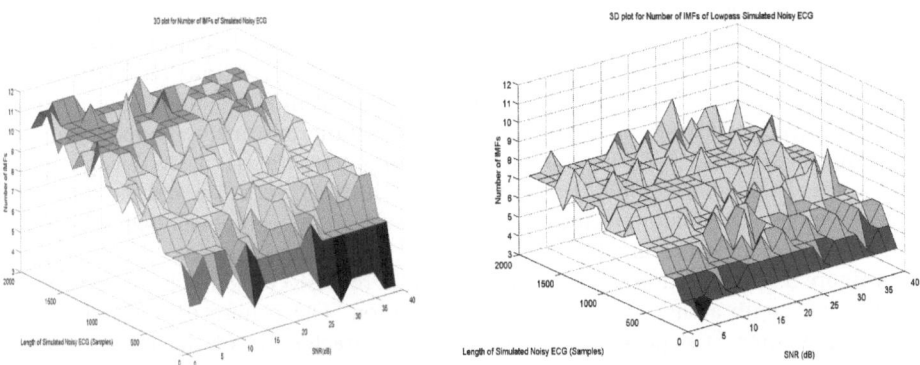

Fig. 2. 3D plots of the number of IMFs as a function of the SNR and the time series length for a simulated White Gaussian Noise corrupted ECG without the filtering with lowpass filter (left figure) and at the right figure with the application of the lowpass filter

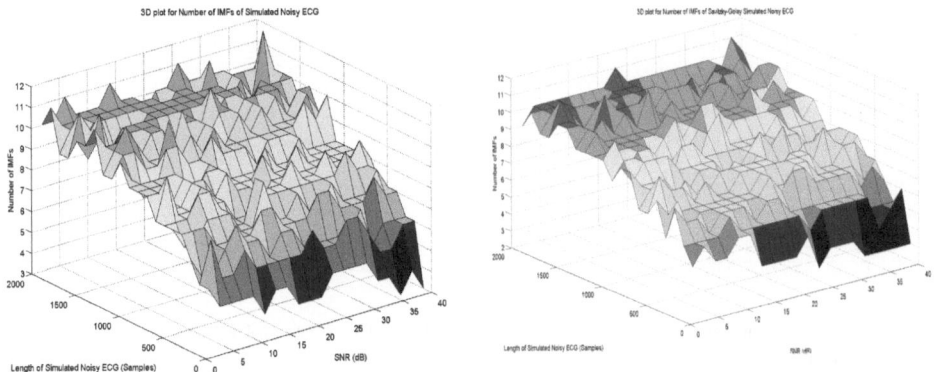

Fig. 3. 3D plots of the number of IMFs as a function of the SNR and the time series length for a simulated White Gaussian Noise corrupted ECG without filtering with Savitzky-Golay (left figure) and at the right figure with the filtering of Savitzky-Golay

An indirect way to estimate computation time is through the number of extracted IMFs. Specifically, computation time is monotonically increasing as the IMF set is growing and the fashion of this relation is quasi proportional. It is also affected by the total number of iterations required for the extraction of the IMF set. This goes down to implementation issues concerning the EMD algorithm and the thresholds used in termination criterion and even in the maximum number of iterations allowed.

For the simulated ECG time series, the length and SNR are controlled independent variables whilst for the experimental ECG the level of noise superimposed in the signal is generally unknown. The independent variable in real ECG records is the time series length.

Multiple time series lengths of simulated ECG are studied providing an overview of the computation time variation as a function of the length for various filtered time series. For demonstration reasons the minimum and maximum number of samples (1000, 8000) are depicted in figure 4. Due to the improvement of signal to noise ratio, noise levels are decreased and the number of noise samples superimposed to ECG time series is reduced. Spline interpolation scheme produces less uniform waveforms for the EMD envelopes resulting in significant increase of iterations required for the IMFs decomposition. The increase of computation time in 8000 samples time series with the increase of SNR is significant in lowpass fitltered time series compared to the corresponding increase in computation times monitored in Savitzky-Golay filtered time series. The combination of two components, the SNR variation and the impact of filtering in the peaky nature of the time series results in the composite behavior of the time series depicted in figure 4.

In figure 5, the variation of computation time in real ECG records is presented as a function of length along with the standard deviation. The pattern of the variation in computation time is dependent on the specific characteristic of the record sample (possible pathologies or ECG distortions) and its spectral characteristics. There is a tendency of computation time to increase as the time series length increases but the pattern of this tendency is not common in every ECG record.

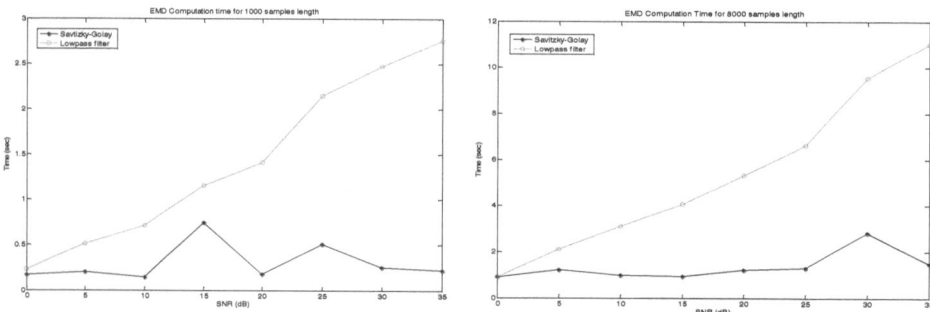

Fig. 4. Comparison results of EMD Computation Time for 1000 and 8000 samples of Simulated ECG time series

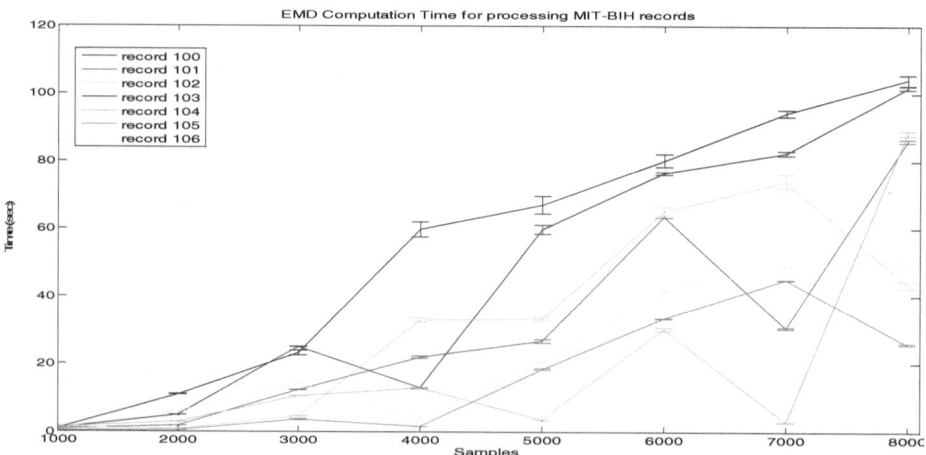

Fig. 5. EMD Computation Time in experimental MIT-BIH ECG time series for various time series lengths

4 Discussion – Conclusions

The introduction of a filtering stage before EMD application is studied and the effects of this scheme are investigated. Simulation results reveal that according to the type of filtering performed on data sets, variations are observed in the total number of IMFs reflecting to changes in total processing time as well. Filtering stage affects the spectral characteristics of the input signal and distortion of the time series' statistical and spectral content have an effect in the performance of EMD algorithm. Based on the inherent properties of the time series to be processed, one may select an appropriate pre-processing stage in order to achieve smaller number of IMFs and optimized processing time without changing in a significant degree the physical content of IMFs.

Total computation time is an essential aspect in transferring EMD algorithm from units with adequate processing power to embedded level in an efficient programming way. In multiple time series lengths, it is observed that computation time is monotonically increasing with the increase of SNR values. It is expected that the time series length is another significant parameter with a quasi proportional relation to the total computation time in simulation approach. However, this is partially verified in experimental ECG time series due to the involvement of various factors such as pathological situations in the signal and artifacts that seriously affect the application of EMD algorithm. Nevertheless, the increase tendency of computation time with the increase of length still exists.

EMD implementation takes into account the termination criterion, a significant parameter to be optimized in order to avoid numerous iterations for the extraction of IMFs. Research effort is still to be undertaken to investigate in what degree tight restrictions in number of iterations drain the physical content of IMFs. An optimization procedure for both termination criterion and number of iterations is an open issue in this field.

In low SNR levels, noise is prevalent in the time series, reflecting in a smoother spline and generally faster extraction due to smaller number of iterations. In high SNR values, it is observed a clear tendency towards the increase of computation time raising the issue of the magnitude of noise to be added in the signal in noise assisted data analysis methods.

References

1. Daubechies, I.: Ten Lectures on Wavelets. CBMS-NSF Series in Applied Mathematics 61, 357 (1992)
2. Mallat, S.: A Wavelet Tour of Signal Processing, p. 637. Academic Press, London (1998)
3. Wigner, E.P.: On the quantum correction for thermodynamic equilibrium. Phys. Rev. 40, 749–759 (1932)
4. Cohen, L.: Time-Frequency Analysis, p. 299. Prentice Hall, Englewood Cliffs (1995)
5. Gabor, D.: Theory of Communications. J. IEE 93, 429–457 (1946)
6. Diks, C.: Nonlinear Time Series Analysis, p. 220. World Scientific Press, Singapore (1999)

7. Huang, N.E., Shen, Z., Long, S.R., Wu, M.C., Shih, H.H., Zheng, Q., Yen, N.-C., Tung, C.C., Liu, H.H.: The empirical mode decomposition and Hilbert spectrum for nonlinear and nonstationary time series analysis. Proc. R. Soc. London 454, 903–995 (1998)
8. Hahn, S.: Hilbert Transforms in Signal Processing, p. 442. Artech House, Boston (1995)
9. Huang, N.E., Wu, M.C., Long, S.R., Shen, S.S.P., Qu, W., Gloersen, P., Fan, K.L.: A confidence limit for the empirical mode decomposition and Hilbert spectral analysis. Proc. R. Soc. A 459, 2317–2345 (2003), doi:10.1098/rspa.2003.1123
10. Echeverría, J.C., Crowe, J.A., Woolfson, M.S., Hayes-Gill, B.R.: Application of empirical mode decomposition to heart rate variability analysis. Med. Biol. Eng. Comput. 39(4), 471–479
11. Torres, A., Fiz, J.A., Jané, R., Galdiz, J.B., Gea, J., Morera, J.: Application of the Empirical Mode Decomposition method to the Analysis of Respiratory Mechanomyographic Signals. In: Proceedings of the 29th Annual International Conference of the IEEE EMBS Cité Internationale, Lyon, France
12. Blanco-Velasco, M., Weng, B., Barner, K.E.: ECG signal denoising and baseline wander correction based on the empirical mode decomposition. Comput. Biol. Med. 38(1), 1–13 (2008)
13. Nimunkar, A.J., Tompkins, W.J.: R-peak detection and signal averaging for simulated stress ECG using EMD. In: Conf. Proc. IEEE Eng. Med. Biol. Soc., pp. 1261–1264 (2007)
14. Charleston-Villalobos, S., Gonzalez-Camarena, R., Chi-Lem, G., Aljama-Corrales, T.: Crackle Sounds Analysis by Empirical Mode Decomposition. Engineering in Medicine and Biology Magazine 26(1), 40–47 (2007)
15. Krupa, B.N., Mohd Ali, M.A., Zahedi, E.: The application of empirical mode decomposition for the enhancement of cardiotocograph signals. Physiol. Meas. 30, 729–743 (2009)
16. Andrade, A.O., Nasuto, V., Kyberd, P., Sweeney-Reed, C.M., Kanijn, F.R.V.: EMG signal filtering based on Empirical Mode Decomposition. Biomedical Signal Processing and Control 1(1), 44–55 (2006), doi:10.1016/j.bspc.2006.03.003
17. Zhang, Y., Gao, Y., Wang, L., Chen, J., Shi, X.: The removal of wall components in Doppler ultrasound signals by using the empirical mode decomposition algorithm. IEEE Trans. Biomed. Eng. 54(9), 1631–1642 (2007)
18. Yeh, J.R., Sun, W.Z., Shieh, J.S., Huang, N.E.: Intrinsic mode analysis of human heartbeat time series. Ann. Biomed. Eng. 38(4), 1337–1344 (2010)
19. Karagiannis, A., Constantinou, P.: Noise components identification in biomedical signals based on Empirical Mode Decomposition. In: 9th International Conference on Information Technology and Applications in Biomedicine, ITAB 2009 (2009), 10.1109/ITAB.2009.5394300
20. Karagiannis, A., Loizou, L., Constantinou, P.: Experimental respiratory signal analysis based on Empirical Mode Decomposition. In: First International Symposium on Applied Sciences on Biomedical and Communication Technologies, ISABEL 2008 (2008), 10.1109/ISABEL.2008.4712581
21. http://www.physionet.org/physiobank/database/mitdb
22. Mark, J.B.: Atlas of Cardiovascular Monitoring, p. 130. Churchill Livingstone, New York (1998)

Session 6

Implantable and Wearable Biomedical Devices

Design of a Novel Miniaturized Implantable PIFA for Biomedical Telemetry

A. Kiourti[1], M. Christopoulou[1], S. Koulouridis[2], and K.S. Nikita[1]

[1] National Technical University of Athens, School of Electrical & Computer Engineering
[2] University of Patras, Department of Electrical & Computer Engineering
{akiourti,mchrist}@biosim.ntua.gr, koulouridis@ece.upatras.gr,
knikita@cc.ece.ntua.gr

Abstract. A broadband, circular, double-stacked, implantable planar inverted-F antenna (PIFA) is proposed for biomedical telemetry at f_0= 402 MHz. Both patches are meandered and a high permittivity substrate material is used to limit the radius and height of the antenna to 3.6 mm and 0.7 mm, respectively. The tuning and radiation characteristics as well as the specific absorption rate (SAR) distribution induced by the proposed antenna implanted inside a skin-tissue simulating box and inside the skin layer of a three-layer spherical human head model are evaluated. Simulations based on both finite-difference time-domain (FDTD) method and finite-element-method (FEM) are carried out. The feasibility of the communication link between the proposed antenna implanted in the spherical head model and an exterior $\lambda_0/2$ dipole antenna is also examined.

Keywords: Biomedical telemetry, implantable antenna, meanders, planar inverted-F antenna (PIFA), shorting pin, specific absorption rate (SAR).

1 Introduction

Recently, biomedical telemetry between antennas implanted inside the human body and exterior equipment has drawn great attention for both medical diagnosis and therapy [1], [2]. In the most common scenario, the signals are wirelessly transmitted at the medical implant communication service (MICS) band of $402-405$ MHz, which is allocated for ultra-low-power active medical implants [3]. Miniaturization and biocompatibility of the antenna, bandwidth broadening to avoid frequency shift effects and optimization of the radiation performance are the main design considerations of the antenna [4], [5]. Furthermore, regulating the power delivered to the antenna to satisfy the specific absorption rate (SAR) limitations [6], [7] in the surrounding tissue in order to ensure patient safety is a critical issue.

In this paper, a novel circular, stacked planar inverted-F antenna (PIFA) is initially designed to be implanted inside a skin-tissue simulating box and operate at f_0= 402 MHz, with a broad bandwidth of 59 MHz. The proposed antenna is subsequently implanted inside the skin-layer of a three-layer spherical human head model. The resonance characteristics and radiation pattern of the antenna, as well as the required net input power to satisfy the IEEE C95.1-1999 [6] and IEEE C95.1-2005 [7]

J. Lin and K.S. Nikita (Eds.): MobiHealth 2010, LNICST 55, pp. 127–134, 2011.
© Institute for Computer Sciences, Social Informatics and Telecommunications Engineering 2011

SAR basic restrictions are evaluated in both scenarios. Finally, the performance of the communication link between the antenna implanted in the spherical head model and an exterior $\lambda_0/2$ dipole receiver is examined. A reduced antenna size is achieved as compared to previous related works [4], [5], [8]-[12]. Simulations have been carried out using the finite-difference time-domain (FDTD) technique and the finite-element-method (FEM) [13].

The paper is organized as follows. Section 2 presents the design of the proposed antenna. In Section 3, simulation results of the antenna implanted inside a skin-tissue simulating box as well as inside the skin-layer of a three-layer spherical human head model are presented. In Section 4, the performance of the communication link between the proposed antenna implanted in the spherical head model and an exterior $\lambda_0/2$ dipole antenna is evaluated. The paper concludes in Section 5.

2   Antenna Design

The geometry of the proposed antenna is shown in Fig. 1(a)-(d). The antenna consists of a circular ground plane (R_1 = 3.6 mm) and two vertically-stacked, circular, meandered patches (R_2 = 3.5 mm) used as the radiating elements. Meandering and stacking of the patches increase the length of the current flow and reduce the size of the antenna [14]. Each of the radiating patches is printed on an 0.3 mm-thick Roger 3210 substrate (ε_r = 10.2). To ensure biocompatibility and robustness of the antenna, an 0.1 mm-thick Roger 3210 superstrate layer covers the structure [5]. Both radiating patches are fed by means of a 50 Ohm coaxial cable with an inner radius of 0.2 mm (placed at d_f = 2.9 mm from the centre of the ground plane), while a shorting pin with a radius of 0.2 mm connects the ground plane with the lower patch to achieve a further reduction in size (placed at d_s = 3 mm from the centre of the ground plane) [15]. The meander lengths of the lower patch are given in Table 1. The meander numbers start at the top (feed point location) and increase in number to the bottom (shorting pin location) of the patch. The width of the meanders equals 0.5 mm. The upper patch is an inverted version of the lower patch.

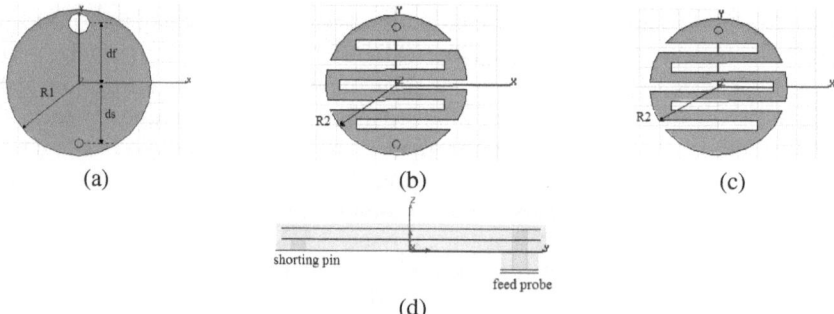

(a)   (b)   (c)

(d)

Fig. 1. Geometry of the proposed implantable antenna: (a) ground plane, (b) lower patch, (c) upper patch and (d) side view

Table 1. Meander lengths of the lower patch

Meander	Length (mm)
1	5.03
2	5.82
3	6.29
4	5.82
5	5.03

The dimensions of the proposed antenna are compared to those of previously reported implantable PIFAs operating at the biomedical frequency band of $402-405$ MHz band in Table 2.

Table 2. Antennas' dimensions comparison

Antenna	Volume (mm^3)
[4]	$24\times32\times4=3072$
[8]	$20\times24\times2.5=1200$
[9]	$18\times22.5\times1.9=769.5$
[5]	$\pi\times7.5^2\times3\approx530.14$
[10]	$10\times10\times1.905=190.5$
[11]	$\pi\times5^2\times1.815\approx142.55$
[12]	$8\times8\times1.905=121.92$
Proposed	$\pi\times3.6^2\times0.7\approx28.50$

3   Antenna Implanted in Skin-Tissue

Two skin-tissue implantation scenarios are examined for the proposed antenna. The antenna is initially designed and simulated while implanted at the center of an 100 mm-edge cubic box filled with skin-tissue simulating material, as shown in Fig. 2(a). The antenna is subsequently simulated while implanted inside the skin-layer of a three-layer spherical human head model consisting of skin, skull and brain (grey matter) tissues, as shown in Fig. 2(b) [16]. The spherical head model has a radius of 10 cm, while the thicknesses of the skin and skull layers are assumed to be equal to 0.5 cm. Table 3 summarizes the dielectric properties of the tissues used for the simulations at 402 MHz [17]. Free space is assumed for the exterior of the skin-tissue simulating box and the sphere, respectively.

Table 3. Electric properties of the tissues used in the simulations at 402 MHz

Tissue	Permittivity (ε_r)	Conductivity (σ, S/m)
Skin (dry)	46.7	0.69
Bone (cortical/skull)	13.1	0.09
Brain (grey matter)	57.4	0.74

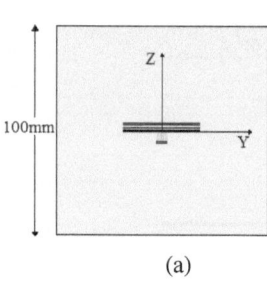
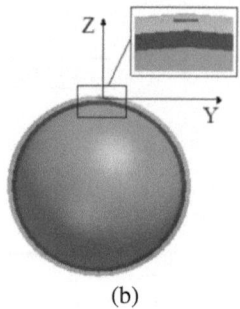

(a)   (b)

Fig. 2. Simulation setup of the proposed antenna implanted (a) inside a skin-tissue simulating box and (b) inside the skin-layer of a three-layer spherical human head model

3.1 Antenna Performance

Assuming that the dielectric properties of the tissues vary negligibly with frequency (inside a small frequency range), the return loss frequency response of the antenna in the scenario of Fig. 2(a) is presented in Fig. 3(a). The antenna resonates at 402 MHz and provides a wide bandwidth of 59 MHz at a return loss less than −10 dB, covering the MICS band under interest. The far-field gain radiation pattern at 402 MHz is shown in Fig. 3(b). Since the antenna is electrically very small, it radiates an omni-directional, monopole-like radiation pattern [18].

The return loss frequency response of the antenna in the scenario of Fig. 2(b) is illustrated in Fig. 4(a). Because of the load effect of the surrounding tissues and the exterior air, the antenna resonant frequency is shifted to 412 MHz and its bandwidth is slightly reduced to 50 MHz at a return loss less than −10 dB. The far-field gain radiation pattern at 402 MHz is slightly modified, but remains omni-directional, as shown in Fig. 4(b).

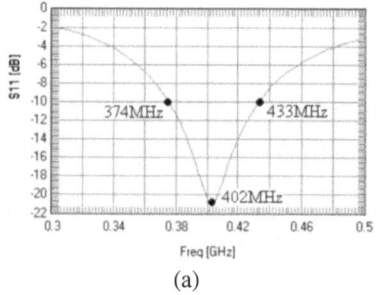
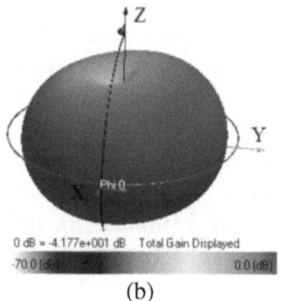

(a)   (b)

Fig. 3. (a) Return loss frequency characteristic and (b) Far-field gain radiation pattern at 402 MHz, for the simulation setup of Fig. 2(a)

3.2 SAR Basic Restrictions

In order to assess the electromagnetic power absorbed by the surrounding tissues, an SAR numerical analysis is performed at 402 MHz for the simulation setups of

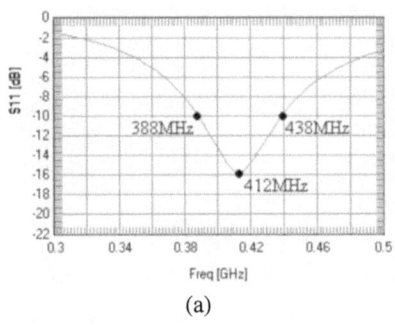
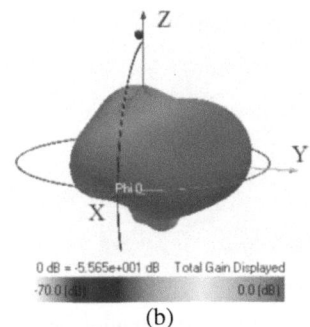

(a)   (b)

Fig. 4. (a) Return loss frequency characteristic and (b) Far-field gain radiation pattern at 402 MHz, for the simulation setup of Fig. 2(b)

Fig. 2(a) and 2(b). Given that the mass density of the skin, bone and brain (grey matter) is equal to $1100 \, kg/m^3$, $1200 \, kg/m^3$ and $1050 \, kg/m^3$, respectively, and assuming that the net input power of the antenna is set to 1 W, the peak 1-g averaged and 10-g averaged SAR values [19] for both scenarios are presented in Table 4.

In order to satisfy the IEEE C95.1-1999 (1-g averaged SAR <1.6 W/kg [6]) and IEEE C95.1-2005 (10-g averaged SAR <2 W/kg [7]) basic restrictions for general public exposure, the power incident to the antenna should not exceed the values of Table 5. Since the peak averaged SAR values for both scenarios were found to be comparable, the maximum allowed power levels for both scenarios are also comparable. Moreover, the IEEE C95.1-1999 standard is found to be stricter, limiting the maximum allowed net input power of the antenna to a value more than ten times lower than that imposed by the IEEE C95.1-2005 standard.

Table 4. Peak 1-g averaged and peak 10-g averaged SAR values for the simulation setups of Fig. 2(a) and 2(b) (net input power 1 W)

Scenario	peak 1-g avg SAR	peak 10-g avg SAR
skin-tissue simulating box	747.7 W/kg	79.76 W/kg
3-layer spherical human head model	739.3 W/kg	76.94 W/kg

Table 5. Maximum allowed net input power of the antenna in the simulation setups of Fig. 2(a) and 2(b) to conform with the IEEE C95.1-1999 and IEEE C95.1-2005 standards

Scenario	IEEE C95.1-1999	IEEE C95.1-2005
skin-tissue simulating box	<2.139 mW	<25 mW
3-layer spherical human head model	<2.164 mW	<25.9 mW

3.3 SAR Distribution

In order to satisfy the strictest limitations set by the IEEE guidelines and be able to compare the SAR numerical results for both scenarios, the net input power of the antenna of Fig. 2(a) and 2(b) is assumed equal to 2.139 mW. Local SAR distributions

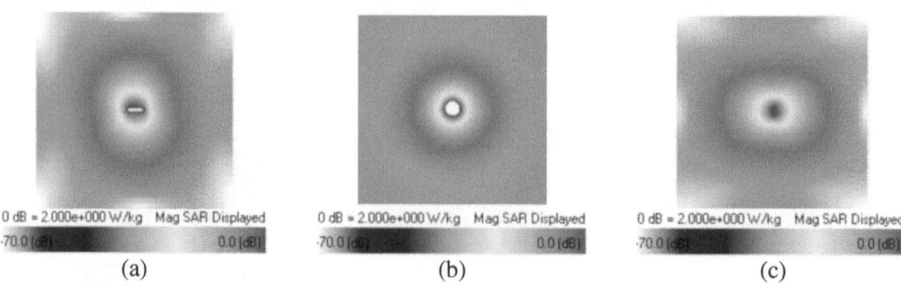

Fig. 5. Local SAR distribution on the (a) yz, (b) xy and (c) xz slices of the simulation setup of Fig. 2(a) where maximum local SAR has been calculated (net input power 2.139 mW)

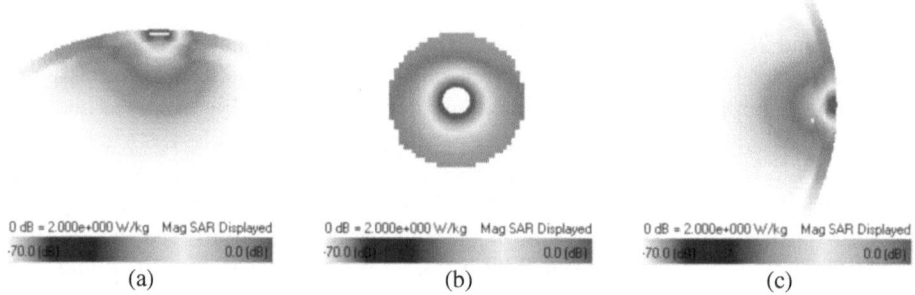

Fig. 6. Local SAR distribution on the (a) yz, (b) xy and (c) xz slices of the simulation setup of Fig. 2(b) where maximum local SAR has been calculated (net input power 2.139 mW)

are presented in Fig. 5 and 6 for the two scenarios, respectively, for the slices where maximum local SAR value has been calculated. For comparison reasons, all SAR results have been normalized to 2 W/kg.

4   Characterization of the Communication Link

Implanted medical devices need a communication link with an exterior monitoring/control unit. In order to characterize the performance of the communication between the proposed antenna when implanted in the spherical head model (transmitter, Tx) and an exterior antenna (receiver, Rx), the simulation setup of Fig. 7(a) is considered. The origin of the coordinate system is located at the center of the implanted antenna's ground plane. A half-wavelength ($\lambda_0/2 \approx 373.14$ mm at $f_0 = 402$ MHz) dipole antenna is placed horizontally above the implanted antenna and symmetrically around the z axis, so that the centers of the Tx and Rx antennas are aligned. A communication link is built between Tx and Rx.

By moving the exterior dipole antenna along the z axis, or equivalently by changing the distance between the implanted and the exterior antenna, the coupling from Tx to Rx is calculated in terms of the coupling coefficient $|S_{21}|$. The S-parameter $|S_{21}|$ quantifies the power transmission in the wireless link, so that $|S_{21}|^2 = P_r/P_t$, where P_t is

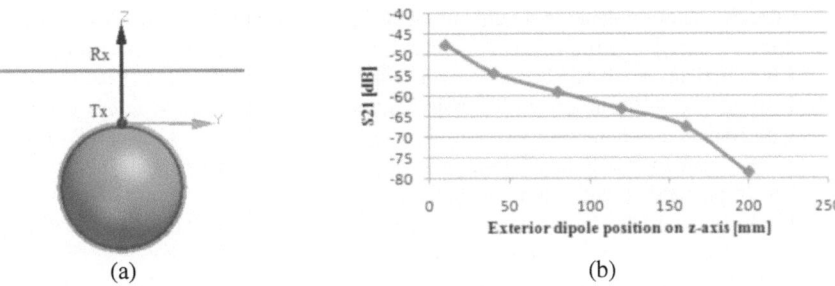

Fig. 7. (a) Simulation setup for characterizing the communication link. (b) Simulated $|S_{21}|$ versus exterior dipole position on the z-axis.

the available power at the Tx, and P_r is the power delivered to a 50 Ohm load terminating the Rx [20]. As seen in Fig. 7(b), there is a large variation in coupling strength with distance, with the lowest coupling being for a distally placed Rx.

5 Conclusions

Through studies with the FDTD and FEM electromagnetic solvers, a novel stacked PIFA was designed considering skin-tissue implantation and biotelemetry communication at $f_0 = 402$ MHz. The antenna was miniaturized to occupy a volume of 28.5 mm^3 and its tuning and radiation characteristics were evaluated while implanted inside a skin-tissue simulating box as well as inside the skin-layer of a three-layer spherical human head model. The maximum net input power in both scenarios was estimated such that the SAR values of the surrounding tissues satisfy the IEEE C95.1-1999 and IEEE C95.1-2005 limitations. Finally, the performance of the communication link between the antenna implanted in the spherical head model and an exterior $\lambda_0/2$ dipole antenna was evaluated. The proposed antenna could be integrated in an active medical device implanted in the human head.

Future work will include numerical calculation of the radiation and SAR characteristics of the proposed antenna while implanted inside an anatomical head model. Subsequent investigations will also include construction of the proposed antenna and experimental validation of the simulation results.

Acknowledgement

The work of AK was supported by the Greek Foundation of Education and European Culture.

References

1. Weiss, M., et al.: RF Coupling in a 433-MHz Biotelemetry System for an Artificial Hip. IEEE Antennas & Wireless Prop. Letters 8, 916–919 (2009)
2. Gosalia, K., et al.: Thermal Elevation in the Human Eye and Head Due to the Operation of a Retinal Prosthesis. IEEE Trans. Biomed. Eng. 51(8), 1469–1477 (2004)

3. FCC, Medical Implant Communications Service (MICS) (FCC) Std. CFR, Part 95 (1999)
4. Kim, J., Samii, Y.: Implanted Antennas Inside a Human Body: Simulations, Designs, and Characterizations. IEEE Trans. Micr. Theory & Techn. 52(8), 1934–1943 (2004)
5. Rucker, D.: A Miniaturized Tunable Microstrip Antenna for Wireless Communications with Implanted Medical Devices. In: Proc. of the ICST 2nd Int. Conf. on BANs (2007)
6. IEEE, Standard for Safety Levels with Respect to Human Exposure to Radio Frequency Electromagnetic Fields, 3kHz to 300GHz (1999)
7. IEEE, Standard for Safety Levels with Respect to Human Exposure to Radio Frequency Electromagnetic Fields, 3kHz to 300GHz (2005)
8. Kim, J., Samii, Y.: Planar Inverted-F Antennas on Implantable Medical Devices: Meandered Type Versus Spiral Type. Micr. & Opt. Techn. Letters 48(3), 567–572 (2006)
9. Lee, C.-M., et al.: Bandwidth Enhancement of Planar Inverted-F Antenna for Implantable Biotelemetry. Micr. & Opt. Techn. Letters 51(3), 749–752 (2009)
10. Liu, W.-C., et al.: Miniaturized Implantable Broadband Antenna for Biotelemetry Communication. Micr. & Opt. Techn. Letters 50(9), 2407–2409 (2008)
11. Liu, W.-C., et al.: Implantable Broadband Circular Stacked PIFA Antenna for Biotelemetry Communication. J. of Electromagn. Waves & Appl. 22, 1791–1800 (2008)
12. Liu, W.-C., et al.: BW Enhancement and Size Reduction of an Implantable PIFA Antenna for Biotelemetry Devices. Micr. & Opt. Techn. Letters 51(3), 755–757 (2009)
13. Sadiku, M.: Numerical Techniques in Electromagnetics. CRC Press, Boca Raton (2001)
14. Wong, K.-L.: Compact and Broadband Microstrip Antennas. John Wiley & Sons, Chichester (2002)
15. Chow, Y.L., et al.: Miniaturizing Patch Antenna by Adding a Shorting Pin Near the Feed Probe - a Folded Monopole Equivalent. In: IEEE Ant. & Prop. Symp., vol. 4, pp. 6–9 (2002)
16. Koulouridis, S., Nikita, K.S.: Study of the Coupling Between Human Head and Cellular Phone Helical Antennas. IEEE Trans. on Electromagn. Compat. 46(1), 62–70 (2004)
17. Gabriel, C., et al.: The dielectric properties of biological tissues. Phys. Med. Biol. 41, 2231–2293 (1996)
18. Abadia, J., et al.: 3D-Spiral Small Antenna Design and Realization for Biomedical Telemetry in the MICS Band. Radioengineering 18(4), 359–367 (2009)
19. IEEE Recommended Practice for Measurements & Computations of RF EM fields with Respect to Human Exposure to Such Fields, IEEE Standard C95.3-2002 (2002)
20. Warty, R., et al.: Characterization of Implantable Antennas for Intracranial Pressure Monitoring: Reflection by and Transmission Through a Scalp Phantom. IEEE Trans. Micr. Theory & Techn. 56(10), 2366–2376 (2008)

Microstrip Antenna Arrays for Implantable and Wearable Wireless Applications

Daniel G. Rucker[1], Haider R. Khaleel[1], Sunny S. Raheem[2], and Hussain M. Al-Rizzo[2]

[1] Department of Applied Science
[2] Department of Systems Engineering
University of Arkansas at Little Rock
2801 South University Ave., Little Rock, AR 72204, USA
{dxrucker,hrkhaleel,ssraheem,hmalrizzo}@ualr.edu

Abstract. Flexible microstrip antenna arrays have become a necessity in today's miniaturized biomedical wireless devices. Implantable and wearable biomedical devices such as pacemakers, drug delivery systems, heart rate monitors, and respiratory monitors need to communicate with exterior base station devices and relayed to healthcare professionals. In this paper, multiple flexible microstrip antenna arrays are designed and simulated for these applications. The frequency bands of 5.2 GHz and 5.8 GHz are utilized to provide a high bandwidth communication link. CST Microwave Studio was used for the modeling and simulation of the antennas. The reflection coefficient, gain, and correlation coefficient for each antenna are presented and discussed. The presented antennas can be utilized together as an array for enhanced gain or independently in a Multiple Input Multiple Output (MIMO) system.

Keywords: Implantable and Wearable Antenna, Microstrip Antenna Array, MIMO.

1 Introduction

Microstrip antenna arrays have enjoyed many uses in today's world of miniaturized wireless devices. The ever increasing demand for smaller and affordable devices with greater operating capabilities has increased the requirements for small microstrip antennas with high efficiencies, gains, and bandwidths [1,2]. In order to meet these needs, the next generation of miniaturized antenna arrays must be developed. Microstrip antennas that function as arrays for either enhanced gain or Multiple Input Multiple Output (MIMO) systems can provide next generation, high data rate wireless systems. For high data rate applications such as wireless local area networks (WLAN), the 5.2 GHz and 5.8 GHz bands are available. The 5.2 GHz band ranges from 5.15 GHz to 5.35 GHz and the 5.8 GHz band ranges from 5.725 GHz to 5.875 GHz.

Today's implantable biomedical systems require wireless links to provide feedback to healthcare professionals. Implantable devices such as pacemakers, drug delivery systems, and in-vivo electroencephalogram (EEG) can utilize wireless links to send data to collection units outside the body thus eliminating hard wire connections [3,4].

J. Lin and K.S. Nikita (Eds.): MobiHealth 2010, LNICST 55, pp. 135–143, 2011.
© Institute for Computer Sciences, Social Informatics and Telecommunications Engineering 2011

Wearable biomedical systems also benefit from wireless links. Applications such as heart rate and respiratory monitors have been used in patient care and sports medicine. By utilizing a wireless link for a wearable system, a runner could utilize a wearable system to provide data on heart rate and respiratory rate while tracking speed and position using a global positioning system (GPS) [5]. A recent growing trend is the integration of wireless connectivity with secure digital (SD) flash memory cards [6]. By using this form factor for the design, antennas and associated circuitry can be integrated with a device's memory all in one package.

Computer modeling and simulation tools provide researchers with the ability to design and fabricate antennas by avoiding the expensive trial and error approach. This allows for many designs to be studied and refined before fabricating the prototypes. CST Microwave Studio (MWS) is a modeling and simulation software package used for antennas and high frequency structures [7]. MWS uses the Finite Integration Technique for time domain simulations.

In this paper, a series of printed microstrip antenna arrays on thin substrates are designed and analyzed. The development of thin, printed arrays is presented as a progression from printed dipoles to square patches then to spiral patches. The simulated S-Parameters, gain, and correlation coefficient results are shown. The antenna arrays are intended for use in Secure Digital (SD) memory card sized, thin, flexible substrates with maximum rectangular dimensions of 32 mm in length by 24 mm in width. The arrays are designed to provide wireless communication links for miniaturized implantable and wearable biomedical devices. The 5.2 GHz and 5.8 GHz frequency bands were selected to reduce the size of the antennas and to serve high data rate applications.

2 Flexible Antenna Design

Flexible microstrip antennas impose multiple design constraints when used for implantable and medical devices. For the prototype antenna arrays in this paper, the two main performance goals are a 5 dB gain and a correlation coefficient of less than 0.2. The arrays must be broadside radiating and nearly omnidirectional with respect to azimuth. The correlation coefficient can be calculated either from the three-dimensional far field radiation pattern (equation 1) which requires extensive calculations or from S-parameters (equation 2). However, in this study, the simulated correlation coefficient has been extracted from the far field analysis which is more accurate than the S-parameter method [8].

$$\rho = \frac{\iint_{4\pi} \bar{G}_1 \, \bar{G}_2{}^* \, d\Omega}{\sqrt{\iint_{4\pi} \bar{G}_1 \, \bar{G}_1{}^* \, d\Omega \iint_{4\pi} \bar{G}_2 \, \bar{G}_2{}^* \, d\Omega}}. \tag{1}$$

$$\rho = \frac{|S_{11}{}^* S_{12} + S_{21}{}^* S_{22}|^2}{(1-(|S_{11}|^2+|S_{21}|^2))(1-(|S_{22}|^2+|S_{12}|^2))}. \tag{2}$$

For two uncorrelated antennas and a reasonable bit error rate, the diversity gain is equal to 10 dB (equation 3).

$$G = 10.\sqrt{1 - |\rho|^2}. \tag{3}$$

2.1 Flexible Printed Dipole Antennas

The printed dipole design was chosen as the initial antenna design for this work. Printed dipoles have been reported in [9,10], among others, and will serve as a basis to compare against other designs. The center frequency of 5.8 GHz will serve high data rate applications while reducing the size compared to 2.45 GHz antennas. Two printed dipoles were modeled on a 100 μm polyamide substrate, with relative permittivity (ε_r) = 3.5, to investigate the use of thin printed dipoles on flexible substrates. The two dipoles were placed on a substrate with a length of 32 mm and width of 24 mm. The dimensions were taken from measurements of a SD memory card commonly used in cameras and other small personal devices. Fig. 1 shows the dipoles located on the thin substrate.

A perfect electric conductor (PEC) is used as the material for the dipole arms to limit the mesh size. The mesh is limited because MWS does not mesh PEC, therefore avoiding a very fine mesh gradient. The substrate does use the MWS default loss tangent of 0.003 for the polyamide. The antenna from Fig. 1 was further developed by adding a microstrip line to feed both antennas. Fig. 2 shows the antenna with the added microstrip line feed. The substrate has been rendered colorless in order to better display both the feed and ground strip. The independently fed dipole antennas required a feed with an input impedance of 72 Ω for correct input matching. The single microstrip line fed dipoles were designed to match to a 50 Ω microstrip line. This allows for the antenna to operate with a standard input impedance common to RF transceiver board SMA connectors.

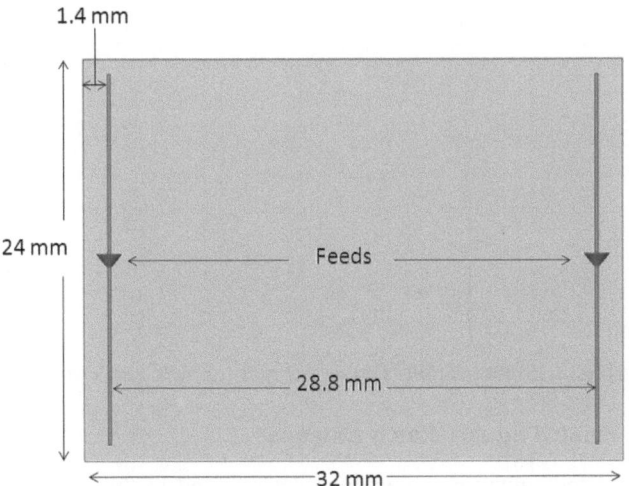

Fig. 1. Printed Dipole Antennas with Independent Feeds

The antenna was simulated using individual feeds and a common microstrip line feed to provide a comparison of the feeding techniques. The S_{11} results compare favorably well within the 5.8 GHz band as seen in Fig. 3. Both antennas share a -10 dB bandwidth of 562 MHz ranging from 5.447 GHz to 6.009 GHz. The far-field gain

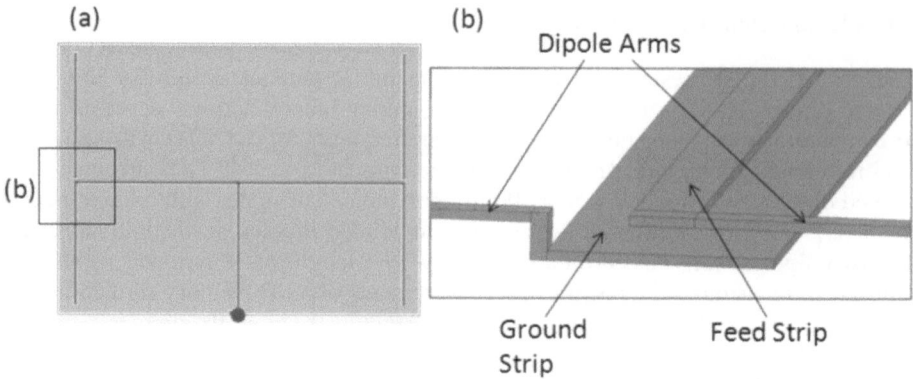

Fig. 2. Printed Dipole Antennas with a Single Feed

pattern of both antennas compares very closely at 5.8 GHz in magnitude and shape. The bore-sight gains of the independent fed and single fed dipoles are 6.6 dB and 6.5 dB, respectively, and both have a half-power beamwidth of 78°. The E-plane and H-plane polar cuts for the single fed dipoles are shown in Fig. 4. Since both dipole gain patterns are approximately equal, Fig. 4 is representative of both arrays. The correlation coefficient calculated from the three dimensional radiation pattern is 0.013. This would allow for the independently fed dipoles to be used for MIMO applications.

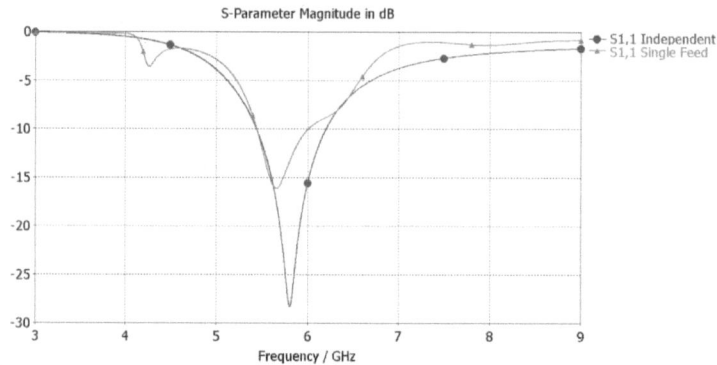

Fig. 3. Printed Parallel Dipole Array S_{11}, Single and Two Feeds

2.2 Flexible Printed Square Patch Antennas

The flexible printed square patch antenna design used in this work consists of a microstrip line feed and square inset patch geometry. The basic patch design for the printed square antenna with an inset fed microstrip line is shown in Fig. 5. W, L, W_f, Y_0 are the four parameters needed to design this patch to operate in the desired resonate frequency of 5.8 GHz. W is the patch width and L is the patch length. W_f is width of the microstrip feed line and also the inset gap width between the feed line and the patch. Y_0 is the adjustable inset length to change the matching impedance of the microstrip line to the patch edge [11].

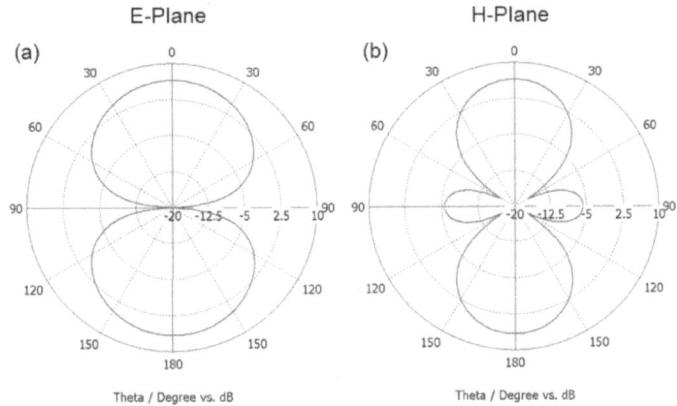

Fig. 4. Parallel Dipole Array, Independent Feeds, Gain E-plane (a) and H-plane (b)

The same flexible polyamide substrate ($\varepsilon_r = 3.5$) as the dipole antennas is used in the design of this square microstrip line fed antenna array. Since this patch is fed through a microstrip line, the width of the microstrip line (W_f) must be calculated in order to match the input impendence. In this design, the input impendence is 50 Ω, thus requiring the width of the microstrip line to be 0.2278 mm. The adjustable inset distance (Y_0) was adjusted to 1.25 mm long resulting in better matching for this antenna to operate at the needed frequency. A parametric sweep was used to determine the appropriate length of the inset. The width of this antenna is 12.00 mm, while the length is 13.752 mm. The distance between the two patches is 6mm (0.217λ). The patch design with dimensions is displayed in Fig. 5. The patch length is adjusted in order to ensure a center frequency of 5.797 GHz with a reflection coefficient of -16 dB, which is displayed in S parameter Fig. 6. The correlation coefficient of 0.204 was calculated from the three dimensional far-field results. Fig. 7 displays the E-Plane and the H-Plane two dimensional graphs of the far-field gain pattern. The main lobe shows the expected radiation pattern of a broadside radiator and has gain 5.3 dB. The angular width (3dB) is 88.5 degrees.

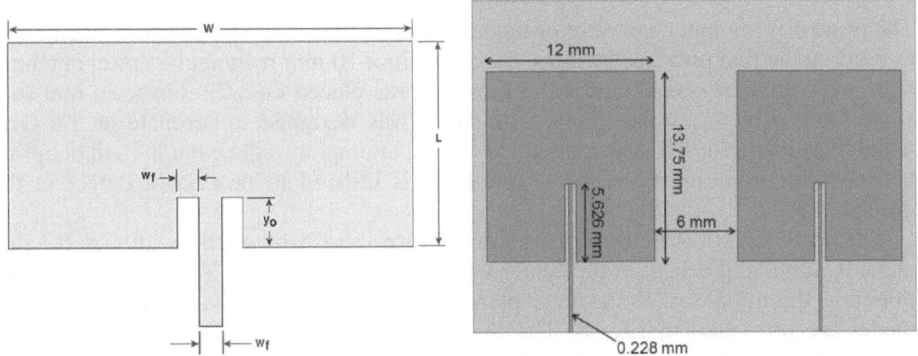

Fig. 5. Square Inset Fed Patch Geometry and Square Microstrip Antenna Array

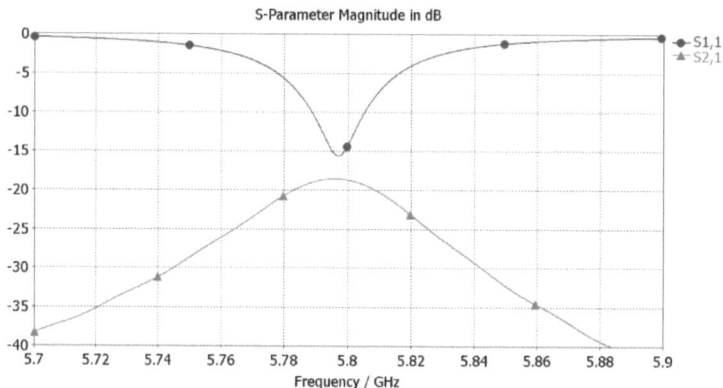

Fig. 6. S-Parameter Results of Double Square Microstrip Fed Patch Antenna

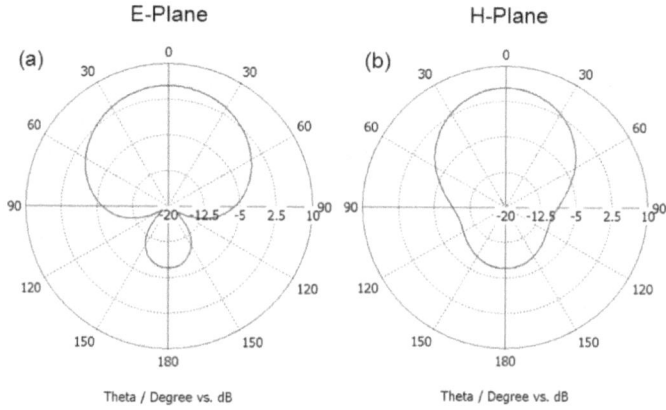

Fig. 7. Square Microstrip Antenna Array

2.3 Flexible Printed Spiral Antennas

The printed spiral antennas were designed to utilize the same SD card form factor size as used on the two previous designs. Two 10 mm × 10 mm rectangular spiral antennas with a 0.7 mm strip width and a 0.5 mm gap was placed on a 22 mm × 30 mm substrate backed by a ground plane. The spiral was designed to resonate at 5.2 GHz which is suitable for WLAN applications. In an attempt to reduce the mutual coupling between the radiating elements, a spiral slit is utilized to produce a defect in the ground plane.

The proposed slit structure consists of a 3-turn spiral with a strip width of 0.4 mm and a 0.5 mm gap except in the center which has a 1.5 mm gap. The structure is positioned at the middle of the ground plane. The front and back views of the antenna model are presented in Fig. 8. The thickness of the substrate is 0.85 mm with a relative permittivity of 5.25 while the inter-element distance is 9 mm (0.36λ). A parametric study was performed for the two coaxial feed locations to achieve optimal impedance matching.

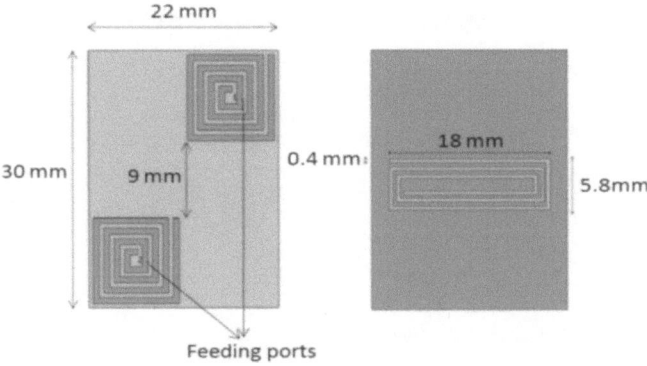

Fig. 8. Microstrip Spiral Antenna Array, Front View (left) and Back View (right)

The simulated S-parameters for the proposed design with and without a ground plane slit are provided in Fig. 9. From the S_{11} results, a return loss of -35 dB at 5.2 GHz is observed for the design without spiral slit. A slight shift in the resonance frequency with a spiral slit is noticed with a return loss of -30 dB. This shift can be compensated for by adjusting the patch length in order to keep the patch resonance frequency identical in both cases. The simulated -10 dB bandwidth is 20 MHz. The mutual coupling between the two spiral elements was analyzed based on transmission coefficient (S_{21}) between the two feeding ports. Obviously, the design with the spiral slit provides further isolation between the radiating elements compared to the conventional design with the same element separation. This behavior can be explained as follows: A portion of surface current is trapped by the spiral ground plane slit between the radiating patch elements which lead to reduced current coupling. This shows that the flow of current from one edge of the ground plane to the other edge is decreased which helps to reduce the mutual coupling between the two radiating elements [12]. Due to this effect, a reduction of 3.3 dB in mutual coupling is achieved.

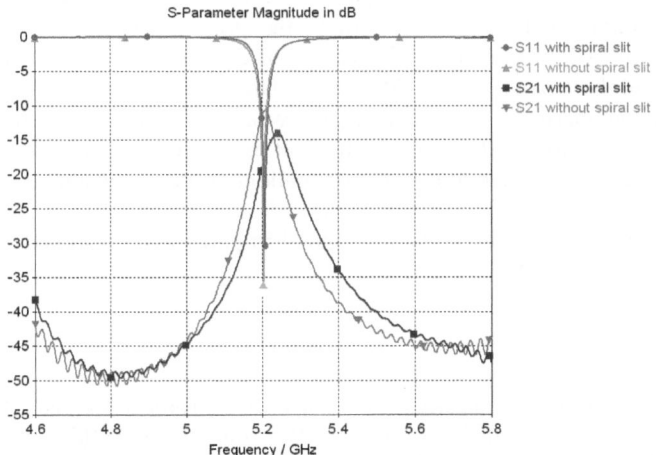

Fig. 9. Simulated S-Parameter for the proposed design with and without spiral ground plane slit

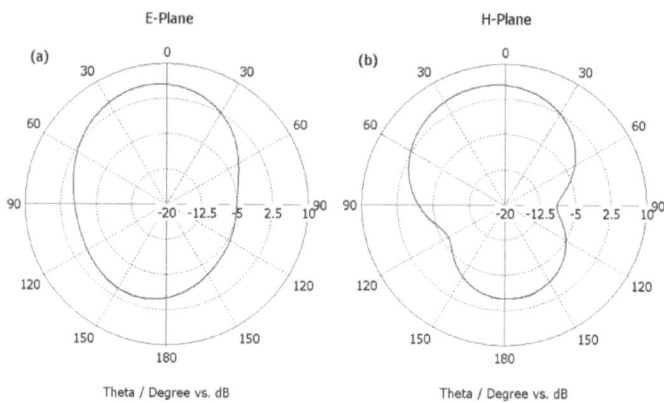

Fig. 10. Microstrip Spiral Array with ground plane slit, Gain E-plane (a) and H-plane (b)

The simulated correlation coefficient is 0.2, along with a diversity gain of 9.8 dB and a 5.7 dB combined elements gain at 5.2 GHz comply with the WLAN technology design requirements. The simulated E-plane and H-plane far field radiation patterns in the presence of the spiral ground plane slit are presented in Fig. 10.

3 Conclusion

In this paper, we presented three antenna arrays to achieve our design goals of SD memory card size, far-field gain, and correlation coefficient for the application of wireless biomedical devices. The printed dipole antenna array provide an effective implementation of a popular design. The microstrip square patch antenna array provides a popular design for comparison. Then, the square spiral microstrip antenna array was designed to achieve a lower resonant frequency while maintaining the same form factor of the dipole and square patch arrays. The results show the spiral array achieved a similar far-field gain pattern to the printed dipoles and square patches while providing a lower resonant frequency of 5.2 GHz. The printed dipole array achieved the highest bandwidth at 562 MHz. The printed dipole array and the spiral array both have merit for implantable and wearable biomedical wireless devices. These antennas will assist 21st century medical professionals to provide better health-care while being less evasive to the hospital patient or the sports athlete.

Acknowledgement. This research was funded in part by the National Science Foundation Grant EPS-0701890.

References

1. Park, S., Jayaraman, S.: Enhancing the Quality of Life Through Wearable Technology. In: IEEE Engineering in Medicine and Biology Magazine. pp. 41–48 (May/June 2003)
2. Rahmat-Samii, Y.: Wearable and Implantable Antennas in Body-Centric Communications. In: The 2nd European Conference on Antennas and Propagation, pp. 1–5 (November 2007)

3. Soontornpipit, P., Furse, C.M., Chung, Y.C.: Design of Implantable Microstrip Antenna for Communication with Medical Implants. IEEE Transactions on Microwave Theory and Techniques 52(8), 1944–1951 (2004)

4. Rucker, D., Al-Alawi, A., Adada, R., Al-Rizzo, H.M.: A Miniaturized Tunable Microstrip Antenna for Wireless Communications with Implanted Medical Devices. In: Proceedings of the 2nd International Conference on Body Area Networks Conference, Florence, Italy (June 2007)

5. Jovanov, E., Milenkovic, A., Otto, C., de Groen, P.: A wireless body area network of intelligent motion sensors for computer assisted physical rehabilitation. Journal of Neuro Engineering and Rehabilitation 2(6) (March 2005)

6. Eye-Fi SD Memory Cards with WiFi (April 2010),
   http://www.eye.fi/products/connectx2

7. CST Microwave Studio (April 2010),
   http://www.cst.com/Content/Products/MWS/Overview.aspx

8. Blanch, S., Romeu, J., Corbella, I.: Exact representation of antenna system diversity performance from input parameter description. Electronic Letters 39, 705–707 (2003)

9. Pozar, D.M.: Analysis of Finite Phased Arrays of Printed Dipoles. IEEE Transactions on Antennas and Propagation 33(10), 1045–1053 (1985)

10. Duffley, B.G., Morin, G.A., Mikavica, M., Antar, Y.M.M.: A Wide-Band Printed Double-Sided Dipole Array. IEEE Transactions on Antennas and Propagation 52(2), 628–631 (2004)

11. Ramesh, M., Yip, K.B.: Design Formula for Inset Fed Microsrtip Patch Antenna. Journal of Microwaves and Optoelectronics 3(3) (December 2003)

12. Chiu, C., Cheng, C., Murch, R.D., Rowell, C.R.: Reduction of Mutual Coupling Between Closely-Packed Antenna Elements. IEEE Transactions on Antennas Propagation 55(6), 1732–1738 (2007)

BER Performance of a BPSK Biomedical Telemetry System under Varying Coupling and Loading Conditions

Asimina Kiourti[1] and Andreas Demosthenous[2]

[1] National Technical University of Athens, School of Electrical & Computer Engineering
[2] University College London, Department of Electronic & Electrical Engineering
akiourti@biosim.ntua.gr, a.demosthenous@ee.ucl.ac.uk

Abstract. Binary Phase Shift Keying (BPSK) is a promising modulation format for downlink data transmission in inductive biomedical telemetry systems, because it achieves high data rates and power efficiencies and requires simple electronics. In this paper, the Bit Error Rate (BER) performance of a BPSK biomedical telemetry system is investigated under Additive White Gaussian Noise (AWGN) and is found to highly depend on the system's coupling and loading conditions. High-level simulations are presented which are indicative of the performance of a real BPSK biomedical telemetry system.

Keywords: Binary phase shift keying (BPSK), biomedical telemetry, bit error rate (BER) performance, inductive link, wireless implants.

1 Introduction

During the last decade, biomedical implanted devices have drawn great attention for both diagnosis and treatment of diseases [1], [2]. Bidirectional communication between the implant and an external control unit for data exchange and power delivery is, most commonly, performed via a wireless, transcutaneous inductive link [3]. This battery-less technique minimizes the size of the implant and eliminates patient discomfort.

The inductive link channel consists of two closely-spaced, mutually-coupled coils, one implanted and one placed outside the human body. The external unit telemeters power and modulated data (commands and stimulation parameters) to the implant (downlink transmission). Depending on the modulation format, several values of data transmission rates, error rates, delivered power and circuit complexity can be achieved. The implant can itself send data (monitoring signals) back to the external unit (uplink transmission), usually by means of load reflectance techniques [4].

Amplitude keying formats (Amplitude Shift Keying, ASK, and On-Off Keying, OOK) were the first to be used for downlink data transmission [5], [6]. However, despite their simple implementation, they were limited to deliver low amounts of power and achieve low data transmission rates. Phase Shift Keying (PSK) techniques have been proved to be the best alternative [7], [8], [9]. Binary Phase Shift Keying (BPSK) is the simplest form of PSK. A single carrier signal is modulated by controlling its polarity according to the binary data signal to be transmitted. The amplitude of

J. Lin and K.S. Nikita (Eds.): MobiHealth 2010, LNICST 55, pp. 144–150, 2011.

the BPSK modulated signal is kept constant, thus increasing the maximum power delivered to the implant. Bit rates as high as 1.12 Mbps for a carrier frequency of 13.56 MHz have been reported in literature [7].

The rest of the paper is organized as follows. In section 2, a BPSK biomedical telemetry system is designed and simulated in Simulink, Matlab [10]. Additive White Gaussian Noise (AWGN) is assumed to distort the signal while propagating in the wireless inductive link channel. In Section 3, the system's Bit Error Rate (BER) performance is evaluated under various noise levels and its dependence on the system's coupling and loading conditions is examined. The paper concludes in Section 4.

2   BPSK Telemetry System Overview

A block diagram of the BPSK biomedical telemetry circuit designed in Simulink, Matlab is illustrated in Fig. 1(a). At the external unit, the binary data are BPSK modulated and driven to a power amplifier to produce an adequate transmitting power. An ideal (theoretic power efficiency of 100%), unity-gain Class-E power amplifier is assumed [11]. Downlink data transmission takes place across the inductive link channel and BPSK demodulation is performed at the implant's side. For simplicity reasons, the implanted electronic system is modeled as an equivalent ac load resistor R_l. Three values are examined, $R_l = 300$, 1000 and 2000 Ohm. In a real system, R_l will be complex and time-varying.

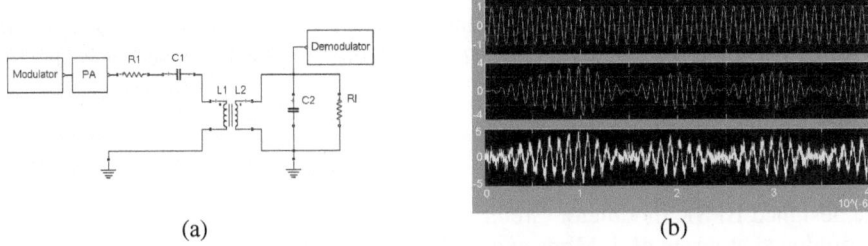

(a)   (b)

Fig. 1. (a) Model of the designed BPSK biomedical telemetry system, (b) Simulated waveforms of the signals at the output of the modulator and input of the demodulator for zero and finite AWGN distortion, respectively

2.1   Inductive Link Channel

To achieve high gain while requiring low input voltages, the inductive link channel consists of a series-external (primary) and a parallel-implanted (secondary) resonant circuits [12], both tuned at the carrier frequency of $f_c = 10$ MHz, according to:

$$2\pi f_c = \frac{1}{\sqrt{L_1 C_1}} = \frac{1}{\sqrt{L_2 C_2}} \, , \tag{1}$$

where L_1, C_1, L_2, C_2 represent the inductor and capacitor values of the primary and secondary circuits. The carrier frequency has been chosen as a compromise between data transfer rate, power efficiency and human safety [13]. The coupling between the coils, or equivalently the proportion of the primary's flux which is linked with the secondary, is described in terms of the coupling factor, k [14]. The coupling factor depends on the geometry and distance between the coils, as well as on the material properties of the coupling medium. The resistor R_1 accounts for the ohmic losses of the external side, while the implanted side's ohmic losses are included in R_I.

The transfer function of the inductive link channel (in the Laplace domain) can be derived from the network equations of the primary and secondary resonant circuits, as:

$$\frac{V_{out}(s)}{V_i(s)} = \frac{sk^2L_1L_2R_I}{\left(sL_2 + s^2R_IL_2C_2 + R_I\right)\left(R_1 + \frac{1}{sC_1} + sL_1\right) - s^2k^2L_1L_2\left(1 + sR_IC_2\right)}, \tag{2}$$

where V_i and V_{out} denote the signals at the input and output of the channel, respectively [7]. The inductive link channel acts as a bandpass filter centered at the resonant frequency [12] and is assumed to add Additive White Gaussian Noise (AWGN), which accounts for coil misalignments, element variations and environmental noise.

The resonant coils are considered to have equal inductances, $L_1 = L_2 = 1.25\,\mu\text{H}$. Three typical values of the coupling factor are examined, $k = 0.03$, 0.06 and 0.1, while $R_1 = 3\,\text{Ohm}$.

Example waveforms of the BPSK modulated signal at the output of the modulator and at the input of the BPSK demodulator, when the channel causes zero and finite AWGN distortion, are shown in Fig. 1(b), respectively, for the case where $k = 0.06$ and $R_I = 300\,\text{Ohm}$.

2.2 BPSK Modulator

The designed BPSK modulator circuit is illustrated in Fig. 2(a). Random binary digits are produced at a rate of 1 Mbps and are converted into a binary bipolar PAM signal, where "1" and "0" bits are represented as $1\,\text{V}$ and $-1\,\text{V}$ voltage levels, respectively. The bipolar PAM signal is subsequently multiplied with a sinusoidal carrier signal of unity amplitude, to produce the BPSK modulated signal:

$$m(t) = \begin{cases} \sin\left(2\pi f_c t\right) & \text{"1" bit} \\ -\sin\left(2\pi f_c t\right) & \text{"0" bit} \end{cases}. \tag{3}$$

Power is delivered to the implant through the energy contained in the incoming BPSK modulated signal, via power rectification and regulation circuits found on the implant's side [15], [16]. As a result, the BPSK modulator serves the dual purpose of data transmission and power delivery. Fig. 2(b) illustrates the simulated waveforms of the first four bits to be transmitted, the carrier signal, and the corresponding BPSK modulated signal, respectively.

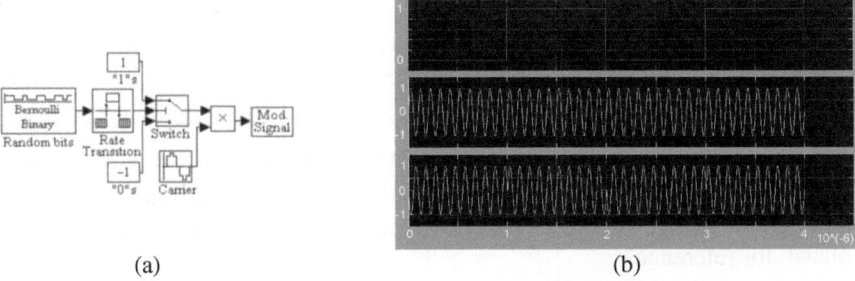

(a)   (b)

Fig. 2. (a) Model of the designed BPSK modulator circuit, and (b) Simulated waveforms of the first four bits to be transmitted, the carrier signal, and the corresponding BPSK modulated signal

2.3 BPSK Demodulator

A simplified coherent BPSK demodulator circuit was designed, as depicted in Fig. 3(a). The received BPSK signal is multiplied with a recovered version of the carrier (most commonly obtained via a Costas loop circuit [17]) and is low-pass-filtered by means of Butterworth low-pass-filter (LPF), with a passband edge frequency of 1 MHz. The resulting signal is driven to a bit recovery circuit which consists of a sample-and-hold and a zero-threshold detector circuits, to recover the received bits.

Simulated waveforms of the signals at the input and output of the LPF and the respective recovered bits for a time period of 6 μsec are illustrated in Fig. 3(b), respectively.

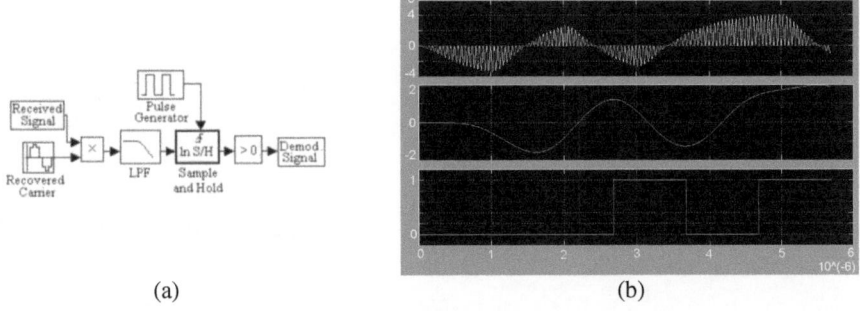

(a)   (b)

Fig. 3. (a) Model of the designed BPSK demodulator circuit, and (b) Simulated waveforms of the signals at the input and output of the LPF and the respective recovered bits for a time period of 6 μsec

3   Simulation Results

Stand-alone C code was generated and executed in Real Time Workshop [18] to simulate the transmission of 1.000.000 bits through the designed BPSK telemetry system under various noise conditions. The transmitted and recovered bits were compared by means of a logical XOR gate and the number of bit errors was calculated.

The effect of coupling and loading conditions on the system's BER performance is shown in Fig. 4(a) and 4(b), respectively. The x-axis of the plots represents the signal-to-noise ratio (SNR) per bit, defined as the E_b / N_0 ratio, where E_b is the energy per bit at the input of the inductive link channel and N_0 is the noise power spectral density, related to the AWGN's variance, σ^2, as $N_0 = 2\sigma^2$. The y-axis indicates the probability of error, or equivalently the BER. The BER performance of an all-pass, unity-gain channel linking the BPSK modulator and demodulator circuits is also depicted, for reference.

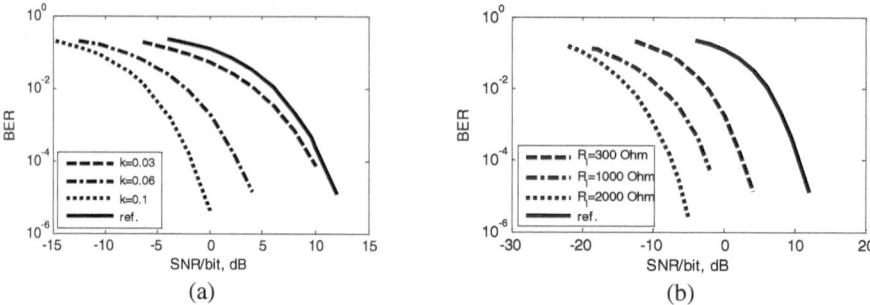

Fig. 4. BER for varying (a) coupling ($R_l = 300\,\mathrm{Ohm}$) and (b) loading ($k = 0.03$) conditions

The results of Fig. 4 can be attributed to the effect of the inductive channel on the BPSK modulated signal at its input. The simulated magnitude transfer functions for the cases under study are illustrated in Fig. 5.

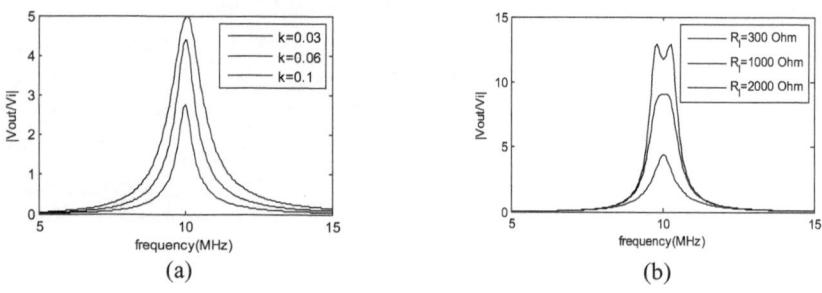

Fig. 5. Inductive link magnitude transfer functions for varying (a) coupling ($R_l = 300\,\mathrm{Ohm}$) and (b) loading ($k = 0.03$) conditions

According to Fig. 5, the inductive link acts as a bandpass filter (as stated earlier), which amplifies the signals at its resonant frequency of 10 MHz. The enhancement of the inductive link's coupling factor, k, (Fig. 5(a)) and the increase of the load resistor, R_l, (Fig. 5 (b)) result in an increasingly amplified output signal. The double-peak phenomenon observed for $k = 0.06$, $R_l = 2000\,\mathrm{Ohm}$ is due to the choice of the design parameters which result in the coupling factor exceeding its critical value [19].

This is indeed the case in the simulated waveforms of Fig. 6. Assuming that the modulated signal at the input of the inductive link channel is given by Eq. (3), Fig. 6(a) shows the signal at the output of the inductive link channel for $R_l = 300$ Ohm and $k = 0.03$, 0.06 and 0.1, respectively, while Fig. 6(b) shows the signal at the output of the inductive link channel for $k = 0.06$ and $R_l = 300$, 1000 and 2000 Ohm, respectively.

As a result, AWGN in the inductive link channel distorts an amplified version of the initial BPSK modulated signal, thus improving the noise performance compared to the case of an all-pass, unity-gain channel. Moreover, when k and/or R_l get higher, AWGN is added to an increasingly amplified version of the initial BPSK modulated signal, thus making the system more tolerant to AWGN distortion.

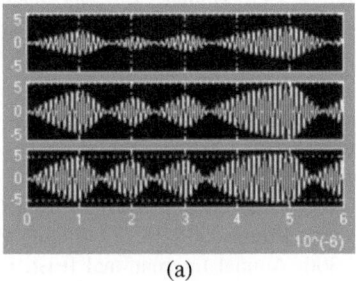 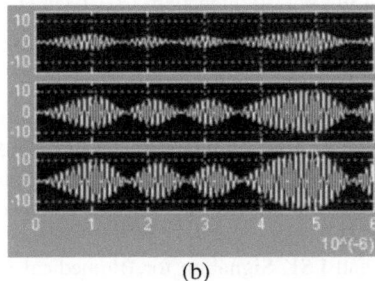

(a)   (b)

Fig. 6. Simulated waveforms of the signal at the output of the inductive link channel for (a) $R_l = 300$ Ohm and $k = 0.03$, 0.06 and 0.1, respectively, and (b) $k = 0.06$ and $R_l = 300$, 1000 and 2000 Ohm, respectively

4 Conclusions

In this paper, the BER performance of a BPSK biomedical inductive telemetry system has been studied under varying coupling and loading conditions using Simulink, Matlab. High-level simulations were presented, yet provide indicative results for a real BPSK biomedical telemetry system. Better-coupled coils and heavier-loaded implants were found to increase the magnitude transfer function of the inductive link at the frequency under interest and improve the system's BER performance. Such a telemetry system can find use in cochlear implants for treatment of motion disorders, spinal canal implants for paraplegics and deep brain stimulation for the treatment of epilepsy.

Future work will include implementation and BER performance comparison with a real BPSK biomedical telemetry system. Subsequent investigations will also include investigation of the simulated BER performance of other two-level or multi-level modulation formats for downlink data transmission in biomedical telemetry systems.

Acknowledgement

The work of AK was supported by the Greek Foundation of Education and European Culture.

References

1. Sodagar, A.M., Wise, K.D., Najafi, K.: A Wireless Implantable Microsystem for Multichannel Neural Recording. IEEE Transactions on Microwave Theory and Techniques 57(10) (2009)
2. Mohseni, P., Najafi, K., Eliades, S.J., Wang, X.: Wireless Multichannel Biopotential Recording Using an Integrated FM Telemetry Circuit. IEEE Transactions on Neural Systems and Rehabilitation Engineering 13(3) (2005)
3. Sawan, M., Hu, Y., Coulombe, J.: Wireless Smart Implants Dedicated to Multichannel Monitoring and Microstimulation. IEEE Circuits & Systems Magazine 5, 21–39 (2005)
4. Tang, Z., Smith, B., Schild, J.H., Peckham, P.H.: Data transmission from an implantable biotelemeter by load-shift keying using circuit configuration modulator. IEEE Transactions on Biomedical Engineering 42(5), 524–528 (1995)
5. Liu, W., Vichienchom, K., Clements, M., DeMarco, S.C., Hughes, C., McGucken, E., Humayun, M.S., de Juan, E., Weiland, J.D., Greenberg, R.: A neuro-stimulus chip with telemetry unit for retinal prosthetic device. IEEE Journal of Solid-State Circuits 35(10), 1487–1497 (2000)
6. Gudnason, G., Bruun, E., Hauglan, M.: A chip for an implantable neural stimulator. Journal of Analog Integrated Circuits and Signal Processing 22(1), 81–89 (2000)
7. Hu, Y., Sawan, M.: A Fully Integrated Low-Power BPSK Demodulator for Implantable Medical Devices. IEEE Transactions on Circuits and Systems 52(12), 2552–2562 (2005)
8. Sonkusale, S., Luo, Z.: A Complete Data and Power Telemetry System Utilizing BPSK and LSK Signaling for Biomedical Implants. In: 30th Annual International IEEE EMBS Conference, pp. 3216–3219 (2008)
9. Deng, S., Hu, Y., Sawan, M.: A High Data Rate QPSK Demodulator for Inductively Powered Electronics Implants. In: IEEE International Symposium on Circuits and Systems, pp. 2577–2580 (2006)
10. The MathWorks, Simulink,
    http://www.mathworks.com/products/simulink/
11. Razavi, B.: RF Microelectronics. Prentice Hall, Englewood Cliffs (1998)
12. Iniewski, K.: VLSI Circuits for Biomedical Applications. Artech House, Boston (2008)
13. Valdastri, P., Menciassi, A., Arena, A., Caccamo, C., Dario, P.: An Implantable Telemetry Platform System for In Vivo Monitoring of Physiological Parameters. IEEE Transactions on Information Technology in Biomedicine 8(3) (2004)
14. Sauer, C., Stanacevic, M., Cauwenberghs, G., Thakor, N.: Power Harvesting and Telemetry in CMOS for Implanted Devices. In: IEEE International Workshop on Biomedical Circuits and Systems, pp. S1.8-1–S1.8-4 (2004)
15. Ghovanloo, M., Atluri, S.: An Integrated Full-Wave CMOS Rectifier With Built-In Back Telemetry for RFID and Implantable Biomedical Applications. IEEE Transactions on Circuits and Systems 55(10), 3328–3334 (2008)
16. Wang, G., Liu, W., Sivaprakasam, M., Kendir, G.A.: Design and Analysis of an Adaptive Transcutaneous Power Telemetry for Biomedical Implants. IEEE Transactions on Circuits and Systems 52(10) (2005)
17. Yuan, H., Hu, X., Huang, J.: Design and Implementation of Costas Loop Based on FPGA. In: 3rd IEEE Conference on Industrial Electronics and Applications, pp. 2383–2388 (2008)
18. The Mathworks, Real Time Workshop,
    http://www.mathworks.com/products/rtw/
19. Baker, M.W., Sarpeshkar, R.: Feedback Analysis and Design of RF Power Links for Low-Power Bionic Systems. IEEE Transactions on Biomedical Circuits and Systems 1(1), 28–38 (2007)

Session 7

Ambient Assistive Technologies

mPharmacy: A System Enabling Prescription and Personal Assistive Medication Management on Mobile Devices

Charalampos Doukas[1,2], Ilias Maglogiannis[2], Panagiotis Tsanakas[3],
Flora Malamateniou[4], and George Vassilacopoulos[4]

[1] University of the Aegean, Greece
doukas@aegean.gr
[2] University of Central Greece, Greece
imaglo@ucg.gr
[3] National Technical University, Greece
panag@cs.ece.ntua.gr
[4] University of Piraeus, Greece
{flora,gvass}@unipi.gr

Abstract. The electronic management of drug treatment can provide means for prescription expenditure control as well as improve the medication process of patients and reduce the risk of adverse drug events. This paper presents the design and implementation details of a mobile platform based on Android OS that can be used for assistive medication management. The presented system is intended for physicians, pharmacists, health managers and patients, enabling not only medication prescribing but personalized treatment monitoring as well, which involves the issuing of alerts and reminders.

Keywords: mobile healthcare, prescription management, mobile medication, assistive application, Android OS.

1 Introduction

Electronic Prescribing and Medication Management has become an important component of the e-health care systems in ambulatory settings ([1] – [5]). Numerous studies report both financial [5] and patient safety benefits ([1], [6]) that may be achievable through the latter applications. The proper management of drug treatment is essential, since modern potent drugs are the cause of hospitalization in 10–16% of internal medicine cases and about half of those could be avoided [2]. Also, considering that the expenditure on drug therapy has been growing faster than any other aspect of health care in many countries ([4] – [6]) the proper control of medicine usage can facilitate in regulating unnecessary expenses. Computerized systems for drug treatment have advanced simultaneously with the development of electronic patient records. With the recent development of telematics, the electronic transfer of medical data has become more common and the good quality of drug treatment achieved with the latter systems may be extended outside the hospital. The use of mobile prescription-assistive technologies have also met great acceptance by medical personnel as

J. Lin and K.S. Nikita (Eds.): MobiHealth 2010, LNICST 55, pp. 153–159, 2011.
© Institute for Computer Sciences, Social Informatics and Telecommunications Engineering 2011

indicated in related studies [14]. Electronic drug treatment has also been associated with the ability to perform medication management and assistance for patients with special needs. It is very common for the elderly or for patients with cognitive impairments (e.g. mild dementia) to neglect taking the appropriate medication on time or make errors during the drug treatment [20]. This paper presents mPharmacy (mobile Pharmacy), a mobile platform based on Android OS that can be used by physicians for prescribing drugs and monitoring patient treatment, pharmacists for implementing prescriptions, health managers for controlling expenses and patients for assistive scheduling of drugs reception. In this paper, we focus on the physician and patient modules, which implement the assistive mobile prescription concept.

2 Related Work

The concept of electronic prescription and medication management is not relatively new. Several platforms and systems ([8] – [13]) have been proposed in the literature for managing electronic prescription that can be either deployed within healthcare organizations or used individually by physicians. Most of the related work utilizes modern interfaces (standalone applications and/or web interfaces) for providing the essential access and management of the medical repositories. Electronic prescriptions can also be forwarded through wireless transmission to in-range pharmacies [8]. The majority of the latter systems are designed for deploying within healthcare environments ([11], [13]).

Regarding personal medication assistance, in [15] a medication reminding service in home environments and its context reasoning method is presented. In order to provide an appropriate medication service depending on the user's situation, authors model and infer the context based on user's condition. Authors in [16] assess the potential value of a home-centered medication reminder system. The system has been conceptualized as a system that uses a television and set-top box, mobile phones and other in-home accessories as a means to set and deliver medication reminders to the elderly. Similarly, in [17] medications are parsed and mapped into event taxonomies and then represented through appropriate displays in a timeline fashion. In [18] technological possibilities for implementing a mobile application to support medication management of elderly vision impaired people are discussed.

All the aforementioned systems address either prescription management or personal medication facilitation individually and do not combine information derived from drug prescription with proper dose and usage. The proposed mPharmacy platform is a novel system that enables both prescription and medication management on mobile devices utilizing the Android OS.

3 Tools and Methods

This section presents the basic tools and method used for enabling the mobile prescription and personal medication management through the mPharmacy system.

3.1 The Android OS Mobile Platform

Android has emerged as a new mobile development platform, building on past successes while avoiding past failures of other platforms. Designed to empower mobile software developers to write innovative mobile applications, Android is an open source platform, allowing developers to enjoy many benefits over other competing platforms. Touted as an innovative and open platform, Android is being positioned to address the growing needs of the mobile marketplace. Android offers an open source software development kit (SDK) that enables developers to utilize extensive and modern application programming interfaces (APIs). The latter provide full access to the mobile device's resources and allow screen drawing, user input, network access (i.e. through WiFi, Bluetooth, 3G), storage, media, graphics and even direct hardware access. Media APIs are available for both playback and recording of audio, video and still images. For storage, developers aren't limited to file-based APIs. SQLite is available for relational data storage, a preferences API is available for simple setting storage and applications can extend the data storage mechanisms available. The latter makes Android suitable for storing healthcare information since it can allow a more structural management of data locally, like prescriptions and medication information. Finally, native support by the SDK is provided for communicated with Web Services.

3.2 Communication through Web Services

Web Services are emerging as a promising technology to build distributed applications. It is an implementation of Service Oriented Architecture (SOA) [7] that supports the concept of loosely-coupled, open-standard, language - and platform-independent systems. The loosely-coupled features allow service providers to modify backend functions while maintaining the same interface to clients. Web Services are accessed through the HTTP/HTTPS protocols and utilize XML (eXtendible Markup Language) for data exchange. This in turn implies that Web Services are independent of platform, programming language, tool and network infrastructure. Services can be assembled and composed in such a way to foster the reuse of existing back-end infrastructure.

Web services provide several technological and business benefits, a few of which include application and data integration, versatility, code re-use and cost savings. The inherent interoperability that comes with using vendor, platform and language independent XML technologies and the ubiquitous HTTP as a transport mean that any application can communicate with any other application using Web services. Web services are also versatile by design. They can be accessed by humans via a Web-based client interface, or they can be accessed by other applications and other Web services. Code re-use is another positive side-effect of Web services' interoperability and flexibility. One service might be utilized by several clients, all of which employ the operations provided to fulfill different business objectives.

4 Proposed System Architecture

This section presents the proposed architecture and the major components of the system that enables the mobile prescription and medication management. As illustrated in Fig. 1, the mobile application consists of two major modules. The physician module that provides all the essential functionality for creating a prescription and the patient module that acquires prescriptions from the system and manages medication through reminders and dose information provision respectively. A local database within the mobile environment is used in order to store and retrieve important information like the submitted prescriptions by a specific physician user or the current drug list that corresponds to the medication prescribed to a patient user. A Web Services Client module provides common functionality to the aforementioned modules for retrieving and uploading information regarding medication and prescription. All the latter modules are hosted by the Android Operating System that runs on the mobile device. The interface for proper data management is implemented through a Web Service that communicates with appropriate database systems hosting prescription and medicine repositories. The Web service implements all the necessary functionality for performing queries in the database based on requests by user for medicines and prescriptions as well as insert new prescriptions into the database created by physicians. A public web-based interface can provide additional access to the information residing into the database and similar functionality. The latter can serve as an alternative portal to manage healthcare information and can be especially utilized by pharmacists in order to acquire and update the submitted prescriptions.

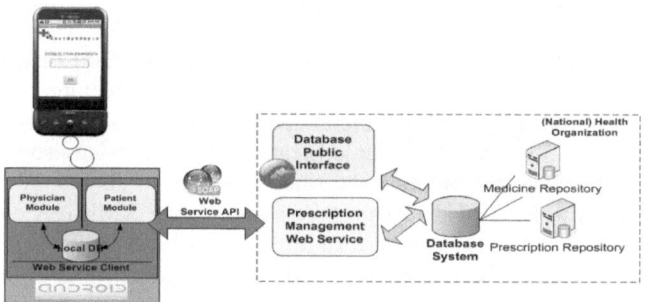

Fig. 1. Illustration of the proposed architecture

5 Mobile Prescription and Medication Management

The main features and processes of the mobile prescription and medication management system are discussed in this section. User access to both physician and patient modules is controlled through appropriate authentication mechanisms. Physicians are authenticated online through credentials that reside on the main database system and are provided only by proper registration. Patients can use credentials that are created and reside locally at the mobile system. Physicians can browse on line the medicine repository and select the appropriate medication based on pathology and retrieve additional information about dose and packaging. Once the appropriate medication is selected, physicians can enter dose and accompanying instructions through appropriate forms (see Fig. 2). The prescription is submitted into the online system and a unique identifier is assigned to each prescription. The latter along with the prescription information is also stored locally, so that it can be retrieved later by the physician.

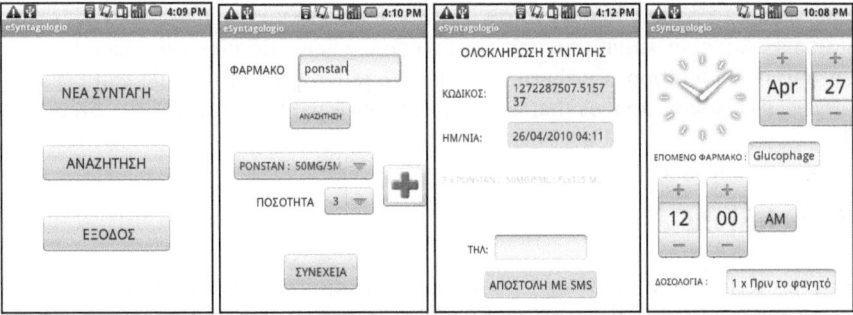

Fig. 2. Screenshots of the mobile application modules featuring main menu screen for physicians, medicine queries, prescription compose and medication management. Text messages are displayed in Greek.

Fig. 2 contains sample screenshots from the physician and patient mobile application modules respectively.

The assigned prescription id can be forwarded by the physician to a patient's mobile phone through text messaging. Patients can use the appropriate mobile application module and retrieve their personal medication list using the provided prescription id. The list contains useful information regarding dose and treatment. A scheduler embedded into the patient application module acts as a reminder for appropriate and on time medication.

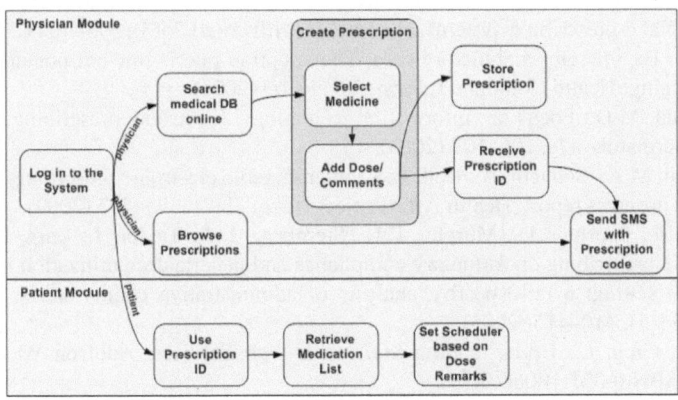

Fig. 3. Data Flow Diagram of the physician prescription management and patient medication module

The process of creating and managing prescriptions from physicians and managing medication from patients is illustrated as a data flow diagram in Fig. 3.

Enabling access to web services along with the advanced wireless connectivity options provided by the Android platform (Bluetooth, WiFi, 3G), the mPharmacy system can easily be integrated with additional external medical information platforms. Collaboration with electronic medical record systems can provide instant and direct mobile access to patient history allowing physicians to take better decisions regarding treatments. Adverse situations can be avoided when allergies on special drugs are taken into consideration. Furthermore, the integrated patient module can easily communicate with smart devices that assist and control medication, like the SmartDrawer [19].

6 Conclusions

Mobile prescription systems and personal medication assistance are promising technologies for addressing financial and personal safety issues that have raised with the current drug treatment process by medical personnel. The proposed mPharmacy platform is a novel system that enables both prescription and medication treatment assistance on mobile devices. Legal, ethical, standardization and interoperability issues need to be resolved before such mobile platforms can be deployed in real environments assisting the management of drug treatment and the medication process. However the proposed implementation proves the feasibility of mobile prescription and assistive medication management systems and exhibits the benefits of such systems.

References

1. Teich, J.M., Marchibroda, J.M.: Electronic prescribing: toward maximum value and rapid adoption. eHealth Initiative, Washington, DC (2004)
2. Grossman, J.M., Gerland, A., Reed, M.C., Fahlman, C.: Physicians' experiences using commercial e-prescribing systems. Health Aff (Millwood) 26(3), 393–404 (2007)
3. Joch, A.: Rx for safer ambulatory care. The adoption rate is low but potential is high for e-prescribing. Health Commun. Inform. 20(11), 60 (2003)
4. Kaufmann, M.D.: Focus on: information technology. Electronic prescribing: an update. J. Drugs Dermatol. 4(1), 106–107 (2005)
5. Friedman, M.A., Schueth, A., Bell, D.S.: Interoperable electronic prescribing in the United States: a progress report. Health Aff. (Project Hope) 28(2), 393–403 (2009)
6. Ross, S.M., Papshev, D., Murphy, E.L., Sternberg, D.J., Taylor, J., Barg, R.: Effects of electronic prescribing on formulary compliance and generic drug utilization in the ambulatory care setting: a retrospective analysis of administrative claims ata. J. Manag. Care Pharm. 11(5), 410–415 (2005)
7. Eric, N., Greg, L.: Understanding SOA with Web Services. Addison Wesley, Reading (2005) ISBN 0-321-18086-0
8. Ghinea, G., Asgari, S., Moradi, A., Serif, T.: A Jini-Based Solution for Electronic Prescriptions. IEEE Transactions on Information Technology in Biomedicine 10(4), 794–802 (2006)
9. Chu, S.: ePrescription: road map from wired to wireless point-of-care order entry, Enterprise Networking and Computing in Healthcare Industry. In: 6th International Workshop on HEALTHCOM 2004, June 28-29, pp. 26–33 (2004)
10. Liu, S., Wei Ma Moore, R., Ganesan, V., Nelson, S.: RxNorm: prescription for electronic drug information exchange. IT Professional 7(5), 17–23 (2004)
11. Puustjarvi, J., Puustjarvi, L.: Automating the coordination of electronic prescription processes. In: 8th International Conference on e-Health Networking, Applications and Services, HEALTHCOM 2006, pp. 147–151 (2006)

12. Costa, A.L., de Oliveira, M.M.B., de Oliveira Machado, R.: An information system for drug prescription and distribution in a public hospital. International Journal of Medical Informatics 73(4), 371–381 (2004)
13. Niinimäki, J., Forsström, J.: Approaches for certification of electronic prescription software 47(3), 175–182 (1997)
14. Oliven, A., Michalake, I., Zalman, D., Dorman, E., Yeshurun, D., Odeh, M.: Prevention of prescription errors by computerized, on-line surveillance of drug order entry. International Journal of Medical Informatics 74(5), 377–386 (2005)
15. Vishwanath, A., Brodsky, L., Shaha, S., Leonard, M., Cimino, M.: Patterns and changes in prescriber attitudes toward PDA prescription-assistive technology. International Journal of Medical Informatics 78(5), 330–339 (2009)
16. Lim, M., Choi, J., Kim, D., Park, S.: A Smart Medication Prompting System and Context Reasoning in Home Environments. In: Fourth International Conference on Networked Computing and Advanced Information Management NCM 2008, vol. 1, pp. 115–118 (2008)
17. Lee Young, S., Joe, T., Nitya, N., Pallavi, K., Engelsma Jonathan, R., Basapur, S.: Investigating the potential of in-home devices for improving medication adherence. In: 3rd International Conference on Pervasive Computing Technologies for Healthcare, PervasiveHealth 2009, pp. 1–8 (2009)
18. Xinxin, Z., Gold, S., Lai, A., Hripcsak, G., Cimino, J.J.: Using Timeline Displays to Improve Medication Reconciliation. In: International Conference on eHealth, Telemedicine, and Social Medicine, eTELEMED 2009, pp. 1–6 (2009)
19. Isomursu, M., Ervasti, M., Tormanen, V.: Medication management support for vision impaired elderly: Scenarios and technological possibilities. In: 2nd International Symposium on Applied Sciences in Biomedical and Communication Technologies, pp. 1–6 (2009)
20. Becker, E., Metsis, V., Arora, R., Vinjumur, J., Xu, Y., Makedon, F.: SmartDrawer: RFID-based smart medicine drawer for assistive environments. In: Proceedings of the 2nd International Conference on PErvsive Technologies Related to Assistive Environments (PETRA 2009), Article 49, 8 pages. ACM, New York (2009)
21. Wessell, A.M., Nietert, P.J., Jenkins, R.G., Nemeth, L.S., Ornstein, S.M.: Inappropriate medication use in the elderly: Results from a quality improvement project in 99 primary care practices. The American Journal of Geriatric Pharmacotherapy 6(1), 21–27 (2008)

AmIVital: Digital Personal Environment for Health and Well-Being

Zoe Valero[1], Gema Ibáñez[1], Juan Carlos Naranjo[1], and Pablo García[2]

[1] Institute for the Applications of Advanced Information and Communication Technologies,
Camino de Vera. sn, 46022 Valencia, Spain
{zoevara,geibsan,jcnaranjo}@itaca.upv.es
[2] Department of Computer Architecture and Computer Technology, ETS. De Ingenierías
Informática y Telecomunicación, University of Granada
pgarcia@atc.ugr.es

Abstract. This work introduces AmIVital, a Spanish project which aims to provide a platform that meets the bases of AAL (Ambient Assisted Living) and facilitates the development of applications and business models for an emerging sector. AmIVital focuses on social needs of first order, and presents the work undertaken in developing the mobile platform. This platform creates a digital personal environment for health and well-being that produces new and innovative e-Health, e-Information, e-Learning, e-Leisure, and e-Assistance services based on Ambient Intelligence (AmI) paradigm. AmI helps make easier the development of services thought to be consumed by elderly, disabled and people with chronic diseases in order to improve their life quality.

Keywords: platform; AAL; mobile computing; OSGi; ESB; SOA; AmI; chronic illness; dependant people; elderly people.

1 Introduction

Current society must face up to the ageing of the world population as one main challenge for the future. According to well-known statistics, the proportion of dependant people will increase substantially in the next years.

One direct consequence of this life enlargement is that it will increase in the same way, the number of adults with disability, people with chronic illness and old people. It is estimated that chronic illness will represent more than 60% of the total illness in the 2020 year. Other study foresees that, in the 2050 year, the third part of the population will be between 65 and 79 years old, in other words a 44% more than at the beginning of this century [1].

Ambient Assisted Living [2] (AAL) pretends to enhance the quality of life of older people by means of the new Information and Communication Technologies (ICT). AAL is an application domain of Ambient Intelligence (AmI) and also includes personal health-related applications.

AmI environments are sensitive and responsive to the presence of people, being aware of the specific characteristics of human presence and personalities, take care of needs and are capable of responding intelligently in an unobtrusive way.

J. Lin and K.S. Nikita (Eds.): MobiHealth 2010, LNICST 55, pp. 160–167, 2011.

To achieve the objectives of AAL concept, services and applications of different nature must be provided, which makes the need arises of using diverse technologies both for the development and the coexistence between them in a same system.

AmIVital [3] is a Spanish project, which aims to provide a platform that meets the bases of AAL and facilitates the development of applications and business models for an emerging sector, concentrated on social needs of first order, solving problems derived from the interconnection between different technologies. This platform is based on the research of a complete and coherent vision of the AmI technological services, and attempting to create a technological background that allows developing services and applications for personal environment of those who need to control their health, life habits and social state. In summary, the result will be an integral and technological proposal for improving the life quality of chronic illness, dependant and elderly people, providing tools for those stakeholders related to the users such as doctors, assistances, relatives and so on.

As starting point, AAL services were selected for covering a wide variety of life aspects such as leisure, health, nutrition, physical exercise, etc. From this selection, common properties from these services were detected, focusing on the non-functional requirements, whether coming from the own services, or being a pre-condition established by the initial project objectives. On the other side, the project analyzed the state of art of new technologies that would enable the development of the final architecture. This analysis was based on the following basis: the selected technologies should facilitate the development, they should make easier the inclusion of new services, they had to be modular and they should improve the deployment capabilities of already-existing services oriented platforms.

Based on the user profiles and the requirements derived from the AAL objectives, AmIVital is divided in three main scenarios with similar architecture that share data model and protocols, being the Coordination Center, Fixed Gateway and Mobile Gateway.

The Coordination Center is in charge of giving support for the professionals and coordinating communications between both platforms, fixed and mobile. It also integrates external service providers, such as social services, emergency services, insurance companies, etc. The Fixed Gateway covers the needs of the user at his home. And finally, the Mobile Gateway covers the same services and those specifics for outdoor environments.

This article is focused on explaining AmIVital project, which is a global architecture that proposes a standardized and interoperable model for improving the life quality to elderly, disabled and people with chronic diseases.

2   Materials and Methods

Services have to be communicated among themselves, regardless the gateway (mobile, fixed or coordination center) where they are deployed. This fact makes the need arises of researching about Enterprise Application Integration approaches (EAI) in order to integrate applications between different organizations, *i.e. a hospital and a service provider*. EAI is a business need to make diverse applications in an enterprise including partner systems to communicate to each other to achieve an objective irrespective of platform and geographical location of these applications. service & event oriented architecture (SOA) [4] and EAI coexist being the prime choice for large scale integration.

SOA represents an architectural paradigm for applications, with Web Services capabilities are implemented, which are available to other applications through application and standard network interfaces and protocols. SOA advocates an approach in which a software component provides its functionality as a service that can be consumed by other software components. Components (or services) represent reusable software building blocks.

The project technological backbone it is SOA architecture applied to an Ambient Intelligence scenario. The most promising technology related to these concepts is OSGi[5], which combined with Web Services[6] are the main architecture foundations. The services are accessible in a transparent way inside the OSGi container; these components are not reachable from or could not access external services, to make this possible the components should publish/consume Web Services. This solution is completed with the use of Enterprise Service Bus (ESB) [7], which is an infrastructure to facilitate the implementation of the SOA approach. It gives API that can be used to develop services and makes services interact with each other reliably.

AmIVital is a distributed architecture based on AmI and SOA 2.0 that is developed through a technological architecture, which main elements are OSGi, Web Services, ESB and Business Process Execution Language (BPEL), providing network connectivity and interoperability among different network environments.

3   AmIVital Architecture

This section presents the AmIVital architecture, giving an overview regarding the three computational nodes deployed on the platform: fixed Gateway (AmI home space), Mobile Gateway (body AmI space) and the Coordination Centre as coordinator of all the services.

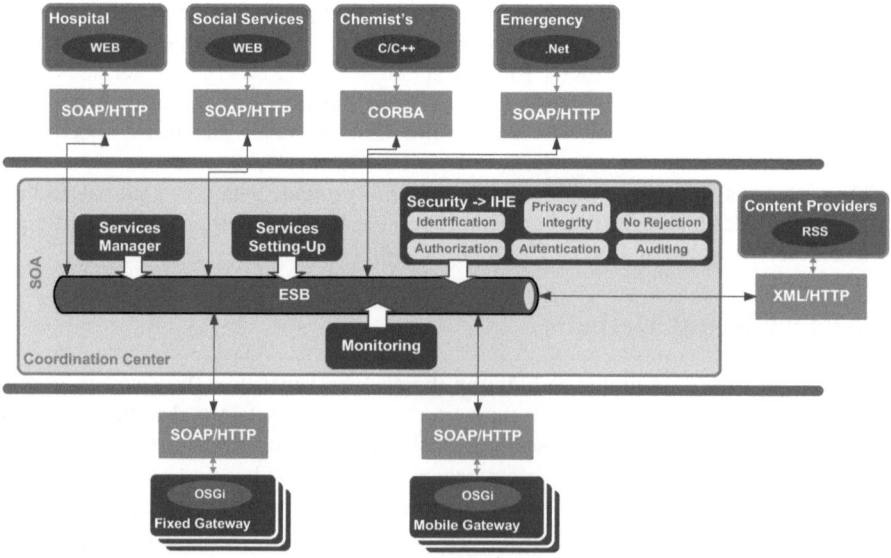

Fig. 1. AmIVital technological deployment

The **coordination center** integrates the mobile and fixed gateways, and communicates both with external service providers. In the following figure can be better appreciated that fixed and mobile gateways are connected through the ESB with the external providers, using as SOAP/HTTP interfaces. Security covers the whole architecture. It is defined by IHE profiles, and it is implemented through WS-Security standard and the SAML assertion language.

The below figure represents the logical reference architecture of the AmIVital platform. This approach is followed by the fixed and mobile gateways.

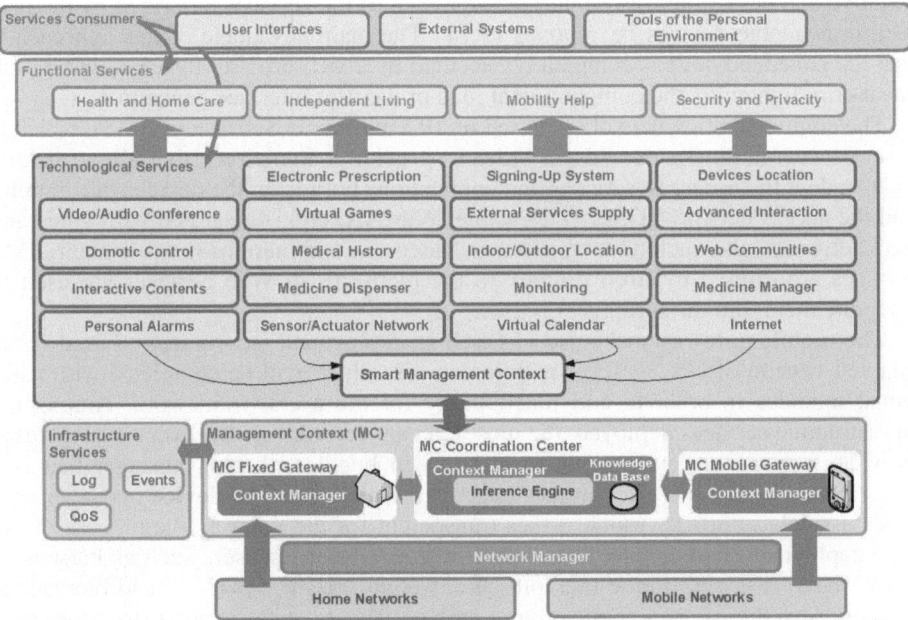

Fig. 2. AmIVital architecture

Fixed and mobile gateways are service oriented, for that categorization of services has been made as functional, technological and infrastructure services.

Functional services are those that arrive to the end user (infarct cerebral prevention service, which control vital signs of patients and send alarms if there appears a risk situation).

Technological services are AmI services and are composed by infrastructure or base services. Each application has underneath a set of technological services that implement its functionalities (infarct cerebral prevention service is composed by monitoring, localization, and contact manager technological services.

Infrastructure services are located in the base of the architecture, and are used to compose technological services, *i.e. the monitoring technological service makes use of the device manager infrastructure service that control sensors connected to the gateway*, the context manager infrastructure service, which is involved in the data evaluation, the persistence infrastructure service for storing data and so on.

Due to resource limitations of mobile devices have been used different technologies for fixed and mobile gateways.

To assure the operation security has been designed and implemented a specific hardware for the **fixed gateway** in order to guarantee the basic services in any moment, including: software, SO, communications and power supplier failure. Some components are worth mentioning such as the context manager, which uses Bossam as reasoning engine and JADE as multiagent platform. Ontologies are in charge of the data model to share all data from inside and outside of AmIVital. OWL-DL is used as ontological language to define the internal ontology.

For the User Graphical Interface has been use GWT [8] technology that provide the intuitive and easy-to-use user interfaces for each of the services described by the project, in available devices *i.e. mobiles or TV*. The main advantage of this approach is that the generated code is completely executed by a web browser through HTML and JavaScript lightening the computational load of the user interface generation.

The communication network is based on IP Multimedia Subsystem (IMS), which is a set of international standards in order to provide a framework that allow making independent the access to services and applications both from the device (PC, mobile) and the access network (DSL, WiFi, cable, WiMAX, etc). Integrated with voice and data networks, also include text, pictures, video or combinations between them. IMS services are offered by itself directly to the platform, so Web Services are used to integrate them into the system.

The **mobile gateway** make use of OSGi as deployment environment, based on an adapted version of eRCP [9] for mobile devices, which will be completed with additional modules in order to add functionality for the users' framework. Among the infrastructure services deployed, the most relevant services are the event manager that provides a communication mechanism between bundles, the log manager that is a general mechanism to write log messages on the platform. The **device manager** provides a single interface, which makes transparent for the gateway the process of device-deployment and enables to connect several types of sensors such as biosensors (ECG, heart rate, respiration rate, pressure, weight, height, SpO2,...) and biomedical clothes. Also the use and application of ambient and presence sensors (location, temperature, activity,...) that operate in a cooperative way.

The **web services manager**, based on Axis [10], which allows consuming mobile gateway services from other platforms. The mobile gateway includes the **persistence** service implemented with db4o [11], which is an object-oriented database engine as well as a graphic user interface that presents the gateway to users (eSWT [12]). Also a **personal alarm manager** has been deployed in order to allow the user asking for help in a fast and easy way. Another deployed service in the gateway is **virtual calendar** service (iCal4j [13]). This service manages programmed events. Finally, the **context manager** is an improved version of 3APL-M [14] inference engine that evaluates information that comes from the mobile gateway.

These *technological services* were selected to be deployed into the mobile gateway. The **monitoring** service provides information of biometric parameters, each measure comes from the sensor devices or manual inputs by means of graphical user interface. Those measures are sent to the context manager, where they will be analyzed in order to determine anomalous states, and to be stored in a persistent way.

If something is wrong, then the **personal alarm manager** will send an alarm to the coordination center and will call to a pre-configured telephone number.

The **virtual calendar** manages appointments and reminders and keeps informed the user about all scheduled events. It is synchronized with the coordination center. The **content manager** is used to download multimedia resources from the coordination center repository. This content teaches how to use available services in the platform with explanatory videos. The **personal agenda** provides access to the patient's favorite telephone numbers. Finally, the **domotic control** service is connected to the fixed gateway, allowing the user to switch off/on lights, control temperature, etc.

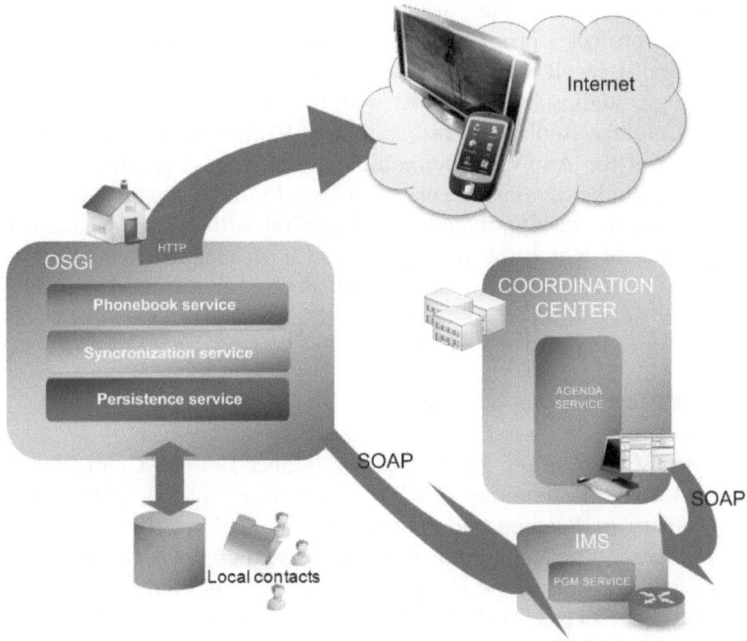

Fig. 3. Contact list service

As example of a functional service of the platform, contact list service is showed in the above figure. It introduces the concept "always connected", by means of the active synchronization of the contacts from the network. The user adds a new contact from a device where the fixed or mobile gateway is deployed. The contact list service interacts with the technological and infrastructure services that it requires, updating the local contact list and doing a synchronization data with the coordination center, where it will keep the master data copy. This synchronization is done through the IMS service.

4   Conclusions and Future Work

AmIVital is oriented especially to sanitary actuations, but applied in a Social Environment, focused on elderly, disabled and people with chronic diseases for improving their life quality. AmIVital asumes available ICT, concentrating the effort in providing a global architecture and propose a standardized and interoperable model to achieve this objective.

The work done proves that the results meet the initial expectations for the coordination center, the fixed and the mobile gateway. In this paper has been explained the work carried out specifically in the mobile gateway, proving that is possible to combine the resource limitations of current devices and services required by the user, providing and robust platform together the rest of AmIVital logical nodes in order to improve the quality of life of end users.

Currently additional services such as videoconference using IMS, and the improvement of security mechanisms are being developed for the mobile gateway. In the last phase of the project a proof of concept will be carried out in a controlled environment with real users. It is prepared in based on interdisciplinary, technical, social and epidemiologic studies (300 patients) with the entire user involved in the project, where COPD Cerebrovascular Disease and Heart Failure is the proposal for the functional validation of the AmIVital technological platform. A positive answer was detected from those studies against the use of personal monitoring devices.

As future work, the results obtained of AmIVital will be used as input in universAAL[15] project, of which the main objective is to make technically feasible and economically viable to conceive, design and deploy innovate new AAL services. Other actions are being done in collaboration with Spanish projects as Inredis [16].

Acknowledgments

The project AmIVital (CENIT 2007-2010), is financed by the Centre for the Development of Industrial Technology (CDTI) which is a Spanish public organisation, under the Ministry of Science and Innovation, whose objective is to help Spanish companies to increase the technological profile of said companies. The authors would like to appreciate the work done by the members of AmIVital consortium, and specially to Telefónica I+D Granada for its involvement together to ITACA in all the process of mobile gateway development, without their contribution it could not have been possible.

References

1. Department of Economic and Social Affairs. World Population Prospects: The 2008 Revision Population Database
2. Ambient Assisted Living, http://www.aal-europe.eu/
3. Entorno Personal Digital para la Salud y el Bienestar, http://www.amivital.es
4. Make way for SOA 2.0,
   http://www.javaworld.com/javaworld/jw-05-2006/
   jw-0517-iw-soa.html
5. Open Services Gateway Iniciative, http://www.osgi.org/Main/HomePage
6. Web Services, http://www.w3schools.com/webservices
7. Chappel, D.A.: Enterprise Service Bus. O'Reilly's, New York (June 2004)

8. GWT: Google, Faster AJAX than you'd write by hand,
   `http://code.google.com/webtoolkit/`
9. eRCP: embedded Rich Client Platform, `http://www.eclipse.org/ercp`
10. Axis, `http://ws.apache.org/axis/java/index.html`
11. db4o Database Engine, `http://www.db4o.com/about/productinformation/`
12. embedded Standard Widget Toolkit,
    `http://www.eclipse.org/ercp/eswt/gallery/gallery.php`
13. ical4j, `http://wiki.modularity.net.au/ical4j/index.php?title=Main_Page`
14. 3APL-M. Inference engine, `http://www.cs.uu.nl/3aplm/index.html`
15. universAAL: UNIVERsal open platform and reference Specification for Ambient Assisted Living, `http://www.universaal.org/`
16. Inredis: Interfaces for relations between environment and people with disabilities, `http://www.inredis.es/Default.aspx`

An Analysis of Bluetooth, Zigbee and Bluetooth Low Energy and Their Use in WBANs

Emmanouil Georgakakis, Stefanos A. Nikolidakis,
Dimitrios D. Vergados, and Christos Douligeris

Department of Informatics, University of Piraeus,
80, Karaoli & Dimitriou St., GR-185 34, Piraeus, Greece
{egeo,snikol,vergados,cdoulig}@unipi.gr

Abstract. A rapid development of services and technologies in the field of health care has been witnessed in the last few years. In this paper we present an analysis and an extensive comparison of radio communication technologies, namely Zigbee, Bluetooth and Bluetooth Low Energy, that have been proposed as likely candidates to provide wireless connectivity between body sensors and the health care system and consequently to lead the development and extended deployment of Wireless Body Area Networks. After the description of their characteristics, we concentrate on the security that these technologies offer since security is extremely important for the sensitive health care clinical information communicated and the protection of patients' clinical information privacy.

Keywords: WBAN, Bluetooth, Zigbee, Bluetooth Low energy, m-Health, security.

1 Introduction

The availability of efficient continuous monitoring of patients can help doctors and trained personnel to provide patients with a series of advanced and effective health care services. These services may include diagnostic procedures, maintenance of chronic conditions or supervising recovery from an acute event or a surgical procedure. These services are typically enabled with the deployment of a Wireless Body Area Network (WBAN).

In this paper we describe the most common wireless technologies that can be used in WBANs. In particular we focus on Bluetooth and Zigbee, which are widely used, as well as on Bluetooth Low Energy (LE), which is an emerging technology. These technologies are presented in detail and they are compared with a focus to their security features.

It is important to note that the available technologies in this field advance rapidly and there is a need for continuous evaluation and comparison of the new features presented by the corresponding standard associations and research forums.

J. Lin and K.S. Nikita (Eds.): MobiHealth 2010, LNICST 55, pp. 168–175, 2011.

2 Wireless Body Area Network (WBAN)

2.1 Overview

A WBAN is a collection of several small devices that are close or attached to the human body. These devices integrate wearable health monitoring systems into a telemedicine system that is able to support the early detection of abnormal conditions and the prevention of its serious consequences. For example a WBAN can alert the hospital, even before a patient has a heart attack, through the measuring of changes in one's vital signs [1, 2].

2.2 Wireless Communications Technologies in WBANs

The most widely used technologies enabling WBANs are Bluetooth and ZigBee. Bluetooth LE is an emerging and very promising technology for WBANs. The use of these technologies is important for the exchange of information that the sensors collect, from the sensor to the monitoring application and vice versa. Thus, there are a lot of parameters and different characteristics that each technology may offer to the health care systems. These characteristics may include the offered applications, the cost, the communication range, the power consumption, the data rate, the frequency band and the security parameters.

3 Bluetooth, ZigBee and Bluetooth LE Functionality and Features

3.1 History and Applications

Bluetooth, which is specified in IEEE 802.15.1, is the widest used wireless technology [3]. It was invented by telecommunications vendor Ericsson in 1994 and was originally conceived as a wireless alternative to RS-232 data cables. It can be used in a variety of applications that include: wireless control and communication between a mobile phone and a hands-free headset, replacement of traditional wired serial communications in test equipment, GPS receivers, bar code scanners, traffic control devices and short range transmission of health sensor data from medical devices to medical computers.

Nokia's research centre, attempted to develop a technology that would successfully address issues that wireless technologies could not manage to carry out successfully. The first guidelines were published in 2004 under the name "Bluetooth Low End Extension" [4]. Following these efforts in 2006 Nokia introduced the Wibree technology as an open industry standard. Bluetooth LE has evolved from the Wibree standard. In July 2010, the Bluetooth SIG announced the formal adoption of Bluetooth Core Specification Version 4.0 with the feature of Bluetooth low energy technology. The Bluetooth LE can be used for the interconnection of small devices like watches and sports sensors as well as in smart energy, home automation and healthcare devices.

In 2004 the IEEE 802.15.4 also known as ZigBee was first defined as a vertically integrated protocol suite that provides a distributed object abstraction for devices on a new low-power wireless link. The broad utility of this link led to the definition of a wide variety of application profiles that include home automation, commercial building automation and smart energy which cut across industry segments and medical monitoring. In December 2006, the ZigBee 2006 specification was released, which was followed in October 2007 by the ZigBee 2007/PRO specification [5].

Bluetooth and Zigbee have already been utilised in healthcare systems that use WBANs in order to offer monitoring services for patients and elderly people that may live alone in their home. Some important of them are the following:

A WBAN System for Ambulatory Monitoring of Physical Activity and Health Status that utilises Zigbee was proposed in [6]. The Improved WBAN communication at mental healthcare system with personalized bio signal devices that uses Bluetooth is proposed in [7].

3.2 Topology

The choice of the appropriate network topology is an important part of the network design. A misconfigured network can result in waste of time, energy and a lot of troubleshooting methods are required to resolve disorders.

The Bluetooth Specification defines a uniform structure for a wide range of devices that connect and communicate with each other. Bluetooth operates primarily using ad hoc piconets, where a master device controls multiple slaves. The slave devices may only communicate with the master device and they do not communicate directly with another slave device. However, a slave device may participate in one or more piconets. Piconets are limited to 8 devices. Figure 1 summarises Bluetooth topology.

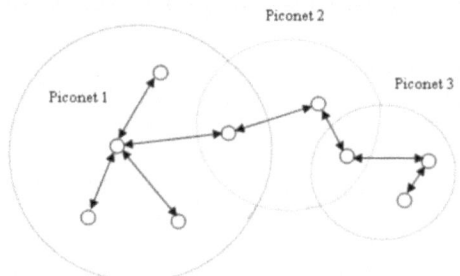

Fig. 1. Bluetooth topology

The topology of the Bluetooth LE is different to Bluetooth. A device is the master in a piconet (represented by the blue dotted area, and known as piconet) with the other devices to be the slaves, The slaves do not share a common physical channel with the master. Each slave communicates on a separate physical channel with the master. Also there are devices that are advertisers and initiators (represented by the red dashed area). Figure 2 presents this topology.

A ZigBee network consists of one coordinator, one or more end devices and, optionally, one or more routers (Figure 3). The coordinator is a Full Function Device (FFD), responsible for the inner workings of the ZigBee network. A coordinator sets up a network with a given PAN identifier which end devices can join. End devices are typically Reduced Function Devices (RFDs) to allow for an inexpensive implementation. Routers can be used as mediators for the coordinator in the PAN, thus allowing

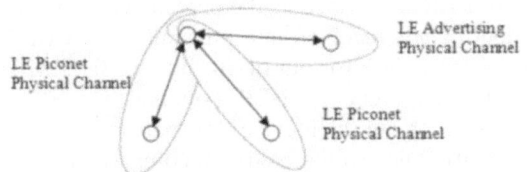

Fig. 2. Bluetooth Low Energy topology

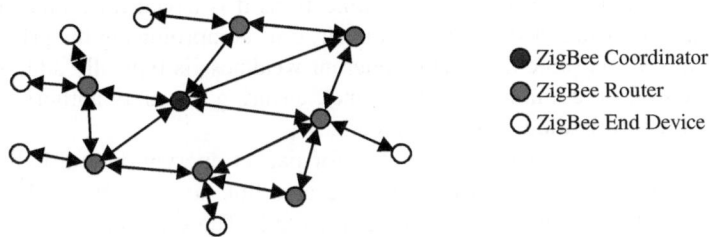

Fig. 3. Zigbee topology

the network to expand beyond the radio range of the coordinator. A router acts as a local coordinator for end devices joining the PAN, and must implement most of the coordinator capabilities. Hence, a router is also an FFD device.

3.3 Power Consumption and Data Rate

ZigBee, was designed to be a low-power alternative to Bluetooth, and indeed offers a significantly improved performance of 30mW compared to the Bluetooth's 100mW. ZigBee can achieve a data rate of 250Kbps at 2.4GHz (16 Channels), 40 Kbps at 915 MHz (10 channels), and 20Kbps at 868Mhz (1 channel).

Bluetooth 1.2 achieves a maximum data rate of 1.2 Mbps and Bluetooth 2.0+EDR (Enhanced Data Rate) achieves up to 3 Mbps. Bluetooth 3.0 supports theoretical data transfer speeds of up to 24 Mbit/s.

The Bluetooth LE enables dual-mode implementations to reuse the Bluetooth RF part and to guarantee ultra low power consumption for devices with embedded stand-alone implementation of the Bluetooth LE specification. The Bluetooth LE has physical layer bit rate of 1 Mbps and may achieve link distance of around 10 meters. Bluetooth LE consumes only 10% of the power consumed by Bluetooth. It can save energy and extend battery life by sleeping and waking up when it needs to send data.

3.4 Error Correction

Bluetooth, ZigBee and Bluetooth LE implement CRCs (Cyclic Redundancy Checks) to protect against errors on communication channels. The error detection capability of a CRC depends on its length. Bluetooth and ZigBee utilise a 16-bit CRC for error control at the link layer. Bluetooth LE implements a 24-bit CRC that provides a higher level of assurance regarding error detection.

The Bit Error Ratio (BER) is defined as the percentage of bits that have errors relative to the total number of bits received in a transmission. A BER of 10^{-6} in a transmission means that one bit is in error out of 10^6 bits (or 0,12 MB) transmitted. A 16 bit CRC can not handle easily very low BER, (smaller than 10^{-6} - 10^{-8}). Hence in the health care applications which are the focus of this paper a 16-bit CRC offers efficient error detection and the difference would be trivial compared to a 24-bit CRC.

3.5   Data Encryption and Authentication

Due to the open nature of Wireless communications it is trivial for an attacker to intercept and acquire data transmitted over the air, thus compromising the privacy of the involved parties at the same time. This inherent weakness is typically addressed with data encryption of the communication channel, ensuring that only authorized entities can decipher the information communicated.

Bluetooth employs the E0 stream cipher for packet encryption and is based on a shared cryptographic secret, a previously generated link key or a master key. A 128-bit key is used in the E0 implementation of Bluetooth. These keys rely upon the Bluetooth PIN which has been entered into the end user devices. The E0 stream cipher has been proven to be susceptible to a number of attacks, degrading the strength of a 128-bit key to that of a 64-bit key [8, 9].

Bluetooth uses algorithms that are based on SAFER+ for key derivation, namely E21 and E22, and authentication as Message Authentication Codes (MACs), called E1. Again attacks against SAFER+ have been demonstrated [10, 11].

ZigBee is based on the security suite specified in the IEEE 802.15.4 standard [12]. The 802.15.4 standard requires the use of the AES (Advanced Encryption Standard) algorithm with 128-bit keys and 128-bit block lengths. AES may be used in several modes, each of which offers either data privacy (encryption), data integrity, authentication or a combination of these functions.

The standard requires that the CCM-64 (Counter with Cipher Block Chaining (CBC)-MAC) mode (encryption plus data integrity, with an 8-byte message integrity code MIC) is supported by the devices. ZigBee supports AES in CCM mode with a 128-bit key, a small variation of the CCM mode. The functionalities of encryption / decryption, authentication and verification / integrity are provided.

Similarly to the Zigbee specification, session confidentiality in Bluetooth LE is provided by the AES encryption, which is used in CCM counter mode. In LE a 128-bit Long Term Key (LTK) is used to generate session keys for encrypted connections. Every time a new LTK is distributed a 64-bit random number (Rand) and a 16-bit encrypted diversifier (EDIV) are generated. Rand and EDIV are used to identify the LTK and establish a previously shared LTK in order to start an encrypted connection among two previously paired devices. Another 128-bit key, called Identity Resolving Key, is used to generate and resolve random addresses, a feature that provides privacy to the communicating parties [4].

Bluetooth LE supports the ability to send authenticated data over an unencrypted channel between two devices with a trusted relationship. This is accomplished by signing the data with a 128-bit Connection Signature Resolving Key (CSRK).

It has to be noted that stream ciphers tend to be faster than block ciphers and the complexity of their implementation in hardware is not high. In addition to that they do not propagate errors, contrary to block ciphers.

However Zigbee and Bluetooth LE that employ variations of AES (block cipher) for encryption and authentication provide high level of assurance with regard to the strength and safety of the deployed algorithm. On the other hand, the encryption (stream cipher) and authentication mechanisms of Bluetooth have been proven to be susceptible to attacks that may undermine the overall security posture of the Bluetooth communication and put at risk the privacy of its users.

3.6 Modulation

Digital modulation techniques can be categorized in three groups: amplitude shift keying (ASK), frequency shift keying (FSK), and phase shift keying (PSK). The data rate and range supported by wireless technologies are directly affected by the modulation scheme adopted.

Zigbee uses PSK modulation, and in particular the BPSK (or 2PSK) and OPSK (or 8PSK). Bluetooth uses both PSK (BPSK and OPSK) and FSK (GFSK) while Bluetooth LE utilises GFSK.

In FSK a binary 0 is transmitted as a frequency f_0 and a binary 1 is transmitted as a frequency f_1. MSK (Minimum Shift Keying) is a form of FSK with a minimum frequency difference between f_0 and f_1 [13]. In Phase Shift Keying the digital information is transmitted by shifting the phase of the carrier among several discrete values. The performance of PSK and FSK is similar, however the bandwidth required by a signal transmitted in PSK is significantly less than in FSK. On the other hand FSK based schemes are considered simpler to implement.

There are many variations of PSK. Some of the more widely used include: binary phase shift keying (BPSK), differential phase shift keying (DPSK), quaternary phase shift keying (QPSK), differential QPSK (DQPSK) and octonary phase shift keying (OPSK). In general the higher order forms of modulation allow higher data rates to be carried within a given bandwidth. Nevertheless, the higher data rates require a better signal-to-noise-ratio (SNR), otherwise the error rates will start to rise and any improvements in the data rate performance will be diminished [13].

4 Conclusions

In this paper, we analysed and compared Bluetooth, Bluetooth LE and ZigBee according to a series of criteria and performance features. Table 1 summarises the advantages and disadvantages of these technologies and Table 2 their similarities and differences.

Bluetooth LE appears to have adopted several key features from Bluetooth and some from Zigbee and it has also introduced several novel ideas. The Bluetooth LE specification improves on the weaknesses and addresses issues that were not resolved in Bluetooth and other wireless technologies. In particular Bluetooth LE appears to have superior features regarding power consumption, scalability, confidentiality, authentication mechanisms and error correction. The improvements in the aforementioned areas have a negative impact on Bluetooth LE data rate transfer and the achievable range. Nevertheless with regards to WBANs a data rate of 1Mbps and a range of 10 meters are acceptable.

However there are several open issues regarding WBANs, the most important aspects that need to be addressed are: interoperability, system devices design, system and device-level security, invasion of privacy, sensor validation, data consistency, sensor resource constrains and the intermittent availability of uplink connectivity.

Table 1. Comparison of Zigbee, Bluetooth and Bluetooth Low Energy

	Bluetooth	ZigBee	Bluetooth LE
Advantages	A widely used technology that is supported by most devices. It is ideal for applications that are requiring high bit rates over short distances.	A low-power alternative to Bluetooth, that offers significantly improved performance of 30mW compared to Bluetooth 100mW.	It offers high spectral efficiency and low power consumption
Disadvantages	Open to interception and attack.	Low data rate.	Not supported by many devices

Table 2. WBAN technologies key features

	Bluetooth	ZigBee	Bluetooth LE
Applications	Computer and accessory devices, Computer to compute, Computer with other digital devices	Home control. Building automation, Industrial automation, Home security, Medical monitoring	Sports and fitness products, watches, smart energy home automation devices, remote controls and healthcare devices.
Frequency Band	2.4 - 2.48GHz	868MHz, 902-928MHz 2.4-2.48GHZ	2.4GHz
Topology	Ad-hoc piconets	Ad-hoc, star, mesh	Ad-hoc piconets
Scalability	Low	High	High
Range	~10 meters	~100 meters	~10 meters
Maximum Data transfer rate:	3 Mbps	20 Kbps 40 Kbps 250 Kbps	1 Mbps
Power Consumption	100 mW	30 mW	~10 mW
Access Method	TDMA	CSMA/CA	TDMA FDMA
Encryption	128-bit encryption E0 stream cipher	128-bit AES block cipher (CTR, counter mode)	128-bit AES block cipher (CCM mode)
Modulation	GFSK, 2PSK, DQSP, 8PSK	BPSK (868/928MHz) OPSK (2.4GHz)	GFSK
Authentication	Shared secret (PIN), SAFER+	AES CBC-MAC (CCM mode)	AES CBC-MAC (CCM mode)
Robustness	16-bit CRC	16-bit CRC	24-bit CRC

References

1. Istepanian, R.S.H., Jovanov, E., Zhang, Y.T.: M-Health: Beyond Seamless Mobility and Global Wireless Health-Care Connectivity. The Proceedings of the IEEE Transactions on Information Technology in Biomedicine, 405–414 (2004)
2. Jovanov, E., Milenkovic, A., Otto, C., de Groen, P.C.: A Wireless Body Area Network of Intelligent Motion Sensors for Computer Assisted Physical Rehabilitation. Journal of NeuroEngineering and Rehabilitation, 6–16 (2005)
3. http://www.bluetooth.com/English/Technology/Building/Pages/Specifcation.aspx
4. http://www.bluetooth.com/English/Products/Pages/low_energy.aspx
5. http://www.zigbee.org/Markets/ZigBeeSmartEnergy/Version20Documents.aspx
6. Jovanov, E., Milenkovic, A., Otto, C., De Groen, P., Johnson, B., Warren, S., Taibi, G.: A WBAN System for Ambulatory Monitoring of Physical Activity and Health Status: Applications and Challenges. In: The Proceedings of 27th Annual International Conference of the Engineering in Medicine and Biology Society, Shanghai, pp. 3810–3813 (2005)
7. Jung, J.Y., Lee, J.W.: Improved WBAN Communication at Mental Healthcare System with the Personalized Bio Signal Devices. In: The Proceedings of 8th International Conference Advanced Communication Technology, Korea, pp. 812–816 (2006)
8. Lu, Y., Vaudenay, S.: Cryptanalysis of an E0-like Combiner with Memory. Journal of Cryptology 21, 430–457 (2008)
9. Lu, Y., Vaudenay, S.: Cryptanalysis of Bluetooth Keystream Generator Two-Level E0. In: Lee, P.J. (ed.) ASIACRYPT 2004. LNCS, vol. 3329, pp. 147–158. Springer, Heidelberg (2004)
10. Vaudenay, S.: On the need for Multipermutations: Cryptanalysis of MD4 and SAFER. In: Preneel, B. (ed.) FSE 1994. LNCS, vol. 1008, pp. 286–297. Springer, Heidelberg (1995)
11. Shihui, Z., Licheng, W., Yixian, Y.: A New Impossible Differential Attack on SAFER Ciphers Computers and Electrical Engineering. Elsevier Computers & Electrical Engineering 36(1), 180–189 (2010)
12. IEEE Std. 802.15.4-2003, IEEE Standard for Information Technology Telecommunications and Information Exchange between Systems Local and Metropolitan Area Networks Specific Requirements Part 15.4: Wireless Medium Access Control (MAC) and Physical Layer (PHY) Specifications for Low Rate Wireless Personal Area Networks (WPANs). IEEE Press, New York (2003)
13. Eren, H.: Wireless Sensors and Instruments: Networks, Design, and Applications. CRC Press, Boca Raton (2005)

Experimental Analysis of RSSI-Based Indoor Location Systems with WLAN Circularly Polarized Antennas

P. Nepa[1], F. Cavallo[2], M. Bonaccorsi[2], M. Aquilano[2],
M.C. Carrozza[2], and P. Dario[2]

[1] Dept. of Information Engineering, University of Pisa,
Via G. Caruso 16, I-56122 Pisa, Italy
p.nepa@iet.unipi.it
[2] ARTS Lab, Scuola Superiore S. Anna
Pisa, Italy
{f.cavallo,m.bonaccorsi,m.acquilano,m.carrozza,
p.dario}@sssup.it

Abstract. Circularly polarized antennas are used in 2.4 GHz ZigBee radio modules to evaluate performance improvement of RSSI (Received Signal Strength Indicator) based location techniques, with respect to conventional linearly polarized antennas. Experimental RSSI measurements in an indoor environment clearly show that multipath fading is significantly reduced when CP antennas are used; this determines a more reliable estimation of the field amplitude decay law as a function of the distance of the mobile node from the fixed access point, and then a higher location accuracy. At the best of authors' knowledge, it is the first time that the circular polarization features are applied to RSSI-based radio location techniques.

Keywords: indoor location, RSSI-based location, circularly polarized antennas.

1 Introduction

In microwave radio links, the effectiveness of the circular polarization (CP) in reducing multipath effects is well known; CP also allows more flexible reciprocal orientation of the transmitter and the receiver antenna. For the above reasons, circularly polarized antennas are used in a number of wireless systems, as for example the GPS (Global Positioning System) system and satellite-to-mobile wideband communication links, as well as most UHF RFID (Radio Frequency IDentification) readers. Moreover, several ATC (Air Traffic Control) radars and SAR (Synthetic Aperture Radar) systems adopt CP antennas, by bringing into play some interesting properties of the polarimetric scattering.

When a circularly polarized wave is incident on a reflecting surface at a small incident angle (near to the normal incidence condition), the handedness of the circular polarization of the reflected wave is reversed: if a right (left) hand CP signal is transmitted, it would become a left (right) hand CP signal after its first reflection; after the second reflection, it would again become a right (left) hand CP signal, and so on. Thus, if the transmitting antenna is circularly polarized and the receiving antenna polarization is also circular with the same handedness as the transmitting antenna,

J. Lin and K.S. Nikita (Eds.): MobiHealth 2010, LNICST 55, pp. 176–183, 2011.

multipath delayed waves after single reflection will be effectively rejected on reception by the receiving antenna. Indeed, it has been shown [1]-[2] that the RMS delay spread for circular polarization is about half of that for linear polarization (in both cases, the same polarization was used for the transmitter and the receiver).

In wireless local area networks (WLANs), circular polarized antennas are suggested for the access points, since a reliable radio links can be obtained independently on the spatial orientation of the mobile node antenna (which often is a linearly polarized antenna).

In the open literature, a comparative analysis between vertical and horizontal linear polarization antennas has been performed, in ZigBee WSNs for localization purposes [3].

Although the superiority of circular polarization over linear polarization for the suppression of the effects of multipath propagation in radio channels is well known, to the best of the authors' knowledge, there has not been a deep investigation on the improvement that can be achieved when CP antennas are used for the fixed/mobile nodes of wireless sensor networks (WSNs), in the context of RSSI (Received Signal Strength Indicator) based indoor location systems. In indoor environments, the performance of RSSI-based location systems is significantly reduced due to the multipath phenomena which determines rapid spatial variations of the electromagnetic field amplitude [4,5]: significant amplitude variations are obtained in short distances [6], which is apparently related to the relatively short wavelength (around 12.5 cm a 2.4 GHz).

It is worth noting that in indoor location systems multipath and Non Line Of Sight (NLOS) conditions make range-free localization methods (like fingerprinting) more reliable than range-based ones [7,8]. Therefore, fading attenuation through the adoption CP antennas can be an effective technique to enhance performance and competitiveness of range-based methods. Furthermore, it should be underlined that the adoption of CP antennas in WLANs, instead of more standard LP antennas, determines a negligible influence on cost and performance of the wireless communication system.

In this paper, preliminary location accuracy measurements for an RSSI-based location technique are shown, when circularly polarized antennas are used at both the anchors and the mobile node of a WSN, and compared with those obtained when conventional linearly polarized antennas are adopted [9]. Measurements with CP antennas have been performed in the same scenario as that for the measurements with conventional linear polarization antennas.

2 Measurement Set-Up

A ZigBee-based wireless sensor network was set-up to measure RSSI over distance in a typical indoor environment and perform a simple localization task in 1-D. The network is composed of ZigBee boards (EM250 from Ember) and is conceived to have three typologies of nodes: coordinator node, mobile node (MN) and anchor node. The coordinator node is USB-connected to a personal computer and is used to create and hold the network, acquire and process data (a graphical interface developed in C# is used for network management and data saving); the MN periodically send messages to anchors to allow for RSSI measurements at each fixed node. Anchors are placed at fixed and known positions, measure the RSSI value and transmit the recorded value to the coordinator node.

In a preliminary experimental set-up, two anchors were placed tree meters apart and a MN mounted on a straightforward aluminium rail has been remotely moved between anchors. A plastic support mounted on the aluminium rail is used to keep nodes 90 cm above the ground (see Fig. 1).

Two types of antennas have been used, to evaluate advantages of using Circular Polarization (CP) instead of Linear Polarization (LP) in RSSI-based indoor location. Murata antennas (ceramic antennas) embedded in EM250 modules were used as LP antennas, while external patch antennas from Hyperlink Technologies (HG2409PCR) were used as CP antennas. The patch antenna is connected to EM250 by means of an MC-CARD external antenna connector and an MC-CARD-to-12-in-N-FEMALE adaptor cable. When the external patch antenna is connected to the EM250 module via MC-CARD connector, an internal switch automatically excludes native Murata antenna from radio module and only the external antenna can radiate. For both polarization cases, transmitting and receiving antennas face each other along their maximum radiation direction, and are at the same height from the floor (they don't rotate during MN translation).

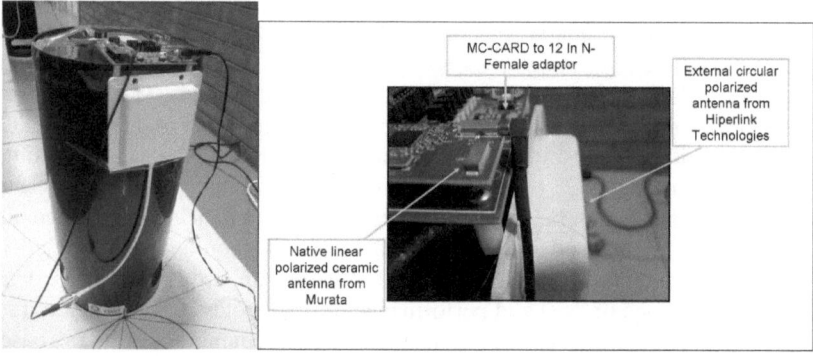

Fig. 1. The plastic support for the wireless node, where the radio module (*on the left*) and both the ceramic and patch antennas (on the *right*) are visible

Measurements were conducted in a repository of ARTS Laboratory. In order to perform RSSI characterization with an adequate spatial resolution, a commercial motion capture system was used, also to guarantee experiment repeatability. A six-camera Vicon 460 system has been installed to capture MN positions. Vicon is a motion capture device based on infrared cameras and IR refractive markers to be attached to the tracked objects. The system is composed of:

1. Six IR digital cameras: cameras are wire connected to Vicon computer workstation, each camera has an autofocus lens (from Sigma) and a ring IR-LED headlight for workspace IR spotting;
2. IR reflective markers: Vicon system can recognize markers thanks to their IR reflectivity and standard dimensions; markers must be attached to the objects for their localization and tracking, and must be visible from at least three cameras simultaneously;

3. An ad-hoc computer station for system calibration, marker tracking, data management and processing;
4. Connection cables and camera/computer interfaces unit for data transfer and cameras power supply.

Stereoscopic vision from at least three cameras is performed to reconstruct 3-D marker location and motion. Every Vicon's camera is on a stable and fixed easel. They spot a piece or the entire workspace in IR bandwidth and illuminate the scene using IR leds. Passive reflective IR markers mounted on monitored objects appear as white spots to the camera. A specific software for marker recognition allows for automatic marker labelling and tracking. A calibration procedure is needed in order to create a common global reference system for all involved cameras and compute the 3-D position of IR markers.

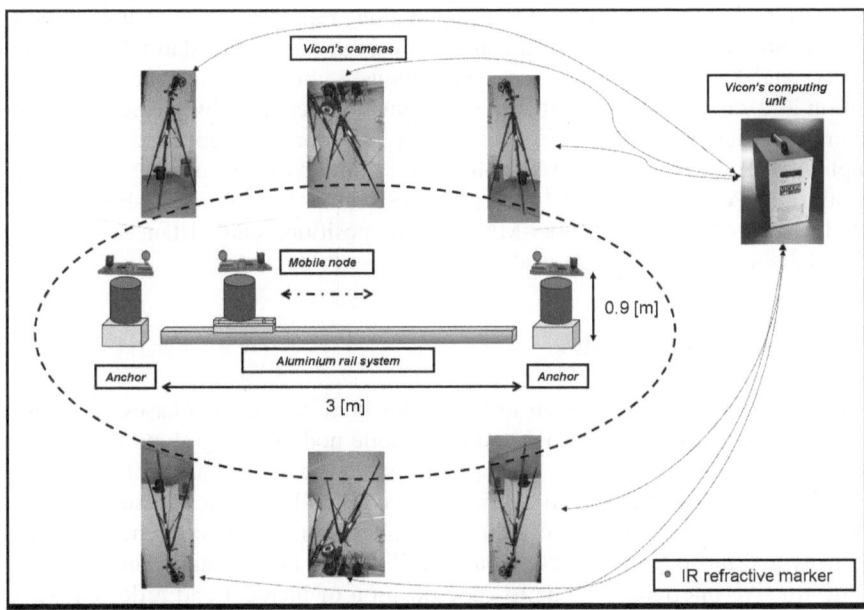

Fig. 2. A schematic description of the whole system made of six IR cameras, two anchors (actually only one has been used to get preliminary results) and a mobile node moving along an aluminium rail

Calibration procedure consists of two steps, a static and a dynamic one:

- Static calibration:
  Static calibration procedure create a prospective projection matrix for each camera to relate camera image reference system coordinate (2-D) with global reference system coordinate (3-D).
- Dynamic calibration:
  Dynamic calibration perform error assessment in IR TAG localization during marker motion along workspace. If large errors occur a new calibration

procedure can be done, otherwise, calibration errors are computed and system is ready for marker tracking task.

After calibration, Vicon is ready for marker localization and tracking. Standard markers are fixed on antennas to reconstruct antenna position and motion during MN translation. When Vicon acquisition procedure starts, 3-D coordinate are continuously recorded on a txt file. At the end of the acquisition, 3-D trajectories are reconstructed and data can be used for further elaborations. Markers can be manually or automatically labelled in 3-D reconstructed vision to distinguish antennas and save relative position coordinates on a txt file. A system accuracy of less than 1 mm can be achieved after calibration procedure. To achieve a satisfactory experiment reliability, the MN was fixed at an aluminium rail and remotely moved by a wire. The MN moved from about 6cm to 275cm from the anchor during the experimental trial, and speed was maintained as constant as possible to get an uniform spatial sampling rate. MN and anchors were fixed to allow only a translation along rail axis, avoiding any rotation.

MN continuously sent data to the anchors during on-rail translation at a frequency of 10Hz and Vicon capture device synchronously computed and recorded IR TAG position at a sampling rate of 100Hz (data position acquired by means of the Vicon system were decimated at a 10 Hz frequency in order to be conformed to the RSSI sampling rate). A mean spatial sampling of 1.2cm has been reached during experimental trials. Post process of the recorded RSSI-values by using Matlab gave us RSSI spatial characterization. Anchors-MN relative positions and distances were reconstructed thanks to Vicon's data, and used as reference data.

3   Experimental Results

Samples of RSSI traces are given in Fig. 3, for both polarization cases, as a function of the distance between an anchor and the mobile node moving along the aluminium rail. For each polarization case, measurements have been repeated 10 times; the ten curves are almost overlapped, so confirming the reliability of the measurement set-up. When LP antennas are used, the fading generated from the interference between the direct ray and those reflected from walls, ceiling and floor is apparent. Constructive and destructive interferences due to superposition of incident and reflected waves in the environment produce relatively high RSSI spatial fluctuations. On the other hand, reduced oscillations can be observed when CP antennas are used, as expected due to the reduced amplitude of the first order reflections with the same CP handedness as that of the direct ray. A higher amplitude of the RSSI values for CP polarization is related to the higher gain of the CP antennas (8dBi instead of the 0dBi of the ceramic LP antennas). Small fluctuations are still present in RSSI traces for CP polarization. Indeed, multipath delayed waves that have undergone single reflection are not always suppressed effectively due to the fact that the antenna axial ratio, AR, is not ideal (AR>0dB), and it changes in the antenna main beam and impedance bandwidth (typical values are AR<2-3dB). Moreover, far from the normal incidence direction the reflection of a CP signal from a wall or ceiling (which are not perfectly conducting surfaces) gives rise to an elliptically polarized signal rather than a CP signal (with reversed handedness). The latter phenomenon is more evident at grazing incidence. Moreover, it must be considered that in indoor environments higher-order reflections are always present. Nevertheless, the use of circular polarization can still be effective, by considering the fact that the channel fading is primarily caused by first-order reflections, and the field amplitude of singly reflected waves is generally much higher than that of higher-order reflection waves.

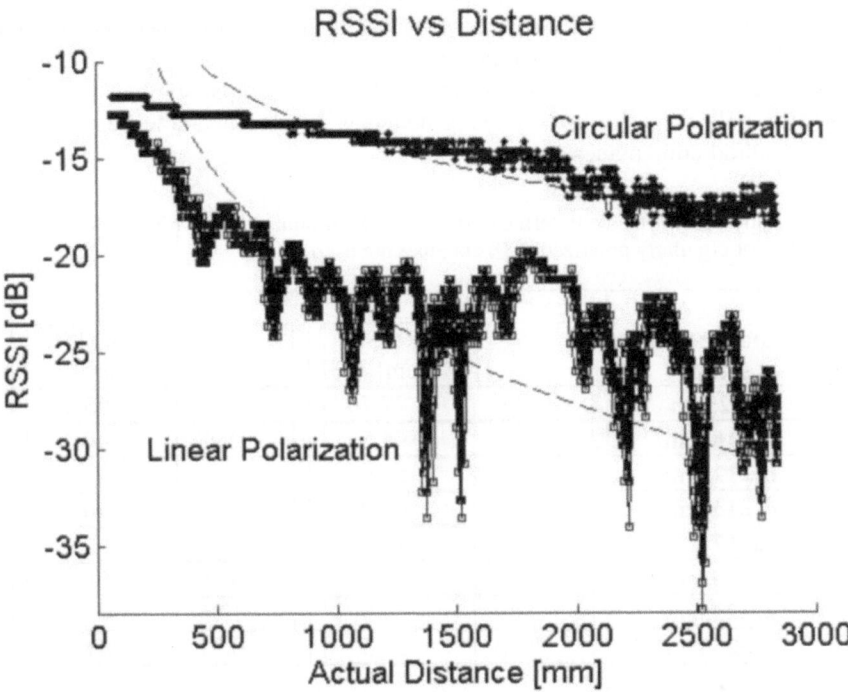

Fig. 3. RSSI as a function of the distance between the mobile node and an anchor, when linearly polarized (LP) or circularly polarized (CP) antennas are used (10 traces for each polarization case). Dashed lines are those obtained by a Hata-like model (see Eq. 1), when d_0=1m and n_p is equal to 1.99 and 0.98, for LP and CP respectively.

The results in Fig. 3 demonstrate that CP could be a useful technique to get a smooth and predictable behaviour of the function RSSI-distance in indoor environments, as required for accurate localization purposes.

As a first tentative to show the effectiveness of CP in improving location accuracy, a standard Hata-like model [10] was implemented to relate measured RSSI and MN-anchor distance:

$$RSSI_{(d)dB} = RSSI_{(0)dB} - 10 \cdot n_p \cdot \log(\frac{d}{d_0}) \ , \tag{1}$$

where n_p is the path loss coefficient (equal to 2 in ideal free-space conditions) and d_0 is a reference distance. For a set of values of the reference distance d_0 (between 25cm and 2.5m), n_p has been chosen to achieve the best fitting between the RSSI Hata-like model and the RSSI measurements. Experimental trials were repeated 10 times using two different antennas configurations.

Localization performance was evaluated by computing the Root Mean Square Error (RMSE) between the estimated distance (using the Hata model) and the actual distance measured by the Vicon system. Numerical results are shown in Table 1. In all experimental trials, n_p values for LP case are always higher than those for the CP case. Minimum localization error (RMSE=40,4cm) is achieved within the CP set-up, by using d_0=1m and n_p=0,98. LP shows worst localization performance because of the higher RSSI spatial fluctuations (see Fig. 3).

Further measurements have been planned, where the comparison between LP and CP antennas will be performed by using antennas with comparable beamwidths in both principal radiation planes.

Table 1. Location performance in terms of the Root Mean Square Error, RMSE, when linearly polarized (LP) or circularly polarized (CP) antennas are used

Experimental setup	LP		CP	
	n_p	RMSE [cm]	n_p	RMSE [cm]
d_0=25cm	1,46	77,7	0,51	65,4
d_0=100cm	1,99	64,5	0,98	40,4
d_0=125cm	2,49	57,6	1,09	42,6
d_0=150cm	3,13	62,9	1,13	46,7
d_0=175cm	3,98	77,5	1,33	60,9
d_0=200cm	3,34	78,7	0,96	43, 7
d_0=225cm	2,69	72,5	1,05	45,4
d_0=250cm	2,90	59,5	0,97	41,2

4   Conclusions

An experimental activity on RSSI measurements in a 2.4 GHz ZigBee-based wireless sensor network has shown that circularly polarized antennas (at both the mobile node and the anchors) can significantly reduce the fading in rich multipath indoor environments. By resorting to a conventional Hata-like model, it has also been shown that the resulting smooth behaviour of the RSSI as a function of the node-distance can guarantee for a better location accuracy when compared to that achievable in the same environment by using linearly polarized antennas. For the measurement set that we considered (linear path with a minimum distance equal to 25cm and maximum distance equal to 250cm), we verified a localization error reduction, going approximately from 60cm to 40cm, when switching from LP to CP. Better location accuracy can be obtained by resorting to advanced RSSI models and increasing the number of anchors, as well as by using data from the accelerometers already available in many commercial radio modules. However, for any network configuration that can be adopted, better performance is expected when CP antennas are used, due to the strong fading reduction that can be achieved.

Future work will be relevant to the extension of this research activity to more complex indoor scenarios and its application to Ambient Assisted Living systems.

Acknowledgment

This work was developed within the ASTROMOBILE experiment project, courteously supported and funded by the ECHORD project.

References

1. Manabe, T., Sato, K., Masuzawa, H., Taira, K., Ihara, T., Kasashima, Y., Yamaki, K.: Polarization dependence of multipath propagation and high-speed transmission characteristics of indoor millimeter-wave channel at 60 GHz. IEEE Trans. on Vehicular Technology 44(2), 268–274 (1995)
2. Rappaport, T.S., Hawbaker, D.A.: Wide-band microwave propagation parameters using circular and linear polarized antennas for indoor wireless channels. IEEE Trans. on Communication 40(2), 240–245 (1992)
3. Huang, X.: Antenna polarization as a complementarities on RSSI Based Location Identification. In: ISWPC 2009, 4th International Symposium on Wireless Pervasive Computing (2009)
4. Potortì, F., Corucci, A., Nepa, P., Furfari, F., Barsocchi, P., Buffi, A.: Accuracy limits of in-room localisation using RSSI. In: IEEE Antennas and Propagation Society International Symposium (APS), Charleston, SC, US (2009)
5. Sathyan, T., Humphrey, D., Hedley, M., Johnson, M.: A wireless indoor localization network-system introduction and trial results. In: International global navigation satellite system society IGNSS Symposium (2009)
6. Bulusu, N., Heidemann, J., Estrin, D.: GPS-Less low cost outdoor localization for very small devices. IEEE Personal Communication Magazine, 7(5), 28–34 (2000)
7. Seco, F., Jimenez, A.R., Prieto, C., Roa, J., Koutsou, K.: A survey of mathematical methods for indoor localization. In: WISP 2009; 6th IEEE Internactional Symposiun on Intelligent Signal Processing (2009)
8. Gezici, S.: A survey on wireless position estimation. Wireless Personal Communication 44(3), 263–282 (2009)
9. Cavallo, F., Aquilano, M., Bonaccorsi, M., Carrozza, M.C., Dario, P.: Preliminary characterization of an indoor localization system using a ZigBee based sensor network and a tri-axial accelerometer. In: AALIANCE Conference, Malaga, Spain, pp. 11–12 (2010)
10. Lymberopoulos, D., Lindsey, Q., Savvides, A.: An Empirical Characterization of Radio Signal Strength Variability in 3-D IEEE 802.15.4 Networks Using Monopole Antennas. In: Romer, K., Karl, H., Mattern, F. (eds.) EWSN 2006. LNCS, vol. 3868, pp. 326–341. Springer, Heidelberg (2006)

Session 8

Mobile Health Technologies, Applications and
Integrated Systems for Chronic Disease
Monitoring and Management

Predictive Metabolic Modeling for Type 1 Diabetes Using Free-Living Data on Mobile Devices

Eleni I. Georga[1,2], Vasilios C. Protopappas[2], and Dimitrios I. Fotiadis[1]

[1] Department of Materials Science and Engineering, University of Ioannina, 45110, Greece
[2] Department of Mechanical Engineering and Aeronautics, University of Patras, 26500, Greece
egeorga@cs.uoi.gr, vprotop@mech.upatras.gr, fotiadis@cc.uoi.gr

Abstract. This study presents a metabolic modeling scheme for glucose prediction of diabetic patients that is intended for use in mobile devices. We investigate the ability to model the multivariate, nonlinear and dynamic interactions in glucose metabolism using free-living data acquired from wearable sensors or inserted through suitable mobile applications. The physiological processes related to diabetes are simulated by compartmental models, which quantify the absorption of subcutaneously administered insulin, the absorption of glucose from the gut following a meal, as well as the effects of exercise on plasma glucose and insulin dynamics. In addition, Support Vector machines for Regression are employed to provide individualized predictions of the subcutaneous glucose concentrations. The proposed scheme is evaluated in terms of its predictive ability using real data recorded from two type 1 diabetic patients. Also, the incorporation of the predictive model in an integrated diabetes monitoring and management system is discussed.

Keywords: glucose prediction, type 1 diabetes, compartmental models and support vector regression.

1 Introduction

Diabetes care has been significantly improved by the development of advanced sensors, mobile devices and information systems that enable the continuous and multi-parametric monitoring and control of the disease. This has also been facilitated by the development of continuous glucose sensing technologies that are available in non- or semi-invasive wearable devices. However, diabetes control further necessitates the monitoring and analysis of all patients' contextual information, such as physical activity and lifestyle. In this direction, data recorded from activity monitoring devices could significantly assist diabetes management systems in the prediction of glucose variations; however, their use remains limited.

An essential component of a diabetes management system concerns the modeling of blood glucose metabolism. Thus, several recent studies have considered advanced data-driven techniques for developing accurate glucose predictive models. The authors in [1], [2] proposed autoregressive models for predicting individual specific glucose concentrations using only the glucose time-series signal. Stahl et al. [3], based

J. Lin and K.S. Nikita (Eds.): MobiHealth 2010, LNICST 55, pp. 187–193, 2011.
© Institute for Computer Sciences, Social Informatics and Telecommunications Engineering 2011

on blood glucose values, food and insulin intake, made an attempt to predict the gly-cemic behavior for the next 2 hours through linear and nonlinear time-series models (i.e. ARMAX and NARMAX). Recently, the effect of free-living data on glucose behavior was taken into consideration [4], [5]. A method based on Wiener models that accurately maps input disturbances concerning food, exercise and stress in blood glucose levels is reported in [4]. Finally, Gaussian Processes were used in [5] in order to model the glucose excursions in response to exercise data.

The aim of this study is to develop and evaluate a predictive metabolic model for type 1 diabetic patients using free-living data. This model will be incorporated in mobile devices as part of the decision support subsystem of an integrated diabetes monitoring and management system, called METABO [6].

2   Materials and Methods

2.1   Materials

The Guardian Real-Time Continuous Glucose Monitoring System (CGMS) (Med-tronic Minimed) is used to record glucose measurements in order to obtain a sufficient fast sampling rate necessary for glucose modeling. The physical activity measure-ments are obtained using the SenseWear Body Monitoring System armband (Body-Media Inc.) which collects data using five sensors: heat flux, skin temperature, near body temperature, galvanic skin response and a two-axis accelerometer. Also, the food ingested the serving sizes and the time of each meal or snack, as well as the type, dose and time of insulin injections are manually notified by the patient. The food composition (i.e. calories, carbohydrates, fat etc.) is post-analyzed by a dietician.

2.2   Methods

The prediction of the dynamic behavior of glucose metabolic process in time as a function of process input parameters can be considered as a regression problem with a time component. In this study a Support Vector machine for Regression (SVR) [7] is employed for the task of subcutaneous (s.c.) glucose time series prediction. The over-all modeling of glucose dynamics is achieved by combining SVR with compartmental models that describe the absorption of subcutaneously-administered insulin and the ingestion of carbohydrates, as well as, the effects of mild to moderate exercise events on plasma glucose and insulin dynamics.

2.3   Subcutaneous Insulin Absorption

The absorption process of subcutaneously injected insulin is described by the pharma-cokinetic model proposed in [8], which covers all the commercially available insulin classes. The evolution of the exogenous insulin flow, I_{ex} (U/min), is given by:

$$I_{ex}(t) = \int_{V_{sc}} B_d c_d(t, r),$$

(1)

where c_d is the dimeric insulin concentration in the subcutaneous tissue, B_d is the absorption rate constant and V_{sc} is the complete subcutaneous volume. The plasma insulin concentration, I_p (uU/ml), after a subcutaneous injection is estimated as:

$$\dot{I}_p = \frac{I_{ex}(t)}{V_d} - k_e I_p(t),$$

(2)

where V_d is the plasma insulin distribution volume and k_e is the rate constant of insulin elimination.

2.4 Carbohydrates Absorption

The model by Lehmann and Deutch [9] is used to describe the time course of glucose appearance in plasma due to food intake. The amount of glucose in the gut, q_{gut}, after the ingestion of a meal containing D grams of glucose-equivalent carbohydrates is defined as:

$$\dot{q}_{gut(t)} = -k_{abs} q_{gut}(t) + G_{empt}(t, D),$$

(3)

where k_{abs} is the rate constant of intestinal absorption and G_{empt} is the gastric emptying function. Then, the rate of appearance of glucose in plasma, Ra (mg/min), is given as:

$$Ra(t) = k_{abs} q_{gut}(t).$$

(4)

2.5 Exercise Effects

The effects of the exercise on plasma glucose and insulin dynamics vary according to the exercise intensity and duration. In particular, the plasma glucose variation, G_{exer} (mg/min), due to exercise events is given by:

$$G_{exer} = \left(G_{prod} - G_{gly}\right) - G_{up},$$

(5)

where G_{up} and G_{prod}, represent the rate (mg/min) of glucose uptake and hepatic glucose production (glycogenolysis) induced by exercise, respectively, while G_{gly} denotes the decrease in the rate of glycogenolysis during prolonged exercise due to the depletion of liver glycogen [10].

Furthermore, the insulin dynamics in (2) are modified as:

$$\dot{I}_p = \frac{I_{ex}(t)}{V_d} - k_e I_p(t) - I_e(t),$$

(6)

where I_e (uU/(ml.min)) is the insulin removal from the circulatory system due to the exercise-induced physiological changes [10].

2.6 Glucose Predictive Model

The prediction of the s.c glucose concentration, y, at the time $t+l$, assuming that t is the current time, is described by:

$$y(t+l) = SVR\left(x_1,\ldots,x_d\right), \tag{7}$$

where $x_i = x_i(t),\ldots,x_i(t-n_i\Delta t)$, with $i=1,\ldots,d$, denotes the inputs in the model, $n_i\Delta t$ is the time lag for the input x_i, Δt is the sampling time and l is the prediction length.

The inputs of the model considered in this study include the plasma insulin concentration, I_p, the rate of glucose appearance in plasma after a meal, Ra, the s.c. glucose measurements, gl, as well as a set of exercise-related variables. In particular, we assume two approaches to investigate the dynamic effect of exercise on glucose variation. In the first approach, the Metabolic Equivalent of Task (*MET*), the heat flux (*hf*) and the skin temperature (*st*) variables, as recorded by the SenseWear armband, are used as inputs in the model. However, in the second approach the output from the exercise compartmental models is used.

2.7 Model Training and Evaluation

The SVR is evaluated using data from two type 1 diabetic patients who were monitored over a period of 5 and 11 days, respectively. The training of the SVR is performed individually for each patient by applying a technique called leave-one-day-out. More specifically, the dataset of each patient is divided into two groups. The first group (i.e. test set) contains the data of ith day, with $i=1,\ldots,k$, where k is the total number of days. The second group (i.e. training set) contains the remaining data. The error is measured by testing the SVR on the data of the ith day. The specific evaluation method is repeated k times and, subsequently, the average of the error is calculated. Considering that the performance of the SVR is affected by the value of parameter C, the evaluation procedure is applied for different values of the specific parameter. The value of the parameter C which produces the lowest average error is selected. Regarding the other parameters of the SVR, a linear kernel is employed and the parameter ε in the insensitive loss function is set equal to 0.001.

Time lags of 30 min are considered for the I_p, R_a and gl. Since it is well-known that the effect of the exercise lasts for several hours, the time lag for the exercise-related inputs (i.e. *MET*, *st*, *hf* and G_{exer}) is assumed to be 3 hours. The sampling time, Δt, was 5 min for all the above cases. Predictions are performed for four different values of prediction length l, i.e. 15, 30, 60 and 120 min.

The prediction performance of the proposed method is assessed by calculating the Root Mean Squared Error, *RMSE*, and the correlation coefficient, estimated by r, for each patient's dataset. The Clarke's Error Grid Analysis (EGA) [11] is used to assess the clinical significance of the differences between the predicted and the measured s.c. glucose concentrations. The Clarke's EGA method uses a Cartesian diagram, in which the values predicted are displayed on the y-axis, whereas the values from glucose sensor are displayed on the x-axis. This diagram is subdivided into 5 zones: A, B, C, D and E which are defined in [11]. Briefly, the values that fall within zones A and B represent sufficiently accurate or acceptable glucose results, whereas the values included in the areas C-E indicate potentially dangerous overestimation or underestimation of the actual values.

3 Results

In Table 1, it can be seen that the glucose response is predicted with sufficiently low *RMSE* in the short-term (i.e. for 15 and 30 min), whereas *RMSE* increases for medium-term predictions (i.e. for 60 and 120 min). An important observation is that either using directly the real sensor data to indicate exercise intensity or the simulation output from the exercise compartmental models, the differences in the *RMSE* and the *r* are relatively small.

Table 1. The *RMSE* and the *r* values obtained for both patients

Physical Activity Input	Prediction Length (min)	r	RMSE (mg/dl)	r	RMSE (mg/dl)
		Patient1		*Patient2*	
Sensor Data	15	0.96	12.57	0.95	9.69
	30	0.90	21.36	0.87	16.32
	60	0.75	33.06	0.68	24.52
	120	0.28	62.29	0.37	31.10
Exercise Modeling	15	0.96	12.069	0.96	9.58
	30	0.91	19.93	0.88	15.91
	60	0.80	30.99	0.69	24.06
	120	0.46	55.43	0.42	31.24

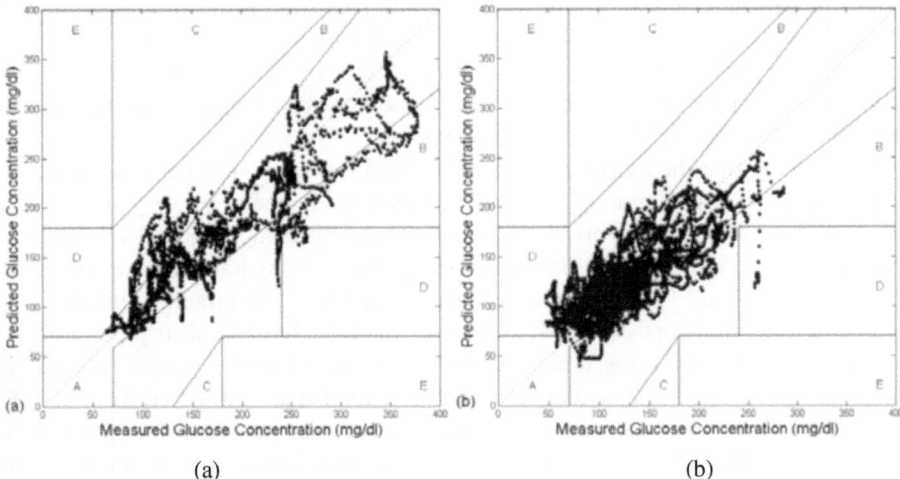

(a)   (b)

Fig. 1. Clarke's-EGA for measured vs predicted s.c. glucose concentrations using sensor data for 60 min prediction length of (a) Patient 1 and (b) Patient 2

The predicted versus measured s.c. glucose concentrations of both patients for one indicative input case are plotted as Clarke's-EGA diagrams in Figs. 1(a) and 1(b), respectively. As shown in Fig. 1, the vast majority of the points for Patient 1 are within zones A (73.84%) and B (24.66%), which indicate clinically acceptable results, whereas a small amount of points (1.5%) are included in zone D. The percentages for Patient 2 are 70.31% for A, 25.78% for B and 3.91% for D. Note that although the predictions for Patient 2 are systematically more accurate than those for Patient 1, more points lie in non-clinically acceptable zones (i.e. D), which was also indicated by the smaller r values for Patient 2.

4 Discussion

A glucose prediction method based on a multi-parametric set of data (i.e. food, insulin, exercise and glucose measurements) was presented. The method employs compartmental analysis and SVR, and was evaluated using a dataset from two type 1 diabetic patients. Training and testing of the SVR was performed individually for each patient by applying a leave-one-day-out technique. The Clarke's-EGA was used to assess the performance of the proposed prediction method from a clinical point of view. The results obtained demonstrate the ability of the method to predict glucose response with a sufficient numerical accuracy and clinical acceptability.

This study makes an innovative use of exercise compartmental models in the sense that (a) feeds the compartmental models with real sensor data to indicate activity intensity and (b) uses the variations in plasma glucose and insulin concentrations induced by exercise as input to predictive modeling. One advantage of exercise compartmental modeling with respect to practical conditions is that even if the patient does not wear the armband continuously, accurate predictions can still be achieved by means of patient's manual notifications for any past exercise events. Similarly, the ability to analyze and predict the effects of exercise on glucose concentrations can be exploited for providing to the patient what-if advice on future hypothetical exercise scenarios. This type of decision support is important for everyday diabetes management and is foreseen in METABO functionalities.

Considering that the dynamics of insulin absorption and intestinal glucose absorption vary significantly among different individuals, it could be very important to estimate the parameters involved in the corresponding compartmental models, individually. Furthermore, we assume that solely the carbohydrates intake affects the glucose metabolism. However, the influence of the fats, the proteins, glucose index and other food nutrients on the dynamics of the digestive and absorptive processes will be also analyzed in the future. In this observational study, patients used a specially designed diary and a dietician analyzed food data. However, in METABO advanced mobile applications and efficient graphical user interfaces have been developed to allow the patient to manually notify of food intake, insulin injections and other information.

When more data will become available from planned observational studies, the validated models will be used in METABO to provide alerts for clinically critical events in both hypoglycemia and hyperglycemia and decision support to assist the patient in the self-management of the disease in daily life.

5 Conclusions

We proposed an innovative modeling methodology which combines compartmental models and SVR for the prediction of glucose concentrations in type 1 diabetic patients. Our future work includes the estimation of the parameters involved in the different compartmental models, as well as the determination of the kernel function and the parameter ε in the insensitive loss function of the SVR. In addition, we will model more individuals to validate the results obtained in this work. The proposed predictive scheme will be incorporated into mobile devices for diabetes management.

Acknowledgments. This work is part funded by the European Union, Project METABO "Controlling Metabolic Diseases Related to Metabolic Disorders", FP7-ICT-2007-1-216270.

References

1. Sparacino, G., Zanderigo, F., Corazza, S., Maran, A., Facchineti, A., Cobelli, C.: Glucose Concentration can be Predicted Ahead in Time from Continuous Glucose Monitoring Sensor Time-Series. IEEE Trans. Biomed. Eng. 54(5), 931–937 (2007)
2. Gani, A., Gribok, A.V., Lu, Y., Ward, W.K., Vigersky, R.A., Reifman, J.: Universal Glucose Models for Predicting Subcutaneous Glucose Concentration in Humans. IEEE Trans. Inform. Tech. Biomed. 14(1), 157–165 (2010)
3. Stahl, F., Johansson, R.: Diabetes mellitus modeling and short-term prediction based on blood glucose measurements. Mathematical Biosciences 217, 101–117 (2008)
4. Rollins, D., Bhandari, N., Kleinedler, J., Kotz, K., Strohbehn, A., Boland, L., Murphy, M., Andre, D., Vyas, N., Welk, G., Franke, W.E.: Free-living inferential modeling of blood glucose level using only noninvasive inputs. J. Process Control. 20(1), 95–107 (2010)
5. Valleta, J.J., Chipperfield, A.J., Byrne, C.D.: Gaussian process modeling of blood glucose response to free-living physical activity data in people with type 1 diabetes. In: 31st Annual International Conference of the IEEE Engineering in Medicine and Biology Society, Minneapolis, pp. 4913–4916 (2009)
6. Georga, E.I., Protopappas, V., Guillen, A., Fico, G., Ardigo, D., Arredondo, M., Exarchos, T., Polyzos, D., Fotiadis, D.I.: Data Mining for Blood Glucose Prediction and Knowledge Discovery in Diabetic Patients: The METABO Diabetes Modeling and Management System. In: 31st Annual International Conference of the IEEE Engineering in Medicine and Biology Society, Minneapolis, pp. 5633–5636 (2009)
7. Smola, A.J., Scholkopf, B.: A tutorial on support vector regression. Statistics and Computing 14, 199–222 (2004)
8. Tarin, C., Teufel, E., Pico, J., Bondia, J., Pfleiderer, H.J.: A Comprehensive Pharmacokinetic Model of Insulin Glargine and Other Insulin Formulations. IEEE Trans. Biomed. Eng. 52(12), 1994–2005 (2005)
9. Lehmann, E.D., Deutsch, T.: A physiological model of glucose-insulin interaction in Type 1 diabetes mellitus. J. Biomed. Eng. 14, 235–242 (1992)
10. Roy, A., Parker, R.S.: Dynamic Modeling of Exercise Effects on Plasma Glucose and Insulin Levels. J. Diabetes Sci. Technol. 1(3), 338–347 (2007)
11. Kovatchev, B.P., Gonder-Frederick, L.A., Cox, D.J., Clarke, W.L.: Evaluating the accuracy of continuous glucose monitoring sensors: Continuous glucose-error grid analysis illustrated by TheraSense Freestyle Navigator data. Diabetes Care 27(8), 1922–1928 (2004)

Architecture for Lifestyle Monitoring Platform in Diabetes Management

A. Martinez[1], W. Ruba[2], A.B. Sánchez[1], M.T. Meneu[1], and V. Traver[1]

[1] ITACA - Health and Wellbeing Technologies, Universidad Politécnica de Valencia,
Valencia, Spain
{anmarmil,absanch,tmeneu,vtraver}@itaca.upv.es
[2] Telemedicine Department of Tromsø University
wru000@post.uit.no

Abstract. Diabetes management has no patterns in the actual health industry. Many models have been presented for monitoring its behavior focusing only in glycemic values and basing patient evolution on diary records. The presented system describes the architecture for fully monitoring diabetes patients through a platform of sensors and a mobile device. Nowadays there is a lack of interoperability standards between sensors and managers, for this, the architecture has been split out into three layers that mask main functionalities and allow adaptation for incoming 11073 standard and certified sensors.

Keywords: Diabetes, eHealth, Sensors, 11073.

1 Introduction

Information from WHO (World Health Organization) reveals the alarming rise in the number of population affected by any type of diabetes mellitus. The fact sheet [1] indicates that in 1985 there were around 30 million people with some type of this metabolic disorder. In 2000, this number increased to 171 million and predictions point that it will reach 366 million people in 2030, drawing this disease as an epidemic.

Nevertheless, some authors have considered the direct cost of diabetes mellitus in Spain oscillating between 2,400 and 2,675 million Euros per year [2]. Hospitalization expenses and the cost of other drug different from insulin figure as the heaviest batches. These studies show the importance of investing in prevention and also affirm the huge cost for managing associated diabetes complications, which can be avoided keeping a good control of the disease [3].

As a matter of fact, rising both micro/nano mobile computing technologies and biomedical sensors development open a wide spectrum for monitoring complex diseases such as diabetes mellitus. Literature has several proposals in this line [4] [5], reporting evidences for improvements in glycemic values.

Diabetes patients are expected to register the results of blood sugar and insulin intake in a notebook diary, which is shown to the specialist each appointment. Compliance and diligence on completing this basic information to the caregiver is variable and erratic. Large data collections would allow physicians to improve their diagnosis and treatment set-up.

J. Lin and K.S. Nikita (Eds.): MobiHealth 2010, LNICST 55, pp. 194–200, 2011.

Healthcare industry is progressively focusing on putting standards for a new era of m-health and e-health systems. But till nowadays it is still missing the real implementation of a full-standardized system. Nonetheless there are many companies working together [8] to overcome this hurdle for the development; but so far only "AND" and Nonin companies offer certified devices compliant with 11073 standard.

This paper presents two monitoring strategies for diabetes patients. On the one hand, it describes the Application Hosting Device (AHD) of the patient station that manages the sensor platform and allows sending IHE-PDC messages that will be compliant with Continua Health Alliance [8] at a WAN level. On the other hand, it also describes a mobile application for monitoring patient lifestyle.

The whole system provides a metabolic profile that integrates information were other systems do not provide. The patient application gathers multiple physiological data from the sensors, for instance, blood pressure, level and duration of performed physical activity, weight, height, consumed energy, values of glucose as well as insulin bolus. In addition patient lifestyle information is recorded in a mobile device.

Evaluation results regarding usability and improvement on the diabetes management will be gathered by two pilots in different focus groups in Spain (Madrid) and Italy (Parma).

2 Methods

The principal purpose was to create a system that gives the opportunity for both the patient and also to physician to check the current status of the disease and its evolution.

The applied methodology that has been used is goal-oriented and carried out in five different stages described below:

2.1 Research Phase

At the beginning of this phase interviews with the different actors involved in the system have been carried out: endocrinology specialized physicians and diabetic patients.

Afterwards, a state of art regarding the selection of sensors used in the system has been made; Chosen sensors are based on the following requirements:

- Fulfillment of European Union regulation.
- Available Application Programming Interface(API)/SDK (Software Development Kit)/Controls
- To be intuitive and user friendly handling.
- Provide data output/interface

The sensors must provide data regarding glycemic values, blood pressure, weight and performed physical activity.

2.2 Modeling Phase

Different types of information acquired from several data sources must be stored in a homogeneous database. The system core must contain the database and the Patient Mobile Device (PMD) should work as a data collector.

The system is classified into three interconnected subsystems:

1. Tablet/UMPC PMD.
2. PDA PMD.
3. Central Server Unit (CSU).

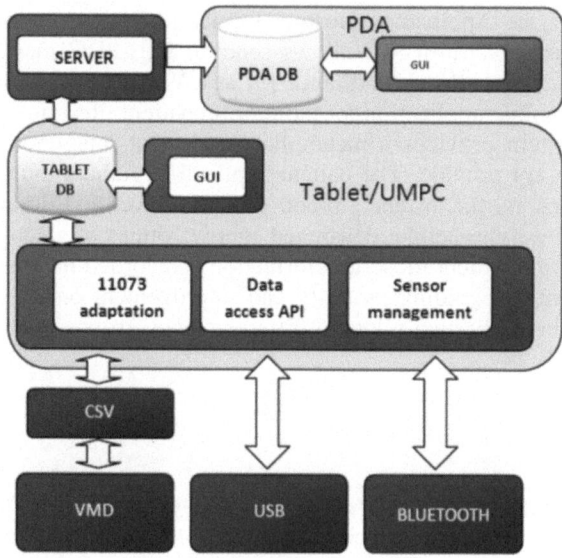

Fig. 1. Stack overview

Tablet/UMPC PMD hosts the subsystem to acknowledge data from medical sensors. PDA PMD subsystem has been modeled as set of forms and questionnaires where the patient will be able to register daily information related to his lifestyle and evolution of the disease. Central Server Unit behaves as a data assembler and service provider. Figure 1 shows the basic structure of the whole system and the access point of each module to its correspondent module.

Regarding the proposed Tablet/UMPC subsystem, an architecture of three modules has been constructed to isolate different functionalities related to Data Access Layer (DAL) and Business Layer (BL). These three modules are 11073 adaptation, Data Access API and Sensor Management.

BL lies into the Sensor Management module. Here, constants and methods are defined for setting up the communication interface over Virtual Medical Device (VMD), USB and Bluetooth physical layer.

Once the sensor has been recognized by the Sensor Management module, Data Access API module retrieves information such measurements and configuration parameters from the device. This module is the layer that masks the methods, protocols and indispensable commands to carry on data exchange between sensors and the system.

After insuring that the data has been received properly, invalid values are discarded and filtered before being stored in the database locally into the Data Storage Unit (DSU) named Tablet DB. Thus, values can be shown as feedback for the patient using graphs and been transferred to the CSU using web services whenever internet connection is available through x73 WAN messages.

11073 adaptation module was designed to encapsulate stored data into x73 WAN messages compliant to Continua Guidelines v1.5 that may be sent to the upper layer in the CSU.

2.3 Requirements Phase

Due to the limitations found during research phase and explained in Results chapter, it has been mandatory to add a Tablet/UMPC device to the architecture to host the module that enables collecting data from the sensors.

The portable device persists in the system because it is the simplest way the user can introduce real-time notifications regarding insulin intake, food ingestion as well as, the daily life events related to the diabetes.

2.4 Development Phase

Both resident tool in the portable device [Compact Edition] and the application that works on the Tablet/UMPC, has been developed using Visual Studio 2008 environment with C# and Framework 3.5, since it provides Web Service support and easy access to Windows Operative System resources. In addition, SQLServer 2008 has been selected for data base engine.

Design and performance for GUI elements have been developed using Photoshop CS4.

2.5 Evaluation of the Test

Two pilots still taking place in Spain and Italy to tests the system. The idea is to have an individual diagnosis of a group of selected patients before the finalization of the implementation of the system. These pilot experiences will help to obtain valuable results and adapt the platform to patient and professional needs.

An in-depth interview is carried out to acknowledge the opinion of a focus group; the procedure will consist of a set of open interviews before, during and after the test of the system.

The technique consists of a semi-structured open interview subject that may not necessarily follow a previously set sequence. The sequence will be determined by the response of the patient interviewed. This methodology focuses over the speech analysis, and will address also usability questions.

In the theoretical sampling the number of studied cases will not affect as the potential of each case, to help in the development of theoretical understandings about the study area. After completing interviews with volunteers, the sample will be diversified depending on the type of people interviewed to cover the entire range of perspectives of people in which we are interested.

3 Results

After the research phase, it has been possible to state that the implantation of standard 11073 has not become general in the commercial sensors. In addition, most of the manufacturers are reluctant to share any API or SDK for third party purpose.

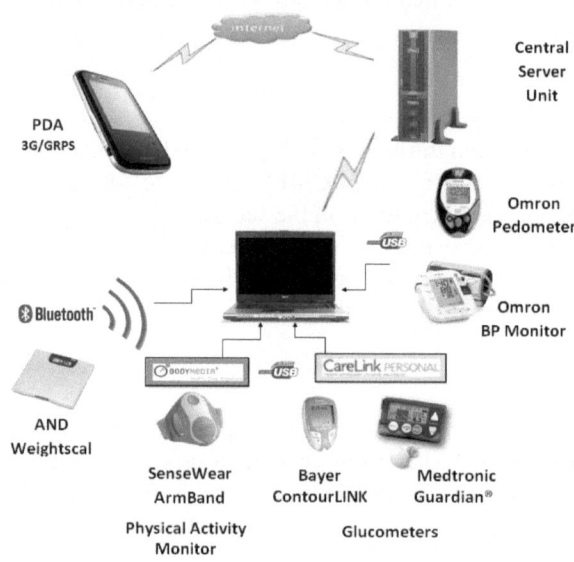

Fig. 2. System overview

Bluetooth interface is available in a quite large number of sensors and PMDs (PDA, Tablet/UMPC) but they may use different Bluetooth stacks depending on the manufacturer. Also to this, most of evaluated PDAs do not support USB hosting, an indispensable capability to enable communication interface of USB sensors.

Figure 2 shows an overview of the complete system.

The sensors of the system are shown in table 1.They have been classified according to their interface to data:

Table 1. Sensors of the System

Sensor	Group
Medtronic Guardian CGMS- Continuous Glycemia Monitoring System	2
Bayer Contour-Link Glucometer	2
SenseWear ArmBand – Physical Activity Sensor	2
OMRON HJ-720IT Pedometer	1
OMRON MT-10T Blood pressure	1
AANDD Weight Scale	3

Group 1: USB-HID access

Communication protocol of the sensor is deployed by a software module that uploads the collection of measurements using USB connection between the device and the Tablet/UMPC. These devices behave as Human Interface Device, a generic group of USB family.

Group 2: VMD access

Virtual Medical Devices (VDM) are devices than cannot be reached directly either through USB and Bluetooth Interface. Through manufacturers own driver, data is exported in a CSV (Comma Separed Value) file. This file is parsed by the VMD software module and measurements are ready for processing.

Group 3: Bluetooth access

Using Bluetooth hardware access libraries, such 32feet, the communication protocol of the sensor is deployed. Then, the measurements are acknowledged by the application.

PDA PMD subsystem consists of a structure of forms based con custom User Controls performed for this purpose. The patient will be capable to register:

- Physical Activity events, describing the activity carried out, the level and the duration.
- Food intake events, specifying the menu and CHO quantities.
- Blood pressure, weight and glycemia measurements manually.
- Medication intakes such insulin and other drugs.
- Special events such stress at work, holiday and birthday party.

These records are gathered in a Diary application that allows seeing all-day events sorted by date.

```
- <MESSAGE>
 <Packet="[..]OBX|3||150020^MDC_PRESS_BLD_NONI
NV^MDC|1.0.1|||||||X|||20100426170613+0000
OBX|4|NM|150021^MDC_PRESS_BLD_NONINV_SYS^MD
C|1.0.1.1|123|266016^MDC_DIM_MMHG^MDC||||||R
OBX|5|NM|150022^MDC_PRESS_BLD_NONINV_DIA^MD
C|1.0.1.2|85|266016^MDC_DIM_MMHG^MDC||||||R
OBX|6|NM|149546^MDC_PULS_RATE_NON_INV^MDC|1.
0.0.1|55|264864^MDC_DIM_BEAT_PER_MIN^MDC||||||R
|||20100426170613+0000" />
 </MESSAGE>
```

Fig. 3. BP Encapsulated Message Sample

Data which comes from the sensors it's gathered and stored for reviewing whenever patient or doctor wants to do it. Also it gives the possibility of introducing commentaries and sending the report to the physician.

Measurements are encapsulated on x73 WAN messages according to Continua Guidelines v1.5. In figure 3 an example of a blood pressure message is shown.

This schema is based on HL7 v2.6 Unsolicited Observation Result and IHE-PCD public standard.

4 Discussion and Conclusion

The work presented in this paper shows the first approach for diabetes monitoring system split out in modules. Each of these modules may be replaced as technology and the implantation of standards and interoperability rules takes over in health care industry. The new generation of healthcare systems must be based on user-transparent platforms and Machine to machine protocols (M2M), and also provide a continuous stream of data from patient squeezing ICT possibilities. Healthcare sensors interfaces to transmit data and manufacturers policy regarding the communications protocols have been two of the mos important limitations for the realization of this study.

Acknowledgement

The current diabetes monitoring system is part of METABO Project (Personal Health Systems for Monitoring and Point-of-Care Diagnostics – Personalised Monitoring) an EU-funded VII Framework ICT Project. Authors wish to appreciate the METABO consortium for their valuable contribution to this work.

References

1. World Health ORganization Fact Sheets,
   http://www.who.int/diabetes/facts/world_figures/en/
   (last access: April 2010)
2. May, P., Ehrlich, H.C., Steinke, T.: ZIB Structure Prediction Pipeline: Composing a Complex Biological Workflow through Web Services. In: Nagel, W.E., Walter, W.V., Lehner, W. (eds.) Euro-Par 2006. LNCS, vol. 4128, pp. 1148–1158. Springer, Heidelberg (2006)
3. Koro, C.E., Bowlin, S.J., Bourgeois, N., Fedder, D.O.: Glycemic Control From 1988 to 2000 Among U.S. Adults Diagnosed With Type 2 Diabetes. Diabetes Care 27, 17–20 (2004)
4. Gómez, E.J., Hernando, M.E., et al.: The INCA System: A Further Step Towards a Telemedical Artificial Pancreas. IEEE Transactions on ITB (470-479), 1089–7771 (2008)
5. Gómez, E.J., Hernando, M.E., Garcia, A., del Pozo, F., Corcoy, R., Brugués, E., Cermeño, J., de Leiva, A.: Telemedicine as a tool for intensive management of diabetes: the DIABTel experience. Computer Methods and Programming in Biomedicine 69, 163–177 (2002)
6. Continua Health Alliance site, http://www.continuaalliance.org/home/ (last access: April 2010)

CLAP: Cross-Layer Protocols for Phealth

Pantelis Angelidis[1,2]

[1] MIT Media Lab
[2] University of W. Macedonia, Greece
pantelis@media.mit.edu

Abstract. We present a low cost, low power, backbone free quality of life monitoring solution, suitable for rural areas of countries under development. CLAP is an MIT/VIDAVO initiative that we envision as a turnaround approach on the way health and quality of life in these areas of the world are being addressed.

Keywords: Rural health, Wireless Sensor Networks (WSNs), Personalised Health (pHealth), ad-hoc networks, energy constrained networks.

1 Introduction

Wireless Sensor Networks (WSN) have emerged recently as a new networking environment that provides end users with intelligence and a better understanding and interaction with the environment. For instance, a WSN of wearable wireless vital sign sensors (including electrocardiogram, blood pressure, etc.) and mobile wireless display devices can be employed to monitor patient health in an outpatient environment (e.g. home or care center).This is one application of a research discipline is known as phealth.

Personalised Healthcare (phealth) is a collective term aiming to reflect all modes of patient-centric healthcare delivery via advanced technology means. Personalized health involves the utilization of micro and nanotechnology advances, molecular biology, implantable sensors, textile innovations and information & communication technology (ICT) to create individualized monitoring and treatment plans. pHealth proactively endorses the sense of "one-to-one" communication to elevate healthcare delivery, optimize patient services and ensure seamless from the patient point of view information exchange.

Recent developments in ICT technologies have enabled the creation of electronic communities of educated users in technologically poor or even virgin environments. Such examples may be found in initiatives like OLPC [1] or Moca [2]. Health status on the other hand, together with education, represent the two major challenges for those parts of the developing world that have found (even partial) solutions on drinkable water and nutrition. An interconnected community (even with limited or low-quality access to a backbone network) has the means to support activities aiming at facilitating disease management and health status control within a larger (to the community) population (e.g. a village or a number of adjacent ones). Such activities may include the implementation of pHealth scenarios in which a WSN-like infrastructure supports monitoring, processing and transmitting of personal, ambient and environmental parameters.

J. Lin and K.S. Nikita (Eds.): MobiHealth 2010, LNICST 55, pp. 201–208, 2011.
© Institute for Computer Sciences, Social Informatics and Telecommunications Engineering 2011

Today's pHealth systems assume a technology advanced environment. Mitigating it to the developing world reality should take into account power consumption, network bandwidth and processing limitations. On top of that the community oriented health monitoring is a novel concept, that, to the best of our knowledge, we introduce it here for the first time.

2 Application Framework

Our conceptualized framework consists of four interacting clouds. Wireless sensor networks collect data monitoring QoL parameters, like the environment (water, soil, air, volcano), vital signs, health related human receptors, behavioral patterns. This is referred as cloud A. In this cloud, sensors are deployed in crucial parts of the rural areas, that could range from river banks, geographically challenging parts (for example; hilly areas), schools, gathering places, homes, down to individuals. The sensor networks could collect various critical data (e.g., level of water in the rivers which could help for flood warning, earthquakes etc.) and send them to gateways (sinks is a term widely found in WSN literature as well) referred as cloud B.

Usually each of the villages or rural areas has at least one cloud B installation. A cloud B acts as a store & forward facility for the acquired data. In addition to the data collected by the wireless sensor networks, a cloud B may support the collection of other useful data like demographic data, health care information (for example, swine flu reported cases in the rural areas of Mexico), agricultural information, etc. that could be manually or semi-automatically entered. Different solutions have been proposed in the literature to implement cloud B functionality, ranging from kiosk/truck [3], to satellite stations [1], to mobile phones [4]. **In our framework a cloud B is implemented by networked communities that pre-exist for some other reason or are formed for this particular case.** Examples of such network communities may be found in a OLPC equipped village, a mobile phones carrying community or a hospital on wheels, a vehicle mounted medical facility with wireless access functionality. A cloud B may move around the rural areas and serve many cloud A implementations or may be attached to only one and collect data only from them. As conceptualized here **cloud B is a distributed self-organised collect, store & forward facility.** One implementation approach to materialize a cloud B is to form wireless ad hoc networks based on PCs (or laptops as a matter of fact). Another approach is to form an NFC network based on mobile phones. A third one would be a tagging network based on RFID and spinners [5]. Independent of the implementation approach any cloud B is able to:

    a)   Collect data from cloud A installations
    b)   Store this data and (optionally) additional
    c)   (optionally) process all this data
    d)   Communicate data to the outer world

Data communication from a cloud B to the outer world is performed by facilities referred as cloud C. The major task of a cloud C implementation is to ensure reliable acquisition and delivery of data from the rural areas to a centrally located center referred as cloud D. A cloud C facility is capable of (wirelessly) communicating data acting as a repeater or router. It may additionally have capabilities for incoming data to be stored temporarily and/or processed. Examples of cloud C implementations may range from very simple solutions of one single PDA carried by a mailman or a drinking water distributor, to more complex facilities of satellite-linked equipment or vehicle mounted communication amenities.

A cloud D collects (processed or raw) data from cloud B installations communicated through the corresponding cloud C facilities. A cloud D would combine this data with data from other cloud A data and past records for a particular rural area or a number of selected areas and supply it to a referral center (which could also combine decision and action government powers). In this way, the government gets the timely and processed data from the rural areas and decides on the necessary actions accordingly. This data not only helps the government provide various services to rural areas and make educative strategic decisions and planning (as for example by monitoring behavioral patterns and socio-economic indicators), but could also help in emergency situations as well as for prevention (among the many examples one could think, virus spread, typhoon creation and floods give a sample that speaks for itself).

3   Network Formation Algorithm

We describe a sensor network formation algorithm to exploit the application environment in the framework presented previously. The sensing nodes (we will refer to them as motes in this paper) form Cloud A. The network is formed in four phases with the aid of an existing peer-to-peer WMN (Cloud B). The four phases are summarized in Table 1.

3.1   Phase 1: Assumptions and IEEE 802.15.4 Parameters

Motes self-organize themselves according to IEEE 802.15.4; self-organization implies that all motes have the status of an FFD [6]. In our application scenario an ad-hod clustered-tree multihop topology is supported [7]. Cluster heads and network coordination is assumed by Cloud B nodes. This results in higher energy efficiency and longer lifetime for Cloud A. A beacon mode with a superframe is used.

Parent and child roles are interchangeable. A child to mote X at some instance may become a parent to mote X. This is the result of changes in network topology as nodes of Cloud B enter, leave or move in respect to Cloud A. The phase 1 route formation of Cloud A (IEEE 802.15.4 Cluster - tree) is stored as the default status in every mote. Information regarding children and the parent is stored on the motes to be utilized by "upper layers".

3.2   Phases 2-4: Operation Phases

Once Phase 1 is completed and Cloud A is set to normal operation, Cloud B nodes will associate themselves with that network as sinks. In phases 2-4 of operation, where at least one node is associated with the network we witness the following types of motes at a given instance:

- Hop 0 motes: motes with a neighbor node
- Childless motes: motes without any children; all phase 1 sink motes and all phase 1 childless motes that are not hop 0 motes and only these fall in this category

- Parent/ child motes: motes that have both a parent mote and one or more child motes.

Each mote maintains a look up table of available nodes (nodes in range). As nodes advertise their presence (or leave) the lookup table is updated. The node that serves as a parent to a mote is not part of the table. Whenever more than one nodes are available the look up table contains the Presence Entry information of all of them except the parent node.

3.3 Presence Information

Each node advertises itself as a sink to Cloud A. This is achieved by having each node broadcast a Presence Entry. All motes that receive the Entry and do not have a one-hop relation to another node set the advertising node as their sink. Motes that already have a one-hop relation with a node ignore the invitation In this case the network topology does not change in the child tree branches of these motes.

The motes that decide to accept the node as a cluster head, become hop 0 motes for this cluster. The first node that arrives in the proximity of Cloud A assumes the role of the coordinator of Cloud A (figure 1). All subsequent nodes will form independent clusters. The coordinator could act as a Cloud C gateway as well; other nodes may also act as gateways, that may act as cluster heads or not. The coordinator role may be transferred between nodes.

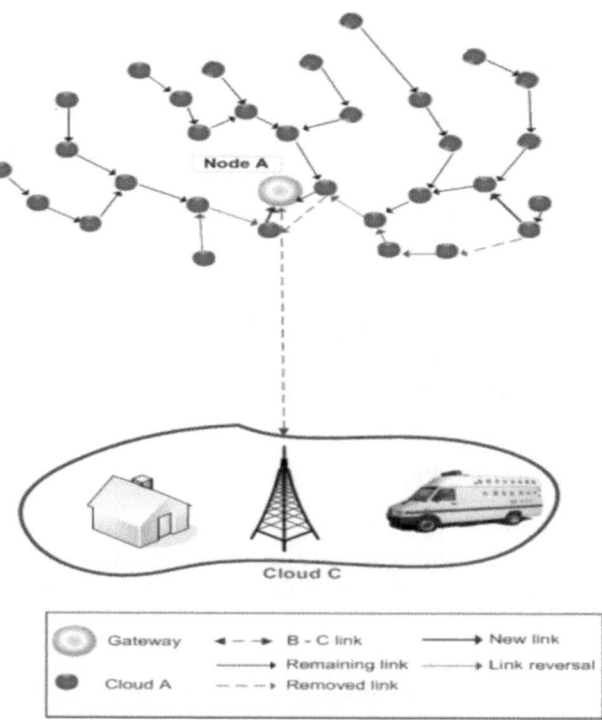

Fig. 1. Phase 2; Network in its infancy

3.4 Clustering

Nodes broadcast Presence Entries as they move. When a mote establishes a direct connection with a node, it informs its neighbors; for this purpose it transmits a Presence Entry itself. In case any of these motes has a 2 or higher hop distance, they transverse their traffic to the mote in question. It may be that the parent of this mote will now become its child (figure 2). In general, whenever a node sends a Presence Entry the following changes in the routing path may occur (in all cases motes disassociate from their past parent node and associate with the new one):

a. Cloud A links broke for the motes that connect directly to the node.
b. Cloud A links reverse for the parent motes that decide to use a (new) route to case a motes.
c. New cloud A links are formed; for each link formed one link disappears.

Motes propagate backwards the new routing status. When any of the above changes occurs a new clustered tree network topology is formed.

4 Discussion

Various routing algorithms have been proposed for WSNs [8]. Among them the Minimum Energy Routing and the Minimum Hop Routing suffer from different inefficiencies, the main ones are that they deplete energy in certain frequently used routes and create congestion. Our assumption is that in our application scenarios all motes are equally important and share the same (energy and storage) characteristics.

Homogeneous approaches are closer to our needs. These mostly work by applying a probabilistic choice of the route to use (or the mote to send the next packet) over a set of routes or motes calculated or determined as of least power consumption or over minimizing a metric like residual battery life. All such approaches consider the network as a general purpose network. WSNs however usually do not fit into that rule; they tend to be application dependent, (almost) unidirectional and of predictable rate and thus data flow. In other words, WSNs tend to be (almost) deterministic, as opposed to general purpose (wireless) nets. This is particularly true for medical WSN application, where each measurement is usually equally (critically) important, but information regarding data type and flow is predictable to a high degree.

Application - based protocol design has been studied mostly for the case of cooperation schemes where measurements are inter-correlated and thus redundancy exist [9]. Our scenarios focus on independent measurements. The uncertainty in our case is "controlled" by the (moving) nodes of Cloud B. So at every transmission instance the mote (of Cloud A) has to find the shortest path to the Cloud B, i.e. to the "closest" node of it.

We define presence as a new way of routing. This approach has recently been demonstrated successfully in a mobile peer-to-peer network setting [10]. Presence information identifies a node or a mote in terms of its participation in a route (tree) in a sensor network.

However, our problem is different from the one in there in various terms:

- Only (cloud B) nodes are mobile
- Only (cloud A) nodes transmit genuine information (nodes only retransmit)

- Broadcasting is not required (at least for data transmission)
- State information about a node or a mote does not contain application or user information; rather the status and it contains type.

Thus, our solution focuses on exploiting the collaboration of the two networks, achieving lower network formation traffic.

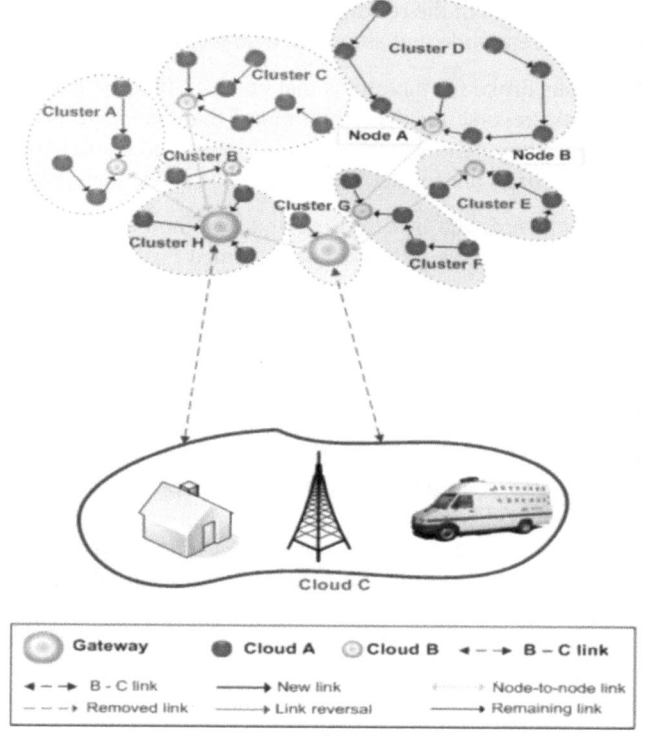

Fig. 2. Phase 3&4; Structured Network and maturity

Another routing algorithm that resembles ours is Low-energy adaptive clustering hierarchy (LEACH) [11]. LEACH adopts a hierarchical approach to organize the network into a set of clusters. Each cluster is managed by a selected cluster head. Simulation results show that LEACH achieves significant energy savings. However, this is only achieved if certain assumptions are valid; these assumptions may evolve to become shortcomings. For example, the assumption that all nodes can reach the base station in one hop may not be realistic, and the length of the steady-state period which is critical to achieving the energy savings may not be suitable for particular applications. Our protocol overcomes these shortcomings by introducing application layer information in the decisions. For example, the rotation of cluster heads appearing in LEACH in order not to exhaust specific motes is irrelevant to us, as the Cloud B nodes are exploited. Furthermore, the steady state period is irrelevant of the protocol and is only dependent on the application features. Finally the cluster tree topology adopted is a direct expansion of the LEACH protocol. Note, that in a simplified case, where enough nodes exist to cover the network area of Cloud A fully, i.e. so as all motes become hop 0 motes, then our protocol operates as a static LEACH network, which is known to have superior energy savings compared to other existing WSN MAC approaches [12].

The network formation protocol described here resembles also design and performance issues of cluster interconnection for beacon-enabled 802.15.4 clusters. Our approach, in which the cluster coordinator is used to bridge clusters is known to be superior in terms of traffic and efficiency and have the drawback that it becomes a single point of failure and a target for security attacks [7]. However, we overcome this drawback by introducing the Cloud B cluster heading instead of a single Cloud A mote. To the best of our knowledge, this is an improvement appearing here for the first time in literature.

5 Conclusion

Costs and effort required for deploying and maintaining a medical sensor network in a rural undeveloped area, have to be justified. There must be a demonstrable and quantified benefit for all participants involved. Quantification examples range from minimizing the required personnel to operate a system, or the required (technological) literacy, to improving the accuracy of an information retrieval service, not to mention realizing a function that would not be possible using other available technology. A wireless sensor network can only be helpful if there is a substantial need.

Therefore, many of successful developed countries applications (e.g. smart aeration and lighting control in apartments, extensive traffic monitoring in large urban areas, or supply-chain monitoring) are ruled out because they lack a broad need in developing countries. A requirements analysis is necessary, albeit a localized one as what is in need in an area may not be the case in another one.

Nonetheless, wireless sensor devices turn out to have a well-suited potential for many application areas in less developed countries. Because of their self-organising characteristics and robustness, wireless sensor networks can be deployed in less benign environments and inaccessible places as well as in places where employing humans is difficult or costly. Although back-end communication infrastructures are needed to interface wireless sensor networks with the Internet or a local area network, they can also function in the absence of any communication infrastructures. This makes them particularly attractive for developing countries where the presence of stable communication infrastructures as a prerequisite for deploying computing systems may not be feasible.

Today, a wireless sensor network is almost the only ICT means we have that can operate independent of any external communication infrastructure or/and electricity network. The CLAP initial results show promising potential in this area. In the near future we are planning a pilot roll-out of the system in a developing country to test it in an actual setting. Different possible candidates are currently being reviewed, many of which are OLPC villages.

Acknowledgements

This work is supported by the EC via grant agreement FP7-234995 -CLAP. Consultation and support from Polychronis Ypodimatopoulos, Michalis Bletsas and Andrew Lippman, all with MIT Media Lab made this work possible.

References

1. http://www.laptop.org
2. http://mocamobile.org/
3. Pathan, A.-S.K., Hong, C.S., Lee, H.-W.: Smartening the environment using wireless sensor networks in a developing country. In: Proc. IEEE International Workshop on Advanced Communication Technology (ICACT 2006), pp. 705–709 (February 2006)
4. Angelidis, P.: Uptake of pHealth: has the time come to become a commodity? In: phealth 2007, June 22 (2007)
5. Malinowski, M., Moskwa, M., Feldmeier, M., Laibowitz, M., Paradiso, J.A.: CargoNet: A Low-Cost MicroPower Sensor Node Exploiting Quasi-Passive Wakeup for Adaptive Asychronous Monitoring of Exceptional Events. In: Proceedings of the 5th ACM Conference on Embedded Networked Sensor Systems (SenSys 2007), Sydney, Australia, November 6-9 (2007)
6. Xiao, Y., Pan, Y. (eds.): Emerging Wireless LANs, Wireless PANs and Wireless MANs. Wiley, Chichester (2008)
7. Misic, J., Udayshankar, R.: Cluster Interconnection in 802.15.4 Beacon-Enabled Networks. In: Boukerche, A. (ed.) Algorithms and Protocols for Wireless, Mobile Ad Hoc Networks. John Wiley & Sons, Chichester (2009)
8. Akyildiz, I.F., Su, W., Sankarasubramaniam, Y., Cayirci, E.: A survey on sensor networks. IEEE Communications Magazine 40, 102–114 (2002)
9. Radeke, R., et al.: On Reconfiguration in Case of Node Mobility in Clustered Wireless Sensor Networks. IEEE Wireless Communications, 47–51 (December 2008)
10. Polychronis Panagiotis Ypodimatopoulos, Cerebro: Forming Parallel Internets and Enabling Ultra-Local Economies, Master of Science in Media Arts and Sciences at the MIT (August 2008)
11. Heinzelman, W.R., Chandrakasan, A., Balakrishnan, H.: Energy-Efficient Communication Protocol for Wireless Microsensor Networks. In: IEEE Proc. Hawaii Int'l. Conf. Sys. Sci., pp. 1–10 (January 2000)
12. Sohraby, K., Minoli, D., Znati, T.: Wireless Sensor Networks: Technology, Protocols, and Applications. John Wiley & Sons, Chichester (2007)

Session 9

Emergency and Disaster Applications

Future Care Floor: A Sensitive Floor for Movement Monitoring and Fall Detection in Home Environments

Lars Klack, Christian Möllering, Martina Ziefle, and Thomas Schmitz-Rode

Human Technology Centre, RWTH Aachen University,
Theaterplatz 14, 52062 Aachen, Germany
{Klack,moellering,ziefle}@humtec.rwth-aachen.de,
smiro@hia.rwth-aachen.de

Abstract. This paper describes the conceptualization and realization of a sensor floor, which can be integrated in home environments to assist old and frail persons living independently at home. Its purpose is to monitor the inhabitant's position within a room, to detect (abnormal) behavioral patterns as well as to activate rescue procedures in case of fall or other emergency events. This floor is part of a living lab ("The Future Care Lab") developed and built within the eHealth project at RWTH Aachen University. The lab, which is part of the European Network of Living Labs (ENoLL), serves as a test environment for user centered design of Ambient Assisted Living (AAL) technologies.

Keywords: sensor floor, position monitoring, fall detection, pattern recognition, living lab.

1 Motivation

In order to minimize daily life health risks for old and frail people and to increase the independency and mobility of an aging society, new concepts for unobtrusive health monitoring within home environments are needed. Implementation and integration of medical technology in living spaces require a new conceptualization of medical device design. Invisibility and unobtrusiveness of technical components combined with high technical reliability have to be major aspects to be respected within the guidelines for the design of future health monitoring devices. In addition to technical features, technology at home also needs to be architectonically integrated in the personal living space and should not change the character of a comfortable and cozy home, respecting individual requirements for intimacy and privacy. For a successful scenario in which both patients and health care institutions profit from home care solutions the technology has to be unobtrusive, affordable and reliable. The Patient has to be and feel as save as in a hospital combined with the comfort and the privacy of his normal home environment.

Many vital parameters like body temperature, weight or blood pressure can be monitored within such an environment [15] but especially the prevention and recognition of falls are important for the elderly. 30% of the persons older than 65 and 50% of the persons older than 80 years suffer from a downfall every year [26]. 20-30% of those downfalls lead to severe injuries [2, 6]. In many cases old people live alone, are

J. Lin and K.S. Nikita (Eds.): MobiHealth 2010, LNICST 55, pp. 211–218, 2011.

not able to call help after a fall and are sometimes not being found for days [4]. The long-term consequences of downfalls are even more dramatic: functional deficits, increased need of care, loss of self-confidence and life quality may lead to morbidity and mortality of persons [18, 19]. A time critical help after a fall or even a preventive identification of atypical movement patterns would represent a considerable improvement for patients and physicians.

The goal of this research is to develop an intelligent floor that may detect characteristic walking patterns, fall events or other abnormal movement behaviors that would indicate an emergency situation for the user. In case that such an emergency situation is detected the system may contact a relative or professional medical personnel. Thus, users do not have to activate the emergency call themselves, which in a lot of cases is not possible, for example when the person is immobile after the downfall or even lost his conscience. Furthermore, older users with high risk for downfalls have an alternative to portable emergency buttons, which are often perceived to be stigmatizing and have a low compliance.

2 State of the Art

The non-invasive monitoring of peoples positions and movements within a limited environment is widely discussed in literature. Technological approaches range from wearable sensors like accelerometers and pressure sensors [20, 21], contact free methods using acoustic (microphone) [11] or visual (video camera) [12, 16, 24] sensors till solutions, which measure the contact forces that are applied to the ground by the users feet [1, 8, 23]. Each approach offers advantages but also drawbacks in certain scenarios. Wearable sensors are mobile and can be used in various locations, however they are not invisible and require a high amount of care and maintenance of the user. Acoustic and visual sensors provide very reliable information but require visible obtrusive technology that may bring up privacy and intimacy concerns. For the research focus of fall detection in a very private environment a ground sensor based approach seems to be the most promising.

Orr et al. created and validated a system for biometric user identification based on footstep profiles [23]. In their approach the ground reaction force of the users foot is measured by load cells and analyzed in order to generate user identification profiles. Addlesee et al. developed a sensor system called Active Floor, which aims at capturing the time varying spatial weight distribution within a given area using the hidden Markov model technique [1]. While the latter approaches are on a prototype level there are commercial projects as well, like the Sensfloor of Future-Shape GmbH [8]. The Sensfloor consists of a pressure sensitive textile layer that can be installed under a carpet. It detects the position of a person on the floor and gives alarms according to predefined scenarios (no movement for a longer period of time, etc.).

3 Future Care Floor

The approach presented in this paper aims not only at detecting a users position on the floor but also at measuring qualitative aspects of moving behaviors, especially downfalls or abnormal patterns which would indicate emergency situations for the user. The following part will explain the systems technical conceptualization and realization.

The basic concept is that of a floor that is equipped with a grid of piezoelectric elements (see Fig. 1). Those elements represent an inexpensive way of measuring forces applied to the ground. When a force is applied to the piezo it will deform and its atomic structure shifts. This causes a charge transfer and a voltage proportional to the applied force is induced within the piezo. This voltage signal we measure between the two poles of the sensor element (red and black cable, Fig. 1).

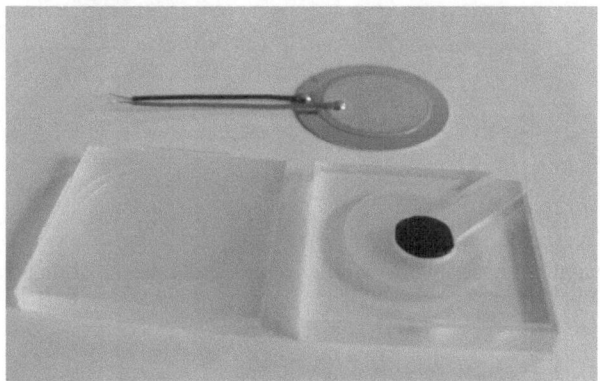

Fig. 1. Piezo sensor and perpex support structure

In order to achieve a good resolution, a net of 240 piezo elements was installed under the 20 m^2 floor surface of the test lab environment. The underlay structure of the floor is a metal grid consisting of steel sections which form squares of 0,6 x 0,6 m^2. At all cross points of this metal grid four piezo elements are installed, they serve as free support for the floor tiles. The floor tiles have a dimension of 0,6 x 0,6 m^2 aswell and a wooden upper surface and a metal basis.

So in each of the four corners of every tile a sensor is positioned and gives information about the force applied to the tile. In order to guarantee good signal quality and safe bedding, the piezo elements are positioned in a custom made perspex support structure. The support structure (Fig. 1) has a height of 5 mm, which makes the actual sensor part very thin and opens the possibility of installing the sensor floor within existing home environments.

Due to the geometry of the support structure primarily bending stress is applied to the piezo element when a user walks on the floor, which result in better signal quality. The voltage signal induced by mechanical deformation of the piezo material changes according to the type of load that is applied to the panel, which is the basis for robust fall detection and pattern recognition.

All sensors are directly wired to operation amplifiers. We use a setup of 15 operation amplifier boards (as shown in Fig. 2) to connect all 240 sensor units. The operation amplifier circuit consists mainly of a logarithmic unit and a voltage adjustment unit (see Fig. 3).

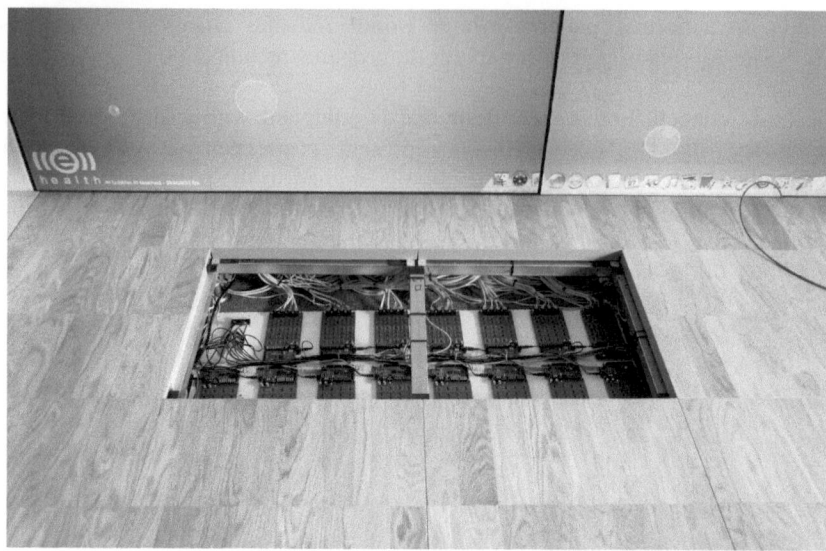

Fig. 2. Operation amplifier and microcontroller boards under the metal support structure for the sensors and the floor tiles

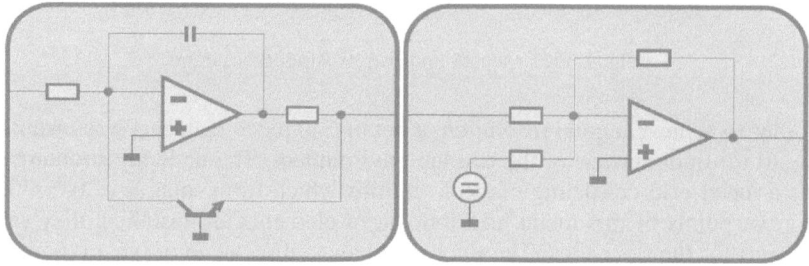

Fig. 3. Circuit diagram of the logarithmic unit (left) and voltage adjustment unit (right)

This setting is used due to the unequally distributed information within the raw voltage signal. Considering the research goal of detecting distinct movement patterns and especially downfalls, we found that the highest information density can be extracted in the voltage range of 20 – 40 Volts. In order to evaluate this range in more detail, without losing the basic signal information of the lower voltage ranges, a logarithmic unit is used. The voltage adjustment unit on the other hand is necessary in order to scale the complete voltage range of the sensor units to the 5V input maximum of the microcontroller boards. The relation of in- and output voltage is defined by the following function, with the virtual zero-point of the output voltage at +2.5 V:

$$U_o = U_T * \ln[U_i / I_{ES} * R]$$

We use 15 Arduino Mega microcontroller boards with serial interface to carry out the analog-digital conversion of the signals. A 10 Bit resolution at a sampling rate of 370 samples per sensor and second can be achieved in the experimental setup.

All further signal processing is done digitally. The data is acquired by a software and gathered in a two dimensional array which represents the structure of the piezos under the floor. This array of raw sensor signals is the basis for the extraction of various features and patterns within the signals. In order to do this, distinct parameters have to be identified and connected to other parameters or sensor information by a superior software entity (context manager). The determined parameters can be for example:

- User enters/leaves the room
- Position of the user within the room
- Pose of the user (standing, sitting, laying)
- Weight of the user

Those parameters combined with the time information provide a relative exact picture of the users movement behavior. For example:

- Velocity of pace
- Movement direction
- User identification

For specific tasks like for example fall detection, the patterns have to be subdivided in different classes, in order to calculate the probability of a fall according to the identified user.

In order to generate robust pattern recognition different machine learning approaches are followed. Supervised learning seems to be the most promising way to structure the signal data. In this approach the users live signal data is constantly compared to previous fall or movement scenarios, evaluated and updated. As the database increases the detection and extraction of different features becomes more and more reliable. In this context the use of Vector Support Machines seems promising. Also other approaches like Hidden Markov Models, Conditional Random Fields or Nearest Neighbor Algorithms [13, 22, 23] are evaluated.

Each signal peak is mathematically analyzed in real time, provided with a time stamp and stored in a database. This opens the possibility of reacting immediately on emergency events like downfalls. As the database is continuously increasing with each step, the systems knowledge about the normal behavior of the user rises constantly.

4 Integration in the Living Lab

The floor is one component of a Living Lab " The Future care Lab" (Member of the European Network of Living Labs [7]) that is being build at the Human Technology Centre of RWTH Aachen University (http://www.humtec.rwth-aachen.de) [27]. In this context the floor is connected with a wall sized interactive multi-touch display (Fig. 4). The overall goal of the research program is to develop adaptive interfaces and novel, integrative prototypes for personal healthcare systems in home environments. This includes new concepts of electronic monitoring systems within ambient assisted living environments. The technological design follows iterative cycles, in which technology development is carefully harmonized and weighted with acceptance and/or usability demands. Patients differing in gender, age, health status, emotional and cognitive factors, and severity of disease will be involved in the design.

To examine how patients communicate with smart homecare environments, how they deal with invisible technology, and how the information is to be delivered such that it meets the requirements of timeliness, data protection, dignity as well as medical demands, an experimental space is necessary, which enables to study patients "life at home". The room consists of a simulated home environment, which enables research-ers to use experimental interfaces with test persons of different ages and health states. Out of validity reasons, the experimental space is of central importance, as patients and care givers need to experience and "feel" the technology to be used, in order to fairly evaluate it [25]. Further, persons might overemphasize their sensitiveness towards privacy violations if their judgments only rely on the imagination of using it [5].

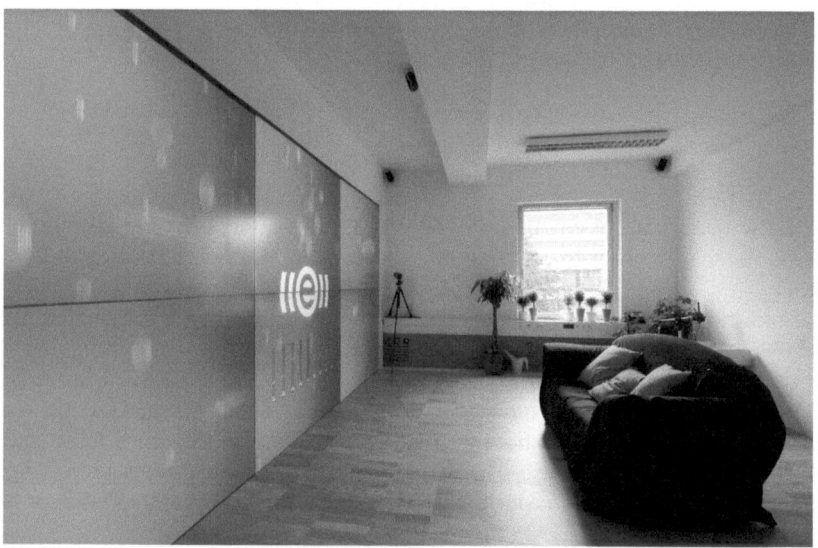

Fig. 4. Future Care Lab. Based on the information provided by the sensitive floor wall applica-tions can react interactively on the users position by zooming in and out or changing perspective.

Medical applications supported by the display wall are life size video consultations with the doctor or physical rehabilitation programs supported by interactive advises or games using the feedback channels of the floor and the wall [14]. One first application realized is a sound game in which the user is able to play music by changing his posi-tion on the floor (not pictured here, http://www.ehealth.humtec.rwth-aachen.de/), encouraging users to move and take exercise. The sound provoked by each step, may enhance patients' compliance and to support medical aftercare.

Another huge advantage of the living lab approach is the expandability of the system, which is interesting from an economic point of view. It is not restricted to medical services, but can be expanded to completely different services, ranging from information and communication services (e.g. getting information from the internet), over entertaining services (cinema, video-phoning with relatives), to social services (virtual meetings, visiting remote family members), to living services (ordering food from the supermarket or drugs from the pharmacy). Also, the digital room components might be used for atmospheric issues: light, tones, music can be integrated, which can have therapeutic or hedonic effects [3].

However, there may be also disadvantages, which need to be carefully addressed. Smart mobile technologies have already fundamentally changed the nature of social, economic and communicative pathways. The omnipresence of information may be perceived as a violation of personal intimacy limits, raising concerns about privacy, and loss of control [9, 17]. So far, we have only limited knowledge about the fragile limits between the different poles: the wish to live independently at home and to feel safe, secure, and fully cared on the one hand and the feeling of loss of control and the disliking of intrusion in private spheres on the other. Future studies aim at an "acceptance cartography" of using motives and barriers, which are assumed to depend on the specific using situation, living contexts and on user diversity. Here, user-centered designs and a consequent inclusion of patients in all phases of system evaluation are needed in order to understand users needs and wants [3, 10].

References

1. Addlesee, M.D., Jones, A.H., Livesey, F., Samaria, F.S.: The ORL Active Floor. IEEE Personal Communications 4(5), 35–51 (1997)
2. Baker, S.P., Harvey, A.H.: Fall injuries in the elderly. Clin. Geriatr. Med., 501–512 (1985)
3. Beul, S., Klack, L., Kasugai, K., Möllering, C., Röcker, C., Wilkowska, W., Ziefle, M.: Between Innovation and Daily Practice in the Development of AAL Systems: Learning from the experience with today's systems. In: 3rd International ICST Conference on Electronic Healthcare for the 21st Century (2010)
4. Campbell, A.J., Reinken, J., Allan, B.C., Martinez, G.S.: Falls in old age: a study of frequency and related clinical factors. Age Ageing 10, 64–70 (1981)
5. Cvrcek, D., Kumpost, M., Matyas, V., Danezis, G.: A Study on the Value of Location Privacy. In: Proceedings of the ACM Workshop on Privacy in the Electronic Society, pp. 109–118. ACM, New York (2006)
6. De Ruyter, B., Pelgrim, E.: Ambient Assisted Living research in CareLab. ACM Interactions 14(4) (2007)
7. European Network of Living Labs, ENoLL (2010), http://www.openlivinglabs.eu
8. Future Shape, Sensfloor (2010), http://www.future-shape.com
9. Fugger, E., Prazak, B., Hanke, S., Wassertheurer, S.: Requirements and Ethical Issues for Sensor-Augmented Environments in Elderly Care. In: Stephanidis, C. (ed.) HCI 2007. LNCS, vol. 4554, pp. 887–893. Springer, Heidelberg (2007)
10. Gaul, S., Ziefle, M.: Smart Home Technologies: Insights into Generation-Specific Acceptance Motives. In: Holzinger, A., et al. (eds.) HCI for eInclusion, pp. 312–332. Springer, Heidelberg (2009)
11. Haines, W.D., Vernon, J.R., Dannenberg, R.B., Driessen, P.F.: Placement of Sound Sources in the Stereo Field Using Measured Room Impulse Responses. In: Computer Music Modeling and Retrieval. Sense of Sounds 2009. LNCS. Springer, Heidelberg (2009)

12. Khan, S.M., Shah, M.: A Multiview Approach to Tracking People in Crowded Scenes Using a Planar Homography Constraint. In: Leonardis, A., Bischof, H., Pinz, A. (eds.) ECCV 2006. LNCS, vol. 3954, pp. 133–146. Springer, Heidelberg (2006)
13. Kim, E., Helal, S., Cook, D.: Human Activity Recognition and Pattern Discovery. IEEE Pervasive Computing 9(1), 48–53 (2010)
14. Klack, L., Wilkowska, W., Kasugai, K., Schmitz-Rode, T.: Die intelligente Wohnung als medizinischer Assistant. VDI Wissensforum "Kunststoffe in der Medizintechnik" (2010)
15. Klack, L., Kasugai, K., Schmitz-Rode, T., Röcker, C., Ziefle, M., Möllering, C., Jakobs, E.-M., Russell, P., Borchers, J.: A Personal Assistance System for Older Users with Chronic Heart Diseases. In: Proceedings of the Third Ambient Assisted Living Conference (AAL 2010), January 26-27. VDE Verlag, Berlin (2010)
16. Kourogi, M., Kurata, T.: Personal Positioning based on Walking Locomotion Analysis with Self-Contained Sensors and a wearable camera. In: Proceedings of the 2nd IEEE/ACM International Symposium on Mixed and Augmented Reality (2003)
17. Lalou, S.: Identity, Social Satus, Privacy and Face-keeping in the Digital Society. Journal of Social Science Information 47(3), 299–330 (2008)
18. Lawrence, R., et al.: Intensity and correlates of fear of falling and hurting oneself in the next year: Baseline findings. Journal of Aging and Health 10, 269–286 (1998)
19. Liddle, J., Gilleard, C.: The emotional consequences of falls for older people and their families. Clinical Rehabilitation 9, 110–114 (1995)
20. Lüder, M., Salomon, R., Bieber, G.: StairMaster: A New Online Fall Detection Device. In: 2nd Congress for Ambient Assisted Living, Berlin (2009)
21. Mann, S.: Smart Clothing: The Wearable Computer and WearCam. Personal Technologies 1(1) (1997)
22. Pirttikangas, S., Suutala, J., Riekki, J., Röning, J.: Footstep Identification from Pressure Signals using Markos Models, Intelligent Systems Group, Infotech Oulu (2002)
23. Orr, R.J., Abowd, G.D.: The Smart Floor: A Mechanism for Natural User Identification and Tracking, Graphics, Visualization and Usability (GVU) Center, Georgia Institute of Technology (2000)
24. Schäfer, R., Müller, W., Ceimann, R., Kleinjohann, B.: A Low-Cost Positioning System for Location-Aware Applications in Smart Homes. In: CHI 2007 Workshop on "Mobile Spatial Interaction" (2007)
25. Woolham, J., Frisby, B.: Building a Local Infrastructure that Supports the Use of Assistive Technology in the Care of People with Dementia. Research Policy and Planning 20(1), 11–24 (2002)
26. World Health Organisation, WHO (2004), http://www.who.int
27. Ziefle, M., Röcker, C., Wilkowska, W., Kasugai, K., Klack, L., Möllering, C., Beul, S.: A Multi-Disciplinary Approach to Ambient Assisted Living. In: Röcker, C., Ziefle, M. (eds.) E-Health, Assistive Technologies and Applications for Assisted Living: Challenges and Solutions. IGI Global, Hershey (2010)

Monitoring and Assessing Crew Performance in High-Speed Marine Craft – Methodological Considerations

Dragana Nikolić[1], Richard Collier[2], and Robert Allen[1]

[1] Institute of Sound and Vibration Research, University of Southampton, Southampton, UK
[2] School of Health Sciences, University of Southampton, Southampton, UK
{d.nikolic,richard.collier,r.allen}@soton.ac.uk

Abstract. This paper proposes a method to monitor and assess human perform-ance specific to high-speed marine craft operation. The high-speed craft crew's ability to efficiently perform their allotted tasks is affected by the manner in which the vessel responds to the variable sea conditions. In general, the reaction of human body to high-speed boat motion and vibration is recognized as the main cause of fatigue during and post transits; whereas random shock repre-sents the most likely cause of injuries during transits. The pilot experiment in-troduced in this paper was designed and performed with the intention to identify and evaluate measures of crew performance during and after a transit in a ma-rine environment that can serve to indicate increasing fatigue, decreased func-tional capabilities and thus possible increased risk of injury.

Keywords: Human performance, Whole body vibration, Muscle fatigue, Sur-face EMG analysis.

1 Introduction

The crew and passengers of high-speed marine craft, such as rigid-hull inflatable boats (RIB), are often exposed to continuous vibrations and shocks and experience high levels of fatigue during and post transits as well as an increased risk of injuries [1]. A study examining the reduction in physical performance post transit demon-strated that performance was reduced by ~30 % for manual dexterity and ~20 % in a step test [2]. As high-speed craft are often used as transit vehicles to delivery person-nel undertaking activities such as search and rescue, it is important that they arrive at the destination in the best possible condition as peoples lives are dependant on their performance. Thus, it is of great importance to identify and examine possible causes of the fatigue and provide effective methods to reduce them.

This paper proposes a method to monitor and assess human aspects during and post high-speed transits at sea. The pilot experiment has been designed and performed with the intention to evaluate measures of fatigue that could be used to assess possible degradation of crew performance. To achieve this, sea trials were undertaken with a RIB instrumented with tri-axial accelerometers and rate gyros to record shocks and boat motion, respectively. In addition, physiological data – surface electromyography (EMG) and electrocardiogram (ECG) – were measured simultaneously during transits

J. Lin and K.S. Nikita (Eds.): MobiHealth 2010, LNICST 55, pp. 219–226, 2011.
© Institute for Computer Sciences, Social Informatics and Telecommunications Engineering 2011

to investigate any effect that could be in association with the exposure to vibration. EMG and ECG signals were also collected during muscle fatigue tests performed instantly before and after each trial to examine the characteristics and effect on theses outcome measures of the high speed transit. Rate of perceived exertion (RPE) using the Borg scale [3] was used to assess subject's level of perceived exertion rated at the point when, during the transit, they perceived they were working hardest.

The paper is organized as follows. A proposed methodology used to measure, process and analyze both physical and physiological data is explained in details in section 2. The results of the experiment are presented and discussed in section 3 followed by the conclusions in section 4.

2   Method Description

2.1   Experimental Procedure

The experiment consisted of a sea trial preceded and followed by a muscle fatigue test. Physical data measured during the trials were: boat LCG (longitudinal centre of gravity), seat and head accelerations and boat motions. Measurements of physiological data were: ECG and surface EMG activities of four spinal muscles (upper fibers of *Trapezius* and *Multifidus* in the lumbosacral region), performed during all phases of the experiment. A scheme of the performance measurement system is depicted in Fig. 1.

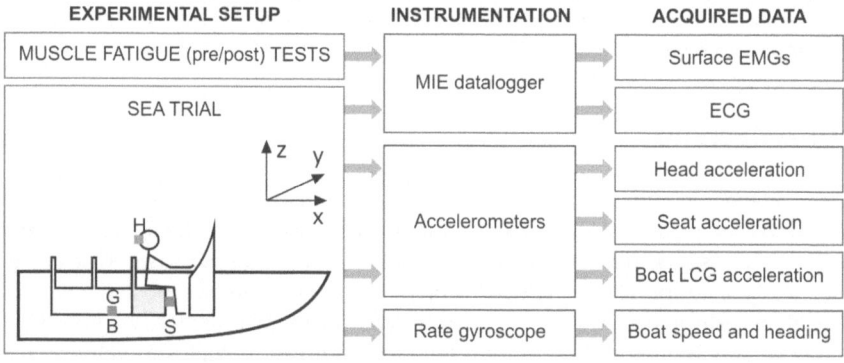

Fig. 1. Performance measurement system (B, H, S and G correspond to the positions of the accelerometers placed at the boat LCG, head and seat and rate gyroscope respectively)

Sea Trials. Three sea trials, each approximately 33 minutes long, were carried out with a RIB-X Expert XT650 at the south coast of England. Each trial was run with one subject sitting on the front left seat next to the driver. Three physically fit male subjects (83±9.6 kg weight, 182±12 cm height, 28.3±3.2 age) participated in this study. The sea conditions were *slight* (sea state 3). The average and maximum boat speed estimated from the GPS recordings for each trial are reported in Table 1 (1 knots≈0.5144 m/s).

Table 1. Boat speed during the sea trials

Trial No.	Trial Duration	Average speed [knots]	[m/s]	Maximum speed [knots]	[m/s]
1	35 min 20 s	20.84	10.72	27.58	14.19
2	27 min 0 s	25.17	12.95	37.73	19.41
3	38 min 50 s	25.58	13.16	36.54	18.80

Muscle Fatigue Test. Before and after the sea trial, a subject performed a standardized isometric back extension test until fatigue [4]. The subject, lying prone, was instructed to maintain the upper body above the floor as long as possible, with his arms aligned with the body and the head in a neutral position looking downward. The test ceased when the subject was no longer able to maintain the trunk in the test position, the time for each test was recorded.

2.2 Instrumentation and Data Acquisition

Tri-axial accelerometers (Crossbox CXL100HF3, range ±100 g) were used to measure boat and human vibrations. The accelerometer positions, denoted as B, H and S in Fig. 1, correspond respectively to: the boat's LCG (accelerometer attached at the floor of the boat), the subject's head (accelerometer attached at the back side of the helmet), and the subject's seat (accelerometer positioned at the front side of the seat). The axes of each accelerometer were referenced according to recommended method such that the x-axis measured fore-aft acceleration, the y-axis measured lateral acceleration, and the z-axis measured vertical acceleration [5]. Acceleration signals were recorded at sampling frequency of 2.5 kHz using a 16-channel logger (IOTECH Logbook 300).

Surface EMG signals were recorded using a differential pair of pre-gelled electrodes attached 3 cm apart over and parallel to the fibers of each muscle using standard SENIAM guidelines [6]. A reference electrode with a built-in 1k gain pre-amplifier was attached at the same distance from the electrodes. Pre-amp cables were fixed to the skin with adhesive tape to reduce potential artifacts caused by movement. Raw signals were amplified, band-pass filtered (3 dB bandwidth: 6-6000 Hz) and recorded with a 1 kHz sampling frequency using a portable data logger (MIE Medical Research ltd).

To synchronize data acquired by two data loggers, tri-axial accelerometer transducers (ranges ±25 g and ±100 g) used by each data logger were mounted close to each other on the back of subject's helmet with the corresponding axes of detection aligned. Thus, the head acceleration signals acquired by two transducers were used in the processing stage to establish an exact match between time scales of the measured signals. All data were stored on memory cards and converted later into a MATLAB format for processing purpose.

2.3 Vibration Data Analysis

In this study, the assessment of the level of exposure to vibration is based on the calculated vibration dose value (VDV). VDV is commonly used as an assessment method when a person is exposed to numerous shocks and represents a cumulative dose of vibration during a total exposure [7],[8]. Two weighting filters – W_d for the horizontal x and y-axes and W_b for the vertical z-axis, were initially applied to the vibration signals measured at the passenger's seat and the boat's LCG in order to estimate exposure level associated with the two positions [5]. In accordance with BS 6841 [7], VDV for each axis is calculated according to the following formula:

$$\text{VDV}_i = \sqrt[4]{\int_0^T a_{iw}^4(t)\,dt}, \ i = x, y, z,\tag{1}$$

where $a_{iw}(t)$ is frequency-weighted acceleration along the i–axis and T is the duration of exposure in seconds, i.e. total period during which vibration occurs.

Total vibration dose in all axes is obtained by summing individual vibration doses for each axis:

$$\text{VDV}_{tot} = \sqrt[4]{\sum_{i=x,y,z} \text{VDV}_i^4}, \ i = x, y, z,\tag{2}$$

where VDV_i is the partial vibration dose value calculated for the i–axis using Eq. (1).

Furthermore, the calculated VDVs can be compared with limit values of vibration exposure standardized to an eight-hour period above which vibration exposure must be controlled or completely stopped. According to [8], exposure action value (EAV) and exposure limit value (ELV) are 9.1 m/s$^{1.75}$ and 21 m/s$^{1.75}$ respectively.

3   Results and Discussion

3.1 Boat Speed and Vibration

Frequency-weighted peaks and root mean squared (rms) amplitudes of the LCG and seat accelerations calculated for each trial are reported in Table 2. For all three trials, the highest impact magnitudes occurred in the vertical direction (z-axis) at the boat's LCG and in the longitudinal (x-axis) or lateral (y-axis) directions at the seat front. (The magnitude and frequency of impacts increased significantly in the second half of each trial.) Overall frequency-weighted rms seat acceleration magnitudes were found to be considerable larger than the rms magnitudes of LCG acceleration. In accordance with BS 6841 [7], vibrations with such frequency-weighted rms magnitudes are indicated as being *uncomfortable*.

Table 2. Vibration parameters of the sea trials

Trial No.	peak [g] x-axis	y-axis	z-axis	rms [m/s^2] x-axis	y-axis	z-axis	total
LCG acceleration (weighted)							
1	0.119	0.109	0.866	0.124	0.083	0.324	0.357
2	0.148	0.162	2.165	0.188	0.103	0.457	0.505
3	1.740	0.212	2.292	0.281	0.191	0.551	0.647
Seat acceleration (weighted)							
1	0.186	0.708	0.799	0.119	0.653	0.248	0.709
2	0.231	1.538	1.363	0.181	1.005	0.347	1.079
3	0.452	1.359	1.490	0.200	1.060	0.352	1.135

3.2 Vibration Dose Values

Partial and total VDVs calculated according to Eqs. (1) and (2) for all three sea trials performed in this study are listed in Table 3. The largest VDVs were reported for the third trial where a higher number of impacts were encountered, especially in the second half of the trial. It can be also seen that the total VDVs calculated at the seat (seated posture) are larger than the total VDVs calculated at the boat's LCG (standing posture) for all three trials. Moreover, a main contribution to the seat's total VDVs is from impacts in lateral direction; while in the case of the boat's LCG it is predominantly the result of vertical impacts. In the second and third trial, even thought the sea state was *slight*, the total VDVs calculated at the seat exceed the EAV of 9.1 m/s$^{1.75}$ standardized for an eight-hour period within 20 minutes.

Table 3. Vibration dose values derived in case of seated and standing postures

Trial No.	VDV (standing posture) [m/s$^{1.75}$]				VDV (seated posture) [m/s$^{1.75}$]			
	x-axis	y-axis	z-axis	total	x-axis	y-axis	z-axis	total
1	1.54	1.19	4.12	4.15	1.40	7.54	3.13	7.60
2	1.92	1.37	8.41	8.41	2.08	12.20	4.92	12.28
3	6.43	2.65	11.37	11.66	2.98	14.73	6.23	14.85

As an example, cumulative effects of the total VDV relative to the frequency-weighted LCG and seat acceleration magnitudes during the third trial are illustrated in Fig. 2 where the exposure action and limit values are marked with the horizontal dotted lines. The EAV is exceeded approximately 18 minutes from the beginning of the trial whilst the magnitude and frequency of impacts increased significantly resulting in a rapid increase of the acceleration magnitudes.

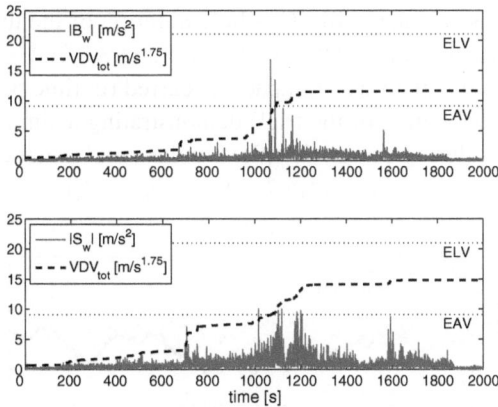

Fig. 2. Frequency-weighted acceleration magnitudes and total vibration dose values calculated from the LCG (top) and seat (bottom) accelerations in the third trial

3.3 Physiological Data

The EMG variables considered in this study are the root mean square (rms) value and median frequency (MDF) [9],[10]. These parameters are calculated from the consecutive 1 s time windows of the bandpass-filtered (10-300 Hz) EMG signals.

All three trials reveal very high correlation between EMG and acceleration rms values. As an example, the normalized running rms values for *Left* and *Right Multifidus* muscles at the level of the lumbar 4th and 5th vertebrae and seat acceleration are shown in Fig. 3, this is zoomed in at the time interval where most impacts occurred. An increase of the EMG magnitudes caused by large impacts in seat acceleration is evident.

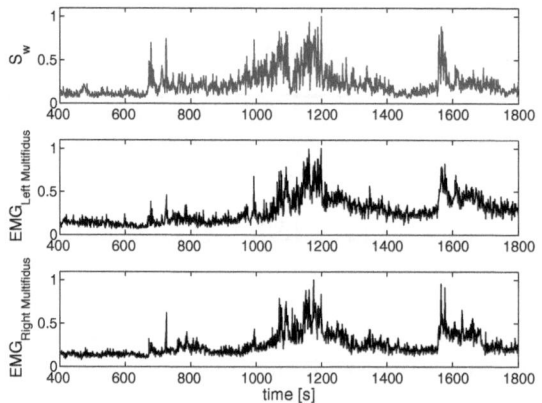

Fig. 3. Normalized rms amplitudes of frequency-weighted seat acceleration (top), *Left Multifidus* EMG (middle) and *Right Multifidus* EMG (bottom)

Median frequencies calculated for the whole duration of the third trial are given in Fig. 4. It can be seen that the MDFs of the *Left* and *Right Multifidus*, decrease by more than 8 Hz when the majority of impacts occurred (in time period between 1070 s and 1200 s from the beginning of the trial) demonstrating a similar effect to that seen when muscle fatigues during an activity [9]. Similar trend is not detected in the upper fibres of *Trapezius*.

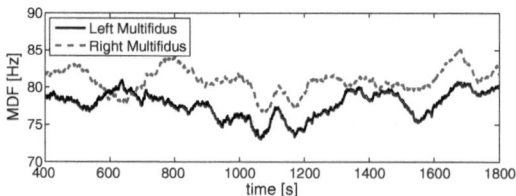

Fig. 4. Median frequencies of *Multifidus* muscles

The results of the Borg RPE test for each trial respectively are 11.5, 12 and 17 indicating that the subjects perception of the sense of effort during the sea trial, when they perceived that they were working at their hardest, was rated between *somewhat hard* (>11) to *very hard* (>15). These results concur with vibration data which illustrates the severity of the trial – as can be seen from Table 2, the vibration parameters increased from the first to the third trial.

The heart rate and MDF values calculated for the EMG and ECG measurements conducted before and after the first trial are given in Tables 4 and 5 respectively. In this pilot study, the results of the muscle fatigue test have not demonstrated general increase of heart rate or decrease of MDF values after the trials. It could be speculated that the effect of the vibration exposure on the muscle fatigue was not significant due to *slight* sea conditions and good fitness levels of the subjects.

Table 4. Comparison of heart rate values for the pre- and post-trial muscle fatigue tests

HR [beats/min]	min		max		mean		st. deviation		range	
	pre-	post-	pre-	post-	pre-	post-	pre-	post-	pre-	post-
	63.8	59.6	95.8	93.1	83.6	77.3	7.2	8.5	32	33.4

Table 5. Comparison of MDF values for the pre-trial and post-trial muscle fatigue tests

MDF [Hz]	min		max		mean		st. deviation		range	
	pre-	post-	pre-	post-	pre-	post-	pre-	post-	pre-	post-
L. Upp. Trap.	64	68.6	75.6	89.2	68.7	79.2	2.6	5.6	11.6	20.6
R. Upp. Trap.	58.8	65	76	88	64.9	73.6	2.4	3.4	17.2	23
L. Multifidus	76.2	84	101.7	104	88.3	94.4	6.7	4.9	25.5	20
R. Multifidus	73	83.8	110	115	91.1	99.1	9.3	7.3	37	31.2

4   Conclusions

In this paper, a method to monitor and assess crew performance in high-speed marine craft transits at sea is proposed and preliminary results of the pilot study are presented. The vibration dose values obtained in this pilot experiment are compared with limit values set by current standards and legislation demonstrating the VDV that can be expected onboard high-speed marine craft. Values would be even larger in more severe sea states and compounded by wind and tide effects. It is shown that the physiological data are highly correlated with vibration magnitudes during sea transits. A decrease in median frequencies of the EMG signals due to an increase in vibration amplitude is demonstrated for lower back muscles. For more thorough analysis of the effects of the trials on the subject's performance during the muscle fatigue tests conducted before and after trial, it would be of interest to collect more experimental data in higher sea states.

Acknowledgments. The authors acknowledge the support of colleagues from the School of Engineering Sciences, University of Southampton, for their help in conducting this experiment. The research was funded by EPSRC (grant no. EP/C525728/1).

References

1. Ensign, W., Hodgdon, J.A., Prusaczyk, W.K., Ahlers, S., Shapiro, D., Lipton, M.: A survey of self-reported injuries among boat operators. Naval Health Research Centre. Tech. Report 00-48 (2000)
2. Hyde, D., Thomas, J.R., Schrot, J., Taylor, W.F.: Quantification of special operations mission-related performance: Operational evaluation of physical measures. Naval Medical Research Institute. NMRI 97-01 (1997)
3. Borg, G.: Borg's Perceived Exertion and Pain Scales, 1st edn. Human Kinetics (1998)
4. Ito, T., Shirado, O., Suzuki, H., Takahashi, M., Kaneda, K., Strax, T.E.: Lumbar trunk muscle endurance testing: an inexpensive alternative to a machine for evaluation. Arch. Phys. Med. Rehabil. 77(1), 75–79 (1996)
5. ISO 2631-1: Mechanical vibration and shock – evaluation of human exposure to whole-body vibration – Part 1: general requirement. International Organization for Standardization, pp. 1–31 (1997)
6. Merletti, R., Hermens, H.: Introduction to the special issue on the SENIAM European Concerted Action. J. Electromyogr. Kinesiol. 10(5), 283–286 (2000)
7. BS 6841: Measurement and evaluation of human exposure to whole-body mechanical vibration and repeated shock. British Standards Institute (1987)
8. Griffin, M.J.: Minimum health and safety requirements for workers exposed to hand-transmitted vibration and whole-body vibration in the European Union; a review. Occupational and Environmental Medicine 61, 387–397 (2004)
9. Merletti, R., Parker, P.: Electromyography – Physiology, Engineering and Noninvasive Applications, 1st edn. John Wiley & Sons, Inc., Hoboken (2004)
10. Cifrek, M., Medved, V., Tonković, S., Ostojić, S.: Surface EMG based muscle fatigue evaluation in biomechanics. Clinical Biomechanics 24(4), 327–340 (2009)

Using Location Information for Sophisticated Emergency Call Management

Lambros Lambrinos and Constantinos Djouvas

Department of Communication and Internet Studies,
Cyprus University of Technology, Limassol, Cyprus
{lambros.lambrinos,costas.tziouvas}@cut.ac.cy

Abstract. It is widely accepted that the faster the response to an incident involving injuries, the higher the probability that lives are saved. Thus, any kind of system that improves the response of the emergency services is expected to be highly beneficial. Improved network connectivity facilities and powerful mobile devices allow the development of smart applications that exploit features such as geographical location identification and Voice over IP. In this paper, we see how we can utilize caller location information to apply policies that enhance emergency call management at both the call originating network and the emergency service call centre; the ultimate aim is to reduce emergency services response times.

Keywords: location based services, VoIP, emergency services, SIP.

1 Introduction

IP-based connectivity via mobile devices is becoming ubiquitous as technologies such as 3G and wi-fi are being widely deployed; the forthcoming 4G will allow for even higher connectivity speeds. Such connections can be utilized by suitable software to enable various applications that users of mobile devices can make the most of. Those applications, allow for much richer information to be exchanged when compared with the standard GSM networks; one such application that is proving quite popular among mobile users is Voice-over-IP (VoIP).

In many situations, people will use their mobile devices to place calls to the emergency services; this is particularly the case for outdoor incidents (e.g. car accidents). In this paper we see how we can utilize caller location information (GPS in particular) to enhance emergency call management at both the calling party gateway as well as at the emergency service call centre.

This paper is structured as follows: after a description of location based services from an emergency management perspective, we present the details of our proposed architecture and call management policies and finish the paper with some concluding thoughts and future work considerations.

2 Background

In this section we present some background information related to our work. First, we describe systems that can be used by mobile devices for location identification and

J. Lin and K.S. Nikita (Eds.): MobiHealth 2010, LNICST 55, pp. 227–232, 2011.
© Institute for Computer Sciences, Social Informatics and Telecommunications Engineering 2011

then present different Location Based Services (LBS) designed for providing different types of assistance during emergency situations. Systems that can be used for mobile device location identification can be divided into three categories: satellite-based, network-based and stand-alone [1].

The satellite-based systems utilize satellites that are in orbit around the earth and send information to terrestrial receivers. One such system is the Global Positioning System (GPS); the GPS receivers can estimate their current position with an accuracy between one and ten meters [2] using the information (the satellite's position and distance from the earth) received from the different satellites.

The network-based systems utilize the service carrier's wireless network infrastructure to identify their location. The simplest but least accurate approach is known as Cell of Origin (COO). Using COO, the location of a mobile device is approximated based on the cell it is currently in and its approximation error can be equal to the cell size; this may be up to 35 kilometers in rural areas. A different and more accurate method is called Angle of Arrival (AOA) and is based on triangulation. Mobile devices can calculate the line-of-sight path to a base station by measuring the strength, time of arrival, and the phase of a signal sent by that base station. Utilizing the signals of two base stations, the mobile phone calculates two paths; the intersection point of these two paths represents the location of the mobile phone. Other similar location identification methods are Time of Arrival (TOA) and Time Difference of Arrival (TDOA).

Stand-alone approaches can only be used for providing location information on designated and small size areas, e.g. buildings. Approaches in this category require special equipment appropriately configured; for example a Bluetooth device that provides location information to mobile devices that enter its coverage area. The accuracy of the resulting location can be controlled by the administrator since it can range from a single office (using Ethernet jacks [3]) up to whole buildings or blocks.

Utilizing location information, different Location Based Services (LBS) can be implemented. From the perspective of emergency management and according to [4], we can define two categories of location-based emergency services:

The first category, regards applications that provide location information. In this category we can assign applications that users use to establish emergency calls; the European Union and the United States have both defined standards (E112 [5] and E9-1-1 [6] respectively) that oblige telecommunication carriers to provide location information for emergency calls. Furthermore, emergency VoIP calls can also belong to this category. Identifying the shift towards IP telephony, an extension of E9-1-1 known as NG9-1-1 [7] is under development and the new standard will extend E9-1-1 with IP based compatibilities. For the dissemination of location information over IP calls, the SIP working group is in the process of defining an extension to the Session Initiation Protocol (SIP [8]), the Location Conveyance for Session Initiation Protocol [9], that can be used for "conveying" location data over a SIP message exchange.

The second category of location-based emergency applications includes applications that propagate emergency related information to users in specific areas; those can be used for informing users in particular areas about an unfolding emergency event. The dissemination of such information can be achieved using different methods with the simplest one being the use of the Short Message Service (SMS); a plain SMS message is sent to all users in a particular area, usually to all phones in the coverage area of one or more base stations [10]. A similar approach that achieves the same results is known as Short Message Service - Cell Broadcast. This method, has a distinct advantage against the plain SMS approach since it achieves the simultaneous delivery of messages to multiple users in a specified cell using broadcasting, preserving resources and bandwidth. In addition to the plain text messages that can be sent using the abovementioned approaches, services like Multimedia Message Service (MMS) [11] can be used for disseminating richer context.

Finally, techniques that allow users in specific areas to receive live streaming are available. For example, the Multimedia Broadcast and Multicast Service (MBMS) [12] facilitates broadcasting of different forms of content to different areas; this allows an unlimited number of users present in the same area to watch the same mobile TV program. Utilizing this technology, users in emergency areas can receive live streaming with the latest information updates on the emergency situation.

3 System Architecture and Call Management Policies

This work aims to create a system that reduces the time required for establishing and handling emergency calls. More precisely, leveraging from the assumption that calls include the caller's location, we concentrate on devising smart call management mechanisms at both the call initiation proxy as well as the call receiving proxy. These mechanisms will efficiently and effectively prioritize emergency calls, resulting in reduced possessing times for such calls.

We concentrate on IP-based telephony which uses the SIP protocol for call establishment. Calls from the User Agents on the mobile devices can include the caller's location in the form of coordinates acquired using GPS; this can be included in the SIP INVITE message. This information will enable the emergency service agents to quickly pinpoint the caller's location and thus emphasize on acquiring incident information.

3.1 System Architecture

The overall architecture proposed for our system is shown in Figure 1. As calls to the emergency services are highly important, it is imperative that they are prioritized over other calls in cases where demand for calls exceeds the capacity available (which is often the case in major incident areas). To facilitate this call handling scheme, we introduce two new entities: the Emergency Call Scheduler (ECS) and the Smart Emergency Call Queue Manager (SECQM).

The Emergency Call Scheduler (ECS) runs on the call initiation proxy and is responsible for handling call requests from mobile users within its coverage area which may include multiple wi-fi access points or mobile base stations. Thus, the prioritization of emergency call requests is the responsibility of the ECS which manages the outgoing call queue and can assign different priorities to pending call requests [13].

At the emergency call centre (PSAP) end, the Smart Emergency Call Queue Manager (SECQM) runs on the call receiving proxy and is responsible for managing the incoming call queue. The SECQM can utilize a number of call distribution and prioritization policies again based on the use of caller location information and call historical data.

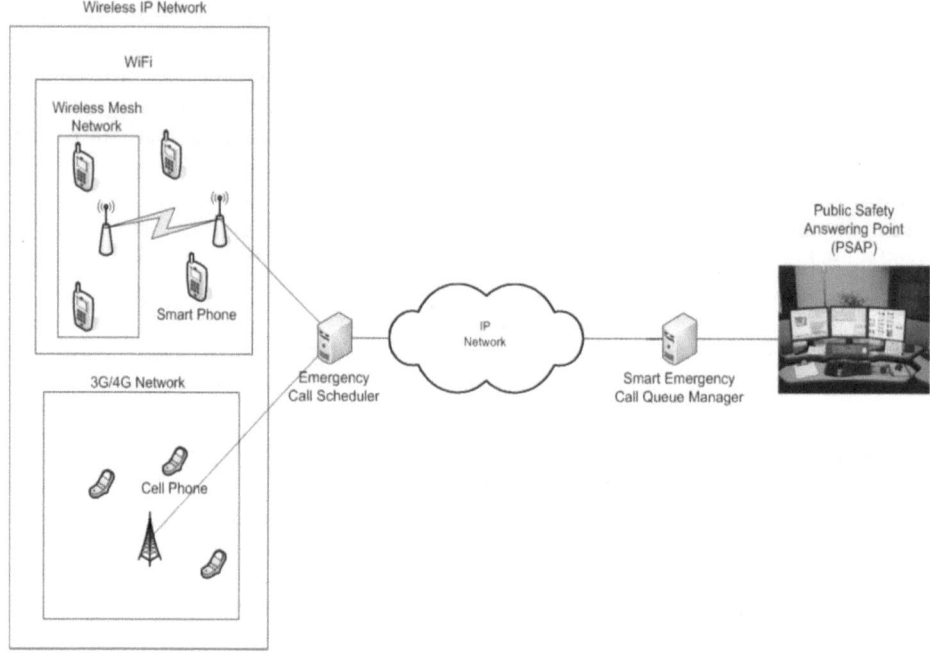

Fig. 1. System Architecture

3.2 Call Management Policies

As already mentioned, in the heart of the proposed system the ECS and SECQM will apply various call management policies to prioritize emergency-related calls; we discuss here some potential prioritization schemes. The elements used to determine a call's priority include: its destination, the caller's location and calling history.

From the point-of-view of the ECS, call requests may be destined for 9-1-1 type numbers or normal telephone numbers with the former having higher priority, as expected. Using calling history information, higher priority (among emergency calls) can perhaps be given to such calls originating from a new location; they are likely to report another incident. Moreover, calls to non-emergency numbers that originate from callers who have previously placed an emergency call may also be prioritized.

Based on the above, the order in a queue of pending calls could be as follows:

a) emergency calls from a new location,
b) emergency calls from a previously reported location,
c) normal calls from users who have previously placed emergency calls or from locations where emergency calls have previously originated and
d) all other calls.

The calls destined for 9-1-1 type services are received by the SECQM whose aim is to reduce call waiting and call handling times; the simple first-come-first-served policy for the calls may not always be appropriate and some call prioritization/allocation may be useful.

Calls with higher probability of reporting a new emergency incident (i.e., originating from regions where no active emergency incidents exist), could be considered as more important than calls originating from regions that the system already knows the existence of an emergency incident. In a more radical note, the queue manager may push calls from callers near a previously reported incident to the end of the queue. Such calls are likely to report the same incident or enquire about the status or location of emergency vehicles and may hence delay the handling of calls regarding new incidents.

The existence of call handling agents can make the operation of the SECQM much more complex. In another scenario, subsequent calls originating from a previously reported location can be directed towards the agent who handled the initial call; this agent (if available) will already be familiar with the incident which can potentially reduce the call completion time.

4 Conclusions and Future Work

It is widely accepted that the faster the response to an incident involving injuries, the higher the probability that lives are saved. Thus, any kind of system that improves the response of the emergency services is expected to be highly beneficial. In this paper we have presented our considerations for such a system that attempts to utilize advances in communication technologies and mobile devices to make emergency call handling mechanisms more sophisticated.

Our immediate plans are to modify an open-source SIP user agent in order to include GPS information in its INVITE messages. To implement the ECS we plan to extend the call scheduling capabilities of the enhanced SIP proxy proposed in [13] and add the ability of processing the additional information in the SIP messages. The acquired info will be passed to the SECQM for further processing.

By allowing the proposed system to manage the incoming call queue, we believe that we can achieve better resource allocation at the emergency call centre which can result in faster response from the emergency services. The implementation of the system will be evaluated under different scenarios to ascertain its effectiveness.

References

1. Zhao, Y.: Vehicle navigation and information systems. In: Webster, J.G. (ed.) Encyclopedia of Electrical and Electronics Engineering, vol. 23, pp. 106–118. Wiley, New York (1999)
2. Hightower, J., Borriello, G.: A Survey and Taxonomy of Location Systems for Ubiquitous Computing. IEEE Computer 34, 57–66 (2001)
3. Mintz-Habib, M., Rawat, A., Schulzrinne, H., Wu, X.: A VoIP Emergency Services Architecture and Prototype. In: 14th International Conference on Computer Communications and Networks, pp. 523–528. IEEE Press, New York (2005)
4. Aloudat, A., Michael, K., Abbas, R.: Location-Based Services for Emergency Management: A Multi-Stakeholder Perspective. In: The Eighth International Conference on Mobile Business (ICMB 2009), pp. 143–148. IEEE Press, New York (2009)

5. European Commission: Commission Recommendation of 25 July 2003 on the processing of caller location information in electronic communication networks for the purpose of location-enhanced emergency call services. Official Journal of the European Union L 189, 49–51 (2003)
6. National Emergency Number Association: NENA Technical Requirements Document On Model Legislation E9-1-1 for Multi-Line Telephone Systems. NENA 06-750, V.2 (2009)
7. The NG9-1-1 Project webpage, http://www.nena.org/ng911-project
8. Rosenberg, J., Schulzrinne, H., Camarillo, G., Johnston, A., Peterson, J., Sparks, R., Handley, M., Schooler, E.: SIP: Session Initiation Protocol, RFC 3261. IETF (2002)
9. Polk, J., Rosen, B.: Location Conveyance for the Session Initiation Protocol, Internet Draft. IETF (2009)
10. Aloudat, A., Michael, K., Yan, J.: Location-Based Services in Emergency Management-from Government to Citizens: Global Case Studies. In: Mendis, P., Lai, J., Dawson, E., Abbass, H. (eds.) Recent Advances in Security Technology, 1st edn., pp. 190–201. Australian Homeland Security Research Centre, Canberra (2007)
11. Mobile networks go broadcast with Ericsson,
    http://www.ericsson.com/thecompany/press/releases/
    2006/04/1043320
12. Multimedia Messaging Service V1.3, http://www.openmobilealliance.org/
13. Lambrinos, L., Djouvas, C.: Applying scheduling policies to improve QoE in wireless Voice-over-IP. In: 28th IEEE International Performance and Communications Conference (IPCCC). IEEE Press, New York (2009)

Session 10

Mobile Devices and Wireless Technologies for Patient Monitoring

Proof of the Accuracy of Measuring Pants to Evaluate the Activity of the Hip and Legs in Everyday Life

Khalil Niazmand, Ian Somlai, Slim Louizi, and Tim C. Lueth

MiMed, Department of Micro Technology and Medical Device Technology
Faculty of Mechanical Engineering, Technische Universität München
Boltzmannstraße 15, D-85748 Garching
khalil.niazmand@tum.de

Abstract. In this paper, an innovative measuring platform for the detection of movements of legs and hips is presented and tested. The system consists of washable pants with built-in acceleration sensors and control and evaluation electronics and is powered by detachable, rechargeable batteries. It measures acceleration at the hip and legs in three directions in space. The movement detection is based on recognizing, by means of the sensors, the posture and acceleration magnitudes usually associated to a specific movement. The raw sensor data are saved on the integrated MicroSD card for posterior analyze in a computer. With the help of mathematical functions presented in this paper, the timely occurrence of a specific movement can finally be detected. The whole system (pants, sensors and electronics) is washable due to component's encapsulation. Thanks to an optimized production process, the system can be affordably reproduced in low volume productions and can be adjusted for multiple purposes.

Keywords: accelerometer / pants / movement.

1 Introduction

Demographic change represents a high burden on the society in Germany and other industrialized countries. The associated costs increase for the social health system might be diminished by means of newly developed assistance systems that focus rather on prevention than on cure.

An important component of Pervasive Care is to collect and analyze health-related data in everyday life. Besides the usual vital parameters, there are also data that permit to get conclusions about the movements of the supervised person.

Sensors for motion detection are continuously becoming smaller, cheaper and more accurate. The evaluation of the data delivered by these sensors is also becoming easier.

By integrating these sensors in garments and subsequently analyzing the data obtained from them, the movements recorded for the user can be detected and documented. Collecting these data over a long period of time allows to characterize the movement habits of the person. Unexpected changes to these patterns can then be used for early detection of potentially disease-related behaviours. As a result, it is possible to initiate appropriate therapy measures.

J. Lin and K.S. Nikita (Eds.): MobiHealth 2010, LNICST 55, pp. 235–244, 2011.
© Institute for Computer Sciences, Social Informatics and Telecommunications Engineering 2011

2 State of the Art

Intelligent assistance systems are already used in telemedicine in the tertiary prevention for the monitoring of chronically ill people. The future of such systems lies in a better integration into daily life and easier usability, so that they can also be implemented for early detection of diseases and for the reduction of risk factors. In 1990, many leading groups in the area of portable integrated sensors predicted the growing integrity of wireless communication as well as the sensor system in everyday clothing [1]. According to [2], the applications of wearable sensors can be divided into six areas: military, civilian (home care and sports), aerospace, public safety (fire fighting), hazardous applications (mine action) and universal (portable mobile applications).

Nowadays, accelerometers are among the most used sensors for these applications. In [3], accelerometers are used in garments in order to carry out localization as well as activity measurement. In [4], acceleration sensors included in garments are used for rehabilitation scopes, where the movements of the upper part of the body are registered and assigned to a particular movement. The same kind of sensors, also attached to the upper part of the body, can be used for respiratory and heart rate measurements [5, 6]. Furthermore, different temperatures can be classified by recognizing tremor [7]. The position of the sensors on the body is of great importance. In [8], 30 accelerometers were distributed all over the body. It became obvious that not only the number of sensors but also their dependence on each other is very important. The challenge of building sensors in garment is that the electronics can't disturb the user and, on the other hand, to provide the necessary stability, so that the electronics aren't harmed during normal daily life movements. This leads to the conclusion that the integrated sensors should not be tight-fitting to the body. In [9], the influence of loose-fitting sensing garments is described in terms of measurement accuracy when a movement is being detected. A comparison of different systems is portrayed in table 1.

Most of the presented systems do not integrate sensors in garments [8, 10], applying them directly on the body. They either have to be attached each time with hook-and-loop fasteners at certain spots or are built in specific, tight-fitting vests. The wearing comfort isn't taken into account.

In order to warrant a long-term recording of data, the measurement garment must be washable, making its production more complicated. There is, on one hand, the possibility of using washable and conductive sensor textiles [11, 4], which increases

Table 1. Summary of the state of the art

Ref.	Sensor	Application	Washable
[1]	NM	None	Yes
[4]	AC	Rehabilitation	Yes
[5]	AC	Heart frequency	No
[6]	AC	Respiration rate	No
[7]	AC	Temperature	No
[8]	AC	Movement	No
[10]	AC	Movement	No
[11]	AC	Movement	Yes

the production costs tremendously. On the other hand, there is the option of an external wiring that has to be removed before washing, which complicates the implementation of such systems in everyday life.

3 Task and Approach

By means of acceleration sensors integrated in a pair of pants, the movements of the hip and legs should be detected. The collected data should be stored on a removable storage medium and analyzed by the user. The electronics should be encapsulated inside a washable unit and the system's power supply should be provided by re-chargeable batteries. It is very important that the whole system doesn't hinder the movements of the user while wearing it. The accuracy of such a garment to determine movements has to be proven. By building this system, the basis for long-term re-cording and analysis of transaction data is created.

4 Dynamic System Concept Description

The pants (Fig. 1, 1) don't differ from a normal garment externally. In its interior, there are five acceleration sensors (2), which measure the movements of the hip and the legs.

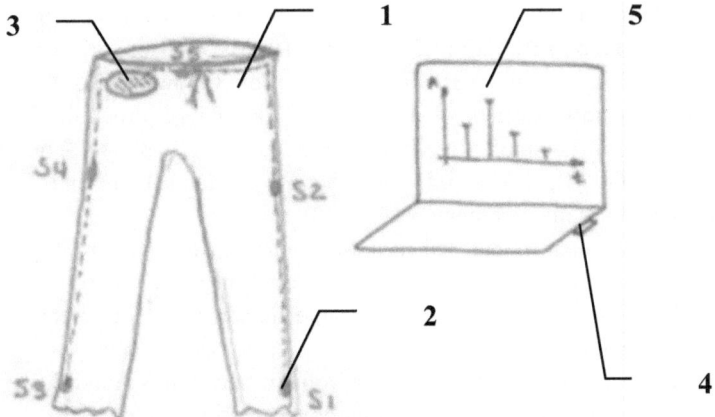

Fig. 1. Description of the system's parts and interfaces

The system is powered by a detachable, rechargeable battery box and the electron-ics installed in the garment are not easily noticeable by the user. The sensors are made washable thanks to encapsulation and connected with a shielded cable network with the electronics unit, which is built in a washable housing and hidden in a pocket. As a result, the measuring pants can be washed whenever necessary without concerns of damaging the integrated electronics.

The pants are dressed just as any other normal ones. The data recording settings, such as time, measurement duration, number of readings per second and software version, are entered in form of a text file on the storage medium (MicroSD card) directly on a computer. The MicroSD card is then inserted into the electronic unit. After the power supply has been ensured by fixing the battery box, the electronic unit reads the saved settings and accordingly sets the desired configurations. The data recording begins then corresponding to the entered settings and the information delivered by the sensors is read and stored on the MicroSD card. At the end of the experience, the battery box is detached and the storage unit can be removed. The data contained in the MicroSD card is subsequently read on a computer, where an algorithm to evaluate the activity of the hip and legs in everyday life can be developed and tested.

The system is characterized by a simple and universal application and a fast and economical production. Additionally, the user is not hindered by the measurement system in his daily life and has the opportunity to wash the garment when needed.

5 Evaluation

5.1 Materials and Methods

In order to define the location of the sensors on certain parts of the body and to protect the cable network, a protective bag made of fabric was sewn in by a tailor along the seam on the garment's inner side. The 3-Axis acceleration sensor (SMB380, Robert Bosch GmbH) delivers digital values that are read over an SPI-interface. Its measuring range can be set to $\pm 2g$, $\pm 4g$ or $\pm 8g$. The five sensors are connected to the electronics unit through a cable network (cross section: 0.1 mm² with PVC isolation).

The electronics unit consists of a nanoLOC module (microcontroller and radio transceiver, Nanotron Technologies GmbH) (Fig. 2, 1), a RV-8564-C2 real-time clock (Micro Crystal AG) (3), a MicroSD-card slot (4), a status LED and the necessary components for power management (2).

The electronics unit is integrated in a washable housing (Polar Electro Oy). The original electrical connections of the housing (press-buttons) are used for plugging the battery-box. The connection between the cable network and the electronics unit is sealed by an encapsulation.

The electronics in this system requires a voltage between 3.5 and 4.5 V. It is provided by a rechargeable battery box (5) that consists of an accumulator with a capacity of 350 mAh, a MAX1555 charging chip (Maxim Integrated Products, Inc.), a USB socket for charging the battery and a charge-status LED.

Each set of data is stored in an individual text file with the name DD_HH-MM.txt, where DD represents the current day of the month, HH the hour and MM the minutes of the measurement recording time. The configuration parameters of the measurement are saved in another file with the name config.txt, where the device number, software version, time, date and number of recordings per second can be set. For this reason, this configuration file has to be updated before valid data recording.

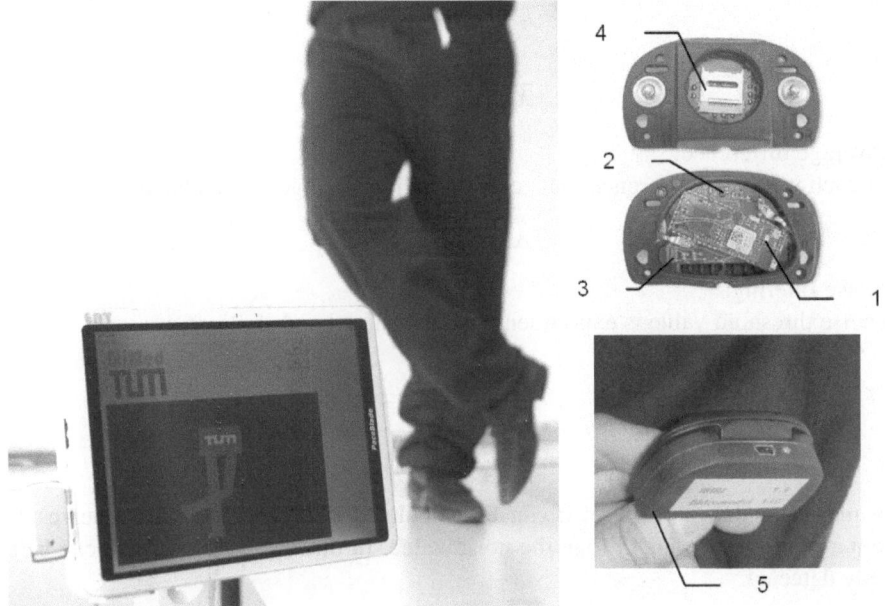

Fig. 2. Left side: Pants being used. Right side, above: electronics unit. Right side, below: battery.

For this experiment, the pants with the number "1" were chosen. The configuration file was set so that the five acceleration sensors should be read 10 times per second with a resolution of ± 4g. In addition, data should be stored every two minutes in a newly generated text file. The obtained raw data in text format could be directly imported into a spreadsheet application such as Microsoft Excel.

Five calculations are then implemented to analyze it. These are:

- Absolute resulting acceleration:
The resulting magnitude of the three coordinates (x, y and z) is calculated as follows:

$$|a| = \left\| \begin{pmatrix} a_x \\ a_y \\ a_z \end{pmatrix} \right\| = \sqrt{a_x^2 + a_y^2 + a_z^2}$$

- Normalization according to Earth's gravity:
The value of Earth's gravitation, g, according to the sensor resolution, is subtracted:

$$(\pm 4g = -512 \ldots +512 \ \rightarrow \ +g \cong 128)$$

$$X = |a| - g$$

- Data average:
The average of the 10 recorded data (recording 10 times per second, $T_0 = 100ms$) is generated as follows:

$$n = 10 \cdot T_0$$

$$\overline{X_{10}[k]} = \sum_{n=k}^{n=k-9} X[k] \Big/ 10$$

- Average difference:
For each value the difference to its corresponding average is calculated:

$$\Delta X[k] = X[k] - \overline{X}[k]$$

- Noise filtering:
A noise threshold value is experimentally determined and applied:
    Noise value = 5 ≅ 0.04 g

$$X = \begin{cases} X & \rightarrow \ |X| \geq 5 \\ 0 & \rightarrow \ |X| < 5 \end{cases}$$

By means of this procedure, it can be calculated if an acceleration value resulting from a movement is larger than the noise value. In this case, a movement can be correctly detected.

5.2 Experiment

An experiment is performed in order to confirm the hypothesis that, by means of the measuring pants, it is possible to detect the occurrence in time of daily life movements of the hip and legs. To assess the effectiveness and accuracy of the proposed method, further experiments with more volunteers are being planned.

A person (male, 30 years old) carried out the following activity five times, after having washed the pants once in a washing machine with a protective laundry bag (Wash settings: 30°C (86°F), max spin cycle 900 rpm). First, the person left the pants on the table for 10 seconds. Next, he puts them on and sits on the chair for another 10 seconds. After this, he stands up, walks slowly for 10 seconds and then stands still for five seconds. Next, he runs for 10 seconds and then stands still again for five seconds. After this, he lies down on the bed for 20 seconds and, finally, sits on the chair for ten seconds.

5.3 Result

The time progression of the gathered data, after being processed with the 5 mentioned calculations, can be seen in fig. 3.

The noise threshold value has to be chosen in such a way so that daily life movements can still be recognized. If it is too high, the movements of the legs aren't detected. If the noise value is too low, a great amount of disturbing additional information is being transferred besides the useful movements. In all five attempts, an alteration of the movement pattern could be detected with every single sensor. In fig. 4, the diagram of sensor SBV (waist in the front) is analyzed as an example.

All signal changes could be attributed to the respective activity. A histogram of the evaluated data confirms that when choosing the noise value, no crucial information that is important for the detection of movements goes astray (fig. 5).

Applying the Fast Fourier Transformation to the analyzed data, it is claimed additionally that a recording frequency of 6 times per second would provide all relevant information.

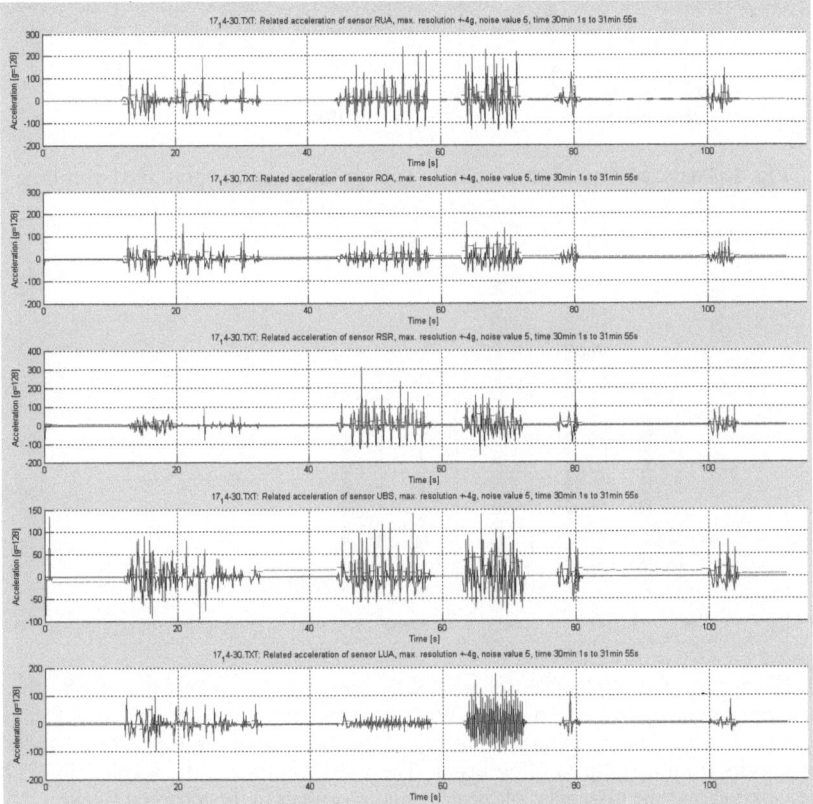

Fig. 3. The recorded data are portrayed according to the sensor location. From the top: RUS= right lower thigh, ROS=right upper thigh, LOS= left upper thigh, LUS= left upper thigh, SBV= waist in the front. The x-axis represents the time in seconds after the beginning of the recording and the y-axis is the registered acceleration amplitude (128 ≙ 1g).

The hypothesis "With the measuring pants, the time occurrence of daily life movements of the hip and legs can be detected" was confirmed in this experiment. The recorded data was subject to five analysis calculations and the obtained values were portrayed in a diagram over the time. The actions carried out in the experiment could be correspondingly assigned in time to the observed data. It was observed that, merely for movement detection, one single sensor (SBV) would be sufficient. However, with five sensors, respective movements of the single body parts can be compared with each other.

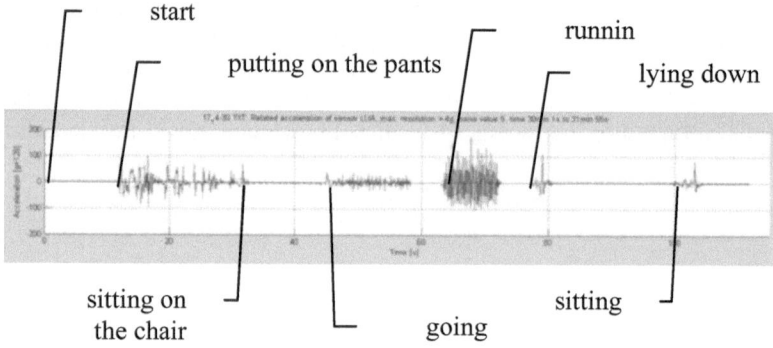

Fig. 4. Analyzed data of sensor SBV (waist in the front) are portrayed over time

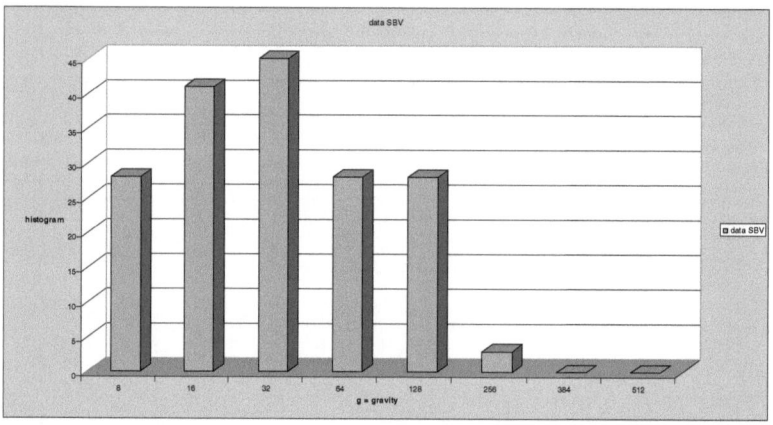

Fig. 5. Histogram of the calculated data of SBV sensor. It is obvious that due to the movements, accelerations up to 2 g can occur. With the elimination of all acceleration values lower that 0,04 g, no crucial information goes astray. If the movements are very slow, usually acceleration sensors from 0,1g up to 0.6 g occur. The x-axis represents the acceleration (128 = g) and the y-axis shows the histogram of the acceleration values in the recorded signal.

As the pants aren't essentially tight-fitting, the sensors don't have an absolute position in terms of the skin surface. Since accurate detection of an activity, such as sitting on a chair, standing or lying, depends largely on the position of sensors, no reliable detection can be implemented applying only one single sensor. An intelligently designed spatial distribution of several sensors could then decrease the error rate and lead to a feasible detection, broadening the field of application.

6 Conclusions

The first prototype of a movement detection system based on measuring pants was presented. It differs from other systems as the sensors are unobtrusively built in the pants and is completely washable. Furthermore, data can be saved on a removable MicroSD card. Functions have been introduced to detect hip and legs movements with a resolution of 0,04g exclusively by means of acceleration sensors. The algorithm was validated in concluding experiments, whose satisfactory results revealed that detection of the timely occurrence of movements is possible with the pants. It was found out that, although the pants are loose-fitting, one single sensor would be sufficient for the detection of movements. However, combining several distributed sensors, certain movements such as e.g. lying, sitting and standing can be detected immediately. Further experiments involving a greater number of volunteers are being planned, in order to assess the effectiveness and accuracy of the proposed method.

Acknowledgment

Within the research consortium of the Bavarian Research Foundation (BFS) „FitForAge" a team of scientists and engineers affiliated to 13 departments of the Bavarian universities Erlangen-Nürnberg, München, Regensburg and Würzburg works together with 25 industrial partners on the development of products and services for the aging society.

The scope of the research consortium is to develop technology based solutions which will help elderly people in their future living environment comprising home and workplace as well as in communication and transportation. Eventually not only elderly people but also all social groups should profit from these solutions.

References

1. Iso-Ketola, P., Karinsalo, T., Myry, T., Hahto, L., Karhu, H., Malmivaara, M., Vanhala, J.: A Mobile Device as User Interface for Wearable Applications, PERMID Munich. LMU Munich, Germany (2005)
2. Sungmee, P., Jayaraman, S.: Enhancing the quality of life through wearable technology. IEEE 22(3) (2003)
3. Lukowicz, P., Junker, H., Stäger, M., von Büren, T., Tröster, G.: WearNET: A Distributed Multi-sensor System for Context Aware Wearables. In: Borriello, G., Holmquist, L.E. (eds.) UbiComp 2002. LNCS, vol. 2498, pp. 361–370. Springer, Heidelberg (2002)
4. Harms, H., Amft, O., Roggen, D., Tröster, G.: Smash: A distributed sensing and processing garment for the classification of upper body postures. In: Third Interational Conference on Body Area Networks (2008)
5. Yoshimura, T., Yonezawa, Y., Maki, H., Ogawa, H., Ninomiya, I., Caldwell, W.M.: An ECG electrode-mounted heart rate, respiratory rhythm, posture and behavior recording system. In: Proceedings of the 26th Annual International Conference of the IEEE EMBS San Francisco, CA, USA, September 1-5 (2004)
6. Reinvuo, T., Hannula, M., Sorvoja, H., Alasaarela, E., Myllyla, R.: Measurement of Respiratory Rate with High-Resolution Accelerometer and EMFit Pressure Sensor. In: SAS 2006 – IEEE Sensors Applications Symposium Houston, Texas USA, February 7-9 (2006)
7. Sung, M., DeVaul, R., Jimenez, S., Gips, J., Pentland, A.S.: A Shiver Motion and Core Body Temperature Classification for Wearable Soldier Health Monitoring Systems. In: IEEE International Symposium of Wearable Computers (2004)

8. Van Laerhoven, K., Schmidt, A., Gellersen, H.-W.: Multi-Sensor Context- Aware Clothing. In: Sixth International Symposium on Wearable Computers, ISWC 2002, pp. 49–57. IEEE Press, Los Alamitos (2002)
9. Harms, H., Amft, O., Troster, G.: Influence of a loose-fitting sensing garment on posture recognition in rehabilitation. In: Biomedical Circuits and Systems Conference (2008)
10. Guler, M., Ertugrul, S.: Measuring and Transmitting Vital Body Signs Using MEMS Sensors, RFID Eurasia, 1st Annual, September 5-6, pp. 1–4. IEEE, Los Alamitos (2007)
11. Noury, N., Dittmar, A., Corroy, C., Baghai, R., Weber, J.L., Blanc, D., Klefstat, F., Blinovska, A., Vaysse, S., Comet, B.: VTAMN - A Smart Clothe for Ambulatory Remote Monitoring of Physiological Parameters and Activity. In: 26th Annual International Conference of the IEEE EMBS San Francisco, CA, USA, September 1-5 (2004)

Nano-coating Protection of Medical Devices

S.R. Coulson and D.R. Evans

P2i Ltd, 127 North, Milton Park, Abingdon, Oxfordshire, OX14 4SA, UK

1 Introduction

Consumer and industrial products are manufactured from a range of materials that are selected for specific bulk properties, cost and/or 'look and feel'. However, many materials chosen in this way do not display the optimum surface properties. This presents an opportunity for surface modifications to apply desirable properties such as fire retardancy, anti-microbial, protein resistance and, water and oil repellency.

It is critical that these modifications do not alter the bulk properties of the product and retain desirable physical attributes. Additionally, they should be ultra-thin and well adhered. For commercial success, the desired effect needs to be a cost-effective and robust industrial process.

Plasmas [1] have long been known for their use for modifying the surface properties of materials [2]. It is widely accepted that fluorinated materials are required for maximizing the levels of liquid repellency [3], [4]. A novel, patented liquid-repellent technology, by P2i, can readily apply a functional nano-coating onto the surface of a wide variety of items made from a diverse range of materials [5]. This is created using a pulsed plasma deposition process at low pressure which allows full penetration of complex products [6].

This liquid repellent effect optimizes the surface properties to radically improve performance and protect items for extended use, adding considerable value to the product in question both as a suitable differentiator and/or a cost saver.

This article provides an overview of the technology and examples of its commercial application.

2 Repellency

PTFE is the benchmark low surface energy material with a surface energy of 18 mN/m. It is very good at repelling water, but low surface tension liquids (such as oil) spread out. In order to create high levels of oil repellency, it is necessary to orientate the fluorinated chains normal to the substrate surface. This can lower surface energies to values as low as 6 mN/m. Fluorinated chains with this particular orientation can readily be created using plasmas.

3 What Is a Plasma?

A plasma is an ionised gas, often referred to as the fourth state of matter. The gas becomes ionised through the application of energy. We create our plasmas by applying radio frequency (RF) electro-magnetic radiation. This lets us control the degree of

J. Lin and K.S. Nikita (Eds.): MobiHealth 2010, LNICST 55, pp. 245–251, 2011.
© Institute for Computer Sciences, Social Informatics and Telecommunications Engineering 2011

ionisation and thus retain key functional groups at the surface, giving rise to the required technical effects.

4 P2i Plasma Process

The process is carried out in a chamber that is pumped to low pressure. The raw materials of gases and vapours are bled into the chamber at this reduced pressure and the plasma is ignited using a RF generator to create the activated state.

As the plasma is a gaseous medium at low pressure, it will readily permeate complex 3D structures and penetrate narrow structures at the sub-micron level. This means a wide range of complex products such as garments and medical devices can be molecularly tailored at the nanometre scale and display desirable properties not shown by the underlying substrate. The technical effect can be applied to a wide range of materials including fibres, plastics, paper, ceramics and glass.

The technology originally used a 0.5 litre chamber, and this has since been scaled through volumes up to 2000 litres. This allows large items or high volumes of small components to be processed.

Plasmas can extensively fragment molecules, but the degree of molecular breakdown can be controlled by reducing the power through pulsing. This creates the required active species to attach to the substrate, and retains the chemical integrity of the starting chemical. This allows specific chemical functionalization at the molecular level.

Critical surface tension of wetting results, on a flat surface, have shown values as low as 4.3 mN/m (cf PTFE ~ 18 mN/m), which explains why high contact angles result with a range of liquids and low liquid retention properties are displayed on a wide number of surfaces.

5 Results and Discussion

Experiment 1: To baseline the liquid repellent technology, 3M repellent test methods were used to determine the level of repellency both before and after processing with the liquid repellent nano-coating technology. Although several materials appear not to repel the highest rating liquids, they do in fact support the droplet due to the specific definitions of the test (it is classed as a fail due to slight surface wetting). Figs. 1 and 2

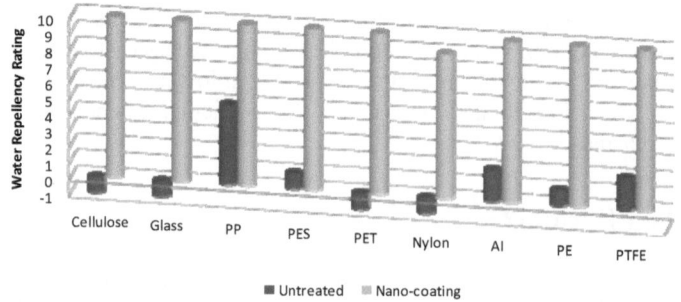

Fig. 1. 3M Water repellency of a variety of uncoated and nano-coated materials

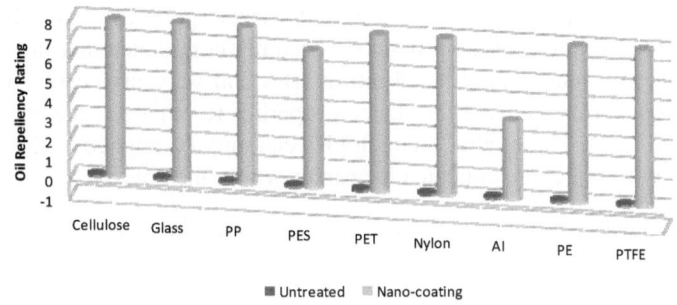

Fig. 2. 3M oil repellency of a variety of uncoated and nano-coated materials

demonstrate the water and oil repellency rating before and after processing on a wide variety of materials.

As can be seen the liquid repellent nano-coating radically improves the liquid repellent performance; no material is inherently oil repellent.

Following the sweat drop test the level of corrosion is assessed visually. As can be seen in Fig. 3, no visible corrosion occurs after the nano-coating process due to its ability to readily penetrate the complex structures.

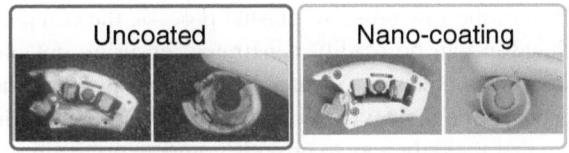

Fig. 3. Uncoated and nano-coated hearing instrument parts after sweat drop testing

Experiment 2– Electronics

P2i's nano-coating technology for the electronics sector is Aridion™, which has been optimized to give the highest throughput for fully constructed electronic devices.

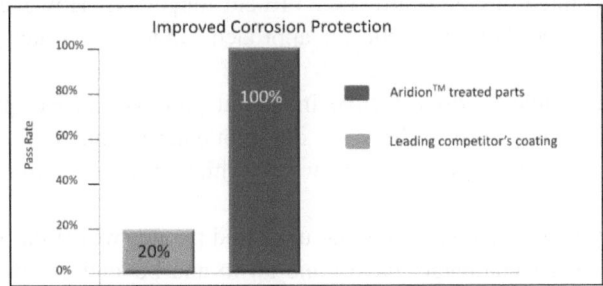

Fig. 4. Improved corrosion protection following Aridion™ treatment is not experienced with other technologies

A much greater proportion of Aridion™ treated products pass corrosion tests (Fig. 4), leading to longer-lived products, consumer confidence that the instrument is working correctly, plus both reduced return rates and warranty costs. Aridion™ also demonstrates superior abrasion resistance properties to other surface coatings used in the industry (Fig 5). These other technologies can only be applied to the plastic housing and so don't protect the delicate electronics within the device.

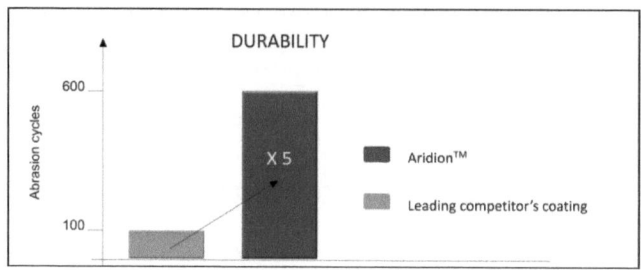

Fig. 5. Aridion™ demonstrates five times higher durability than competitor surface coatings

Further work in electronics has focused on mobile phones, demonstrating the huge benefits from applying a gas phase ionization process to the fully completed unit.

Due to the nature of the low pressure plasma process, the complex construction of a mobile phone handset can be readily penetrated, ensuring not only that the outer casing has an increased protection to water ingress, but also that the water repellent properties are present inside the device, adequately protecting the delicate electronics.

It is well known that the only way to provide compete protection to devices such as mobile phones is to build in a physical barrier with no holes for gas or liquid to penetrate. This can only realistically be delivered by a fully sealable box using an o-ring or gasket seal. That does not provide a market-acceptable solution, since the look and feel of the device are ever more critical in a hugely competitive market.

One of the main failure modes of mobile phones is through water or moisture damage due to ingress of rain water. Incumbent technologies look at providing protection to the internal printed circuit board (PCB) to aid longevity. However, not only can these suffer from poor adhesion, but this approach cannot stop water getting into the device.

By having available a cost effective industrial process that can protect the fully constructed end device, most of the water does not enter the handset in the first place. This meansthere is minimal exposure to water; which translates into longer operating times.

In-house testing has demonstrated that untreated phones which fail within 2-4 minutes of a spray water challenge, have gone up to and beyond 30 minutes of testing without failure, when treated with Aridion™. Equally importantly, the process does not affect the look or feel of the device, and has passed the temperature and humidity cycling tests required to demonstrate efficacy in all operating environments.

This experience and application is directly relevant for the medical device sector, where electronic devices are used either at point-of-care or in retail environments. There is a strong drive towards miniaturizing these devices for a closer resemblance to 'cool' products such as mobile phones and MP3 players. This makes protection from liquid ingress increasingly difficult to achieve. In addition, corrosion and failure problems associated with liquid ingress of point-of-care devices leads to expensive bureaucracy and negative brand impact, due to the open reporting laws.

Experiment 4 – Life Sciences: Under increased pressure to discover new drugs and therapeutics, ever greater levels of precision are required in routine analysis and day-to-day laboratory work. In addition, chemical cocktails or starting samples can be very expensive or minimally available, putting pressure on liquid handling capabilities to maximize utilization. Low retention technologies are highly valued for many applications to maximize recovery and reduce residues. Fig. 6 demonstrates that the nano-coating out-performs standard, untreated tips and other low-retention technologies.

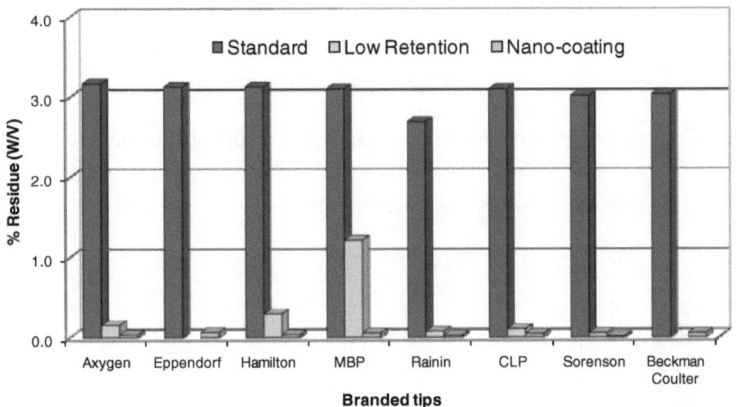

Fig. 6. Nano-coated pipette tips outperform both standard and other low retention tips

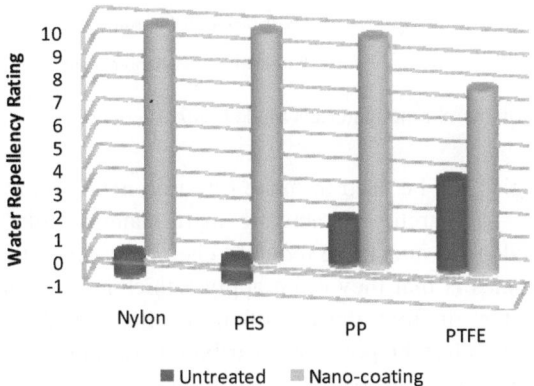

Fig. 7. Common membrane materials made highly hydrophobic using a nano-coating

Experiment 5 – Energy & Filtration: Filtration media rarely display the desired surface properties and will generally benefit from being either highly hydrophilic or highly hydrophobic. Figs. 7 and 8 demonstrate how the liquid repellent nano-coating increases the levels of water and oil repellency allowing the media to perform in harsher environments or out-perform current materials in use.

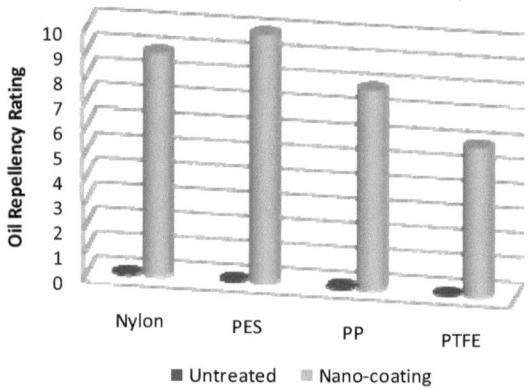

Fig. 8. Common membrane materials made highly oleophobic using a nano-coating

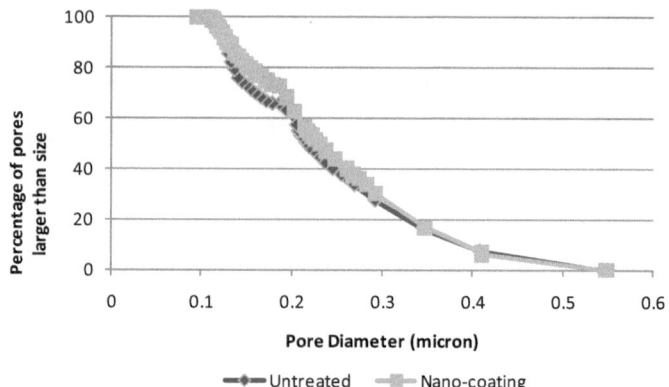

Fig. 9. Common membrane materials made highly oleophobic using a nano-coating

Other technologies can be used to make filtration media more repellent; however, many suffer from an inability to activate inert materials like polypropylene and polytetrafluoroethylene to attach the required chemistry. One other drawback of conventional technologies is that they often apply a thick coating that can block up the pores and change the air-flow and use of the media. Fig. 9 demonstrates how the nano-coating does not alter the pore size distribution, despite the increase in water and oil repellency. This allows it to be used for all intended applications (and many more besides), due to increased performance levels.

6 Conclusions

Imparting a highly water and oil repellent nano-coating has been demonstrated to improve the performance of several everyday commercial and industrial products. The efficacy of the nano-coating has been proven first through laboratory verification, second in production prototyping and third through deployment in cost-effective industrial processes. By providing protection to fully constructed devices, many of the previously encountered issues are overcome, leading to a new opportunity to reduce product return rates, which boosts brand perception and reduces costs.

References

[1] Grill, A.: Cold Plasma Materials Fabrication: From Fundamentals to Applications. Wiley, Chichester (1994)
[2] Biederman, H.: Plasma Polymer Films. Imperial College Press (2004)
[3] Kissa, E.: Fluorinated Surfactants and Repellent. Marcel Dekker, New York (2001)
[4] Kissa, E.: Functional Finishes Part B. In: Lewin, M., Sello, S.B. (eds.) Handbook of Fibre Science', vol. II. Marcel Dekker, New York (1984)
[5] Coulson, S.R., Brewer, S.A., Willis, C.R., Badyal, J.P.S.: GB Pat. Patent: WO 98/58117
[6] Coulson, S.R., Woodward, I.S., Badyal, J.P.S., Brewer, S.A., Willis, C.R.: Ultralow Surface Energy Plasma Polymer Films. Chem. Mater. 104, 2031–2038 (2000)

A UHF Radio Frequency Identification (RFID) System for Healthcare: Design and Implementation

Anastasis C. Polycarpou[1], George Gregoriou[1], Panayiotis Polycarpou[2],
Loizos Papaloizou[1], Aggelos Bletsas[3], Antonis Dimitriou[4], and John Sahalos[4]

[1] Cyprus Academic Research Institute, Metochiou 66, 2407 Nicosia, Cyprus
[2] University of Cyprus, 75 Kallipoleos, Nicosia, 1678, Cyprus
[3] Technical University of Crete, 73100 Chania, Greece
[4] Aristotle University of Thessaloniki, 54124 Thessaloniki, Greece
{polycarpou.a,gregoriou.g}@unic.ac.cy,
{polikarpou.panayiotis,papaloizou.loizos}@ucy.ac.cy,
aggelos@telecom.tuc.gr, antodimi@ee.auth.gr, sahalos@auth.gr

Abstract. This paper presents a customized design of a UHF Radio Frequency Identification (RFID) system to be installed at the Bank of Cyprus Oncology Center (BOCOC) in Cyprus. This is a pilot project that aims at evaluating the effectiveness and overall benefits of UHF RFID technology in the healthcare sector. The purpose of the project is threefold: a) Error-free identification of in-hospital patients through the use of RFID wristbands/cards; b) drug inventory control and monitoring; c) Real Time Location Service (RTLS) capable of locating tagged objects within the premises of the hospital. For the three main pillars of the project, a Graphical User Interface (GUI) was developed in order to run on light-weight medical tablet PCs. The application can access data from a secured central database hosting sensitive information regarding patients, drugs, medical assets, and high-value equipment. The communication between the server and the medical tablet PCs is done over an encrypted wireless local access network.

Keywords: RFID, e-health, patient identification, drug inventory control, RTLS, smart labels.

1 Introduction

RFID technology uses radio frequency signals to identify objects that are equipped with RFID tags. The RFID tags utilized in this project are passive UHF tags composed of a printed antenna and an integrated chip hosting a unique 96-bit identification code. The technology is based on the UHF-band EPC C1 Gen2 data exchange protocol between the tag and the reader (interrogator). The interrogator launches a UHF signal (30dBm) which impinges on a number of RFID tags in its vicinity and, from the modulated backscattered field, the reader is able to read and identify hundreds of these tags per second. Identification of objects is possible when the tagged objects are located within the area of coverage of the interrogator's antenna, even when there is no direct line-of-sight between the two. This is a major advantage of RFID technology over the well-accepted and widely-used barcode technology where

J. Lin and K.S. Nikita (Eds.): MobiHealth 2010, LNICST 55, pp. 252–259, 2011.

the reader must be in contact with the barcode label. The maximum distance between the interrogator and an RFID tag, in order to allow readability, depends on the total link budget between the two devices, which in turn depends on the sensitivities of the interrogator and the tag, the gain of the reader's antenna in the direction of the tag, the sensitivity and input impedance of the chip, the propagation loss, the cable losses, the communication protocol, etc. Our primary objective in this pilot project was to optimize our design in order to achieve maximum RFID coverage in the premises of the hospital at minimum cost. For this purpose, we used ray-tracing algorithms, optimization tools, and electromagnetic simulation software, where several parameters have been taken into consideration, in order to properly design the RFID system. The number of antennas placed in each of the hospital's patient rooms and the precise location and orientation of these antennas were judiciously chosen in order to maximize RFID coverage and reduce the probability of "fail-to-read" a tag.

This project was designed to help medical personnel overcome major problems that are nowadays present in a hospital environment. Routine hospital tasks, like drug prescription or drug administration, are based on paper-bound processes that are prone to human errors thus putting patients in great danger on an everyday basis. The US Institute of Medicine estimates that more than 44,000 deaths occur each year in the US due to in-hospital medication errors [1]. The US Food and Drug Administration (FDA) estimates that medical errors approach 40% in paper-based environments. Simply stated, there are patient mix-up errors due to paper-bound processes which often end up in serious health problems for the hospitalized people. With the launch of an RFID system, in-hospital patients will be given a unique identification code, in the form of an RFID wristband or a plastic card, which will be automatically identified by a handheld UHF RFID reader attached to a light-weight medical tablet PC in the hands of a medical doctor or nurse. Once the patient is uniquely identified, the tablet will upload from the central database the patient's medical profile and relevant information. This is the first major pillar of the pilot RFID project.

The second pillar of the project is drug inventory control and monitoring. Drugs are usually stored in inventory rooms which are extremely difficult to monitor on a daily basis. Drugs may expire without noticing; drugs are sometimes removed from the inventory room without authorization; in other cases, drugs run out without the pharmacist being aware of it. It is estimated that approximately 10% of the inventory drugs are lost every year [2]. Unavailability of certain drugs may certainly put patients in great danger. Tagging each drug with a unique RFID allows the pharmacist to monitor drug inventory at all times.

The third pillar of the project is locating and tracking tagged objects in the premises of the hospital. Such objects may include patient files, infusion pumps, wheelchairs, walkers, expensive medical equipment, and even medical personnel. It is estimated that hospital employees spend approximately 25-33% of their time searching for medical equipment [2]. This translates to a waste of valuable time, inefficiency, and low productivity at workplace. The problem can be effectively solved by tagging objects or equipment with passive RFIDs, and by using the RTLS system with a network of antennas and stationary readers, these objects can be located and tracked everywhere in the premises of the hospital. Of course, a successful implementation of this idea mandates a careful design of the RFID system taking into account all possible factors ranging from the current needs of the medical personnel at workplace to major engineering issues such as electromagnetic coverage, tag readability, electromagnetic interference with other devices, security, privacy of sensitive data, etc. All these have been considered and carefully studied in order to be able to design and implement a system that meets all the specifications and expectations of the research team involved – including, of course, the medical personnel of the hospital.

2   RFID System Design and Implementation

The RFID system under development will be installed in one of the two hospital wards (Ward A) of the Bank of Cyprus Oncology Center in Nicosia, Cyprus. The top view of the hospital ward is shown in Fig. 1. Due to limitations in research funds, the system will provide electromagnetic (EM) coverage only for three patient rooms (Rooms 33-35) and for a drug inventory cabinet sitting in the area of the nurse station (indicated as 14-15 in Fig. 1). Nevertheless, this small-scale installation is deemed sufficient for the purpose of the project as our primary goal is to evaluate the designed RFID system in a realistic hospital environment and to draw valuable conclusions as to the effectiveness and the overall benefits of this technology for the patient and the healthcare system in general. At the time when this paper is being written, the RFID system has been only partially installed at the BOCOC. No measurements or testing has been performed, yet. The only measurements and testing of the system was carried out in a laboratory setting. A number of meetings have been organized between the developers/designers of the system and the medical personnel of the BOCOC in order to obtain feedback and valuable suggestions that can be used toward improving and perfecting the capabilities of the application.

For the design and implementation of the system, the following major devices were acquired: a) Handheld and stationary readers supporting the UHF ETSI (EN 302 208) band of frequencies together with the EPC Class 1 Generation 2 protocol which is characterized by a better anti-collision scheme as compared to previous generation protocols and, therefore, higher percentage of tag readability; b) A network based RFID printer that can support a wide variety of passive inlay tags. This type of printer can program RFID tags before they are attached to objects. The printer communicates with the front application via a local area network (LAN/WLAN) in order to, first, record a specific tag ID to the SQL database and, second, associate this unique ID number to a specific object; c) Tablet PCs for medical applications having specific characteristics including Wi-Fi capabilities, light weight, long-lasting batteries, ease of charging, USB ports, ability to disinfect; d) Wireless Access Points (APs) that will provide adequate coverage at high bit rates everywhere in the hospital ward; e) RFID antennas that are circularly polarized, with low Voltage Standing Wave Ratio (VSWR), high gain, moderate beamwidth, etc.; f) Low-loss coaxial cables to allow transmission and reception without significant attenuation due to cable loss; g) Computer server to host a secured central database housing sensitive information regarding patients, medical personnel, assets, drugs, patient files, etc.; h) Effective RFID tags that can be used for asset tracking as well as drug inventory control. The tags must provide high enough sensitivity in order to support long-range reading capabilities. Fig. 2 illustrates a block diagram of the RFID system design for hospital applications along with the interconnectivity of the devices involved. For example, the RFID printer will be installed at the pharmacy of the hospital and will be networked. Through the use of the application, the pharmacist will be able to access the printer, read an unused RFID label, obtain the corresponding unique EPC code, assign this code to a drug or asset, type his/her comments and/or associated expiration date, and store this information onto the secured database. The label can then be attached to the particular drug or asset and sent to its final destination. Once in the database, the tagged object can be uniquely identified or located if seen by the networked antennas.

In achieving a good RFID system design for a healthcare environment, the research team carefully examined the suggestions and recommendations of the medical personnel of the hospital. A network of highly efficient antennas was designed in order to provide maximum RF coverage inside the patient room, thus allowing a high degree of tag identification. The antenna gain is 7 dBi and the corresponding elevation and azimuth beamwidths are approximately 72 degrees. They exhibit VSWR below 1.3 within the band of interest (865-870 MHz) and the Front-to-Back (F/B) ratio is below -17 dB. They are all Right Hand Circularly Polarized (RHCP) antennas and their physical dimensions are 19cm x 19cm. Even though we could have chosen antennas with higher gain, in order to further improve EM coverage, we decided to use the antennas with 7 dBi gain because of the smaller physical size. The antennas were connected to the ports of the stationary RFID reader using low-loss coaxial cables. As most of the ordinary coaxial cables are characterized by high losses, and since the distance between the antenna and the reader's port was approximately 10 meters, it was important to incorporate into the design coaxial cables that have very low losses, otherwise the system would fail to provide sufficient coverage within the room. The coaxial cables used in the system design are characterized by 1.3 dB/10m attenuation. Cables with lower attenuation may now be found in the market, which can certainly help further improve the performance of the system.

A number of computer simulations using electromagnetic software and ray-tracing models [3] were conducted in order to optimize antenna position and orientation as a function of RF coverage inside a typical room. Measurements were conducted in a laboratory setting in order to verify the simulation results. Tag identification was improved by using spatial and polarization diversity at the expense of using multiple tags per object. This was necessary in cases where the sensitivity of the tags used was not very low. Initially, we were using tags with -14dBm sensitivity, whereas recently we introduced tags with -17dBm sensitivity, thus allowing us to improve readability and system performance. Alternatively, we used a pair of antennas per room, instead of a single antenna, in conjunction with a two-way power splitter/combiner. The position and orientation of the antennas inside the room was optimized using a ray-tracing code [3]. Fig. 3(a) shows the field distribution inside a typical patient room when using a pair of antennas whose position was optimized in order to have maximum EM coverage. As seen in the figure, the two antennas were placed at a close proximity to each other with a certain elevation/azimuth tilt. Using this configuration and assuming tag sensitivity of -14dBm and 3dB power reduction due to the bi-directional power splitter/combiner, we can achieve 93% RF coverage inside the room. In case the two antennas are placed apart from each other, at arbitrary locations/orientations, one may observe in Fig. 3(b) the nulls of the field that are created due to destructive interference between the radiated fields by the two antennas. Thus, a judicious choice of the antenna position and orientation is necessary in order to have constructive interference between the two radiated fields and the surroundings, thus improving EM coverage and tag readability.

The benefits of using the highly sensitive tags were obvious during an experiment we recently performed at the laboratory just before we launched the installation at the BOCOC. We used a room that resembles a patient's room at the hospital and we positioned more than 130 RFID tags (-17dBm sensitivity) inside the room at different locations and heights. The tags were oriented in all different directions. The system was using a pair of antennas with 7 dBi gain along with low-attenuation cables (10m long); the antennas were positioned 2 meters high at an optimized location obtained through multiple numerical simulations using ray-tracing codes. The transmitted power was 30dBm, according to the EU directive. Allowing the stationary reader to scan the room for a maximum of 3 seconds, the system was able to identify 100% of the tags. Consequently, tag diversity may not be necessary in the case of using highly sensitive RFID tags. Note that tag sensitivity improves significantly year after year. Note also that the tags used in the experiment were attached onto a paper type of material. From other experiments performed, it was observed that a tag behaves differently when attached to a bottle filled with liquid or to a metallic container. These are issues that will be addressed at a later stage.

A user-friendly GUI was developed, according to the needs and suggestions provided by the medical staff of the BoC Oncology Center. The GUI has numerous functionalities including adding/deleting patients to/from the system database, interfacing with the handheld RFID reader attached to the USB port of the medical tablet PC, identifying patients equipped with a passive RFID tag, loading patient's medical history and profile, assigning tasks to the nurses and monitoring their tasks, allowing doctors to prescribe drugs to in-hospital patients, allowing pharmacists to monitor drug flow in and out of the inventory room, locating and tracking medical assets everywhere in the hospital ward, and more. Fig. 4(a) illustrates a front view of the GUI with an account icon for nurses, doctors, and pharmacists, an icon for inventory control and monitoring, an icon for medical asset locating and tracking, an icon for printing RFID tags for assets, and an account icon for hospital administrators. Each of the accounts has different capabilities and privileges. For example, the doctor's account allows access to prescription of drugs, whereas all other accounts do not. In addition, the administrator's account has the privilege of adding and removing accounts from the system; however, he/she cannot access patient data as these are encrypted on the database. Fig. 4(b) depicts the top view of the hospital ward indicating all medical assets/equipment that were located. This is part of the RTLS component of the project. As shown in the figure, the system of networked antennas was able to locate 1 wheelchair in room 33 and 2 wheelchairs in room 35. The application card is able to search for other type of equipment or assets such as infusion pumps, walkers, patient files, and medical/surgical equipment. It is very easy to use but very powerful, and that is exactly what makes this application suitable for the healthcare environment. A similar card can be shown for the inventory control and monitoring which tabulates all drugs found in the cabinet or inventory room (see Fig 5 (a)). By double-clicking on a particular item, more information about the drug can be shown, e.g., expiration date, type of drug, etc. Another card, shown in Fig. 5(b), depicts the profile of a patient who was uniquely identified by the system through the use of a wireless tablet PC and a handheld RFID reader. Once the patient is identified, depending on the account, his/her medical history and profile are automatically uploaded onto the screen of the tablet.

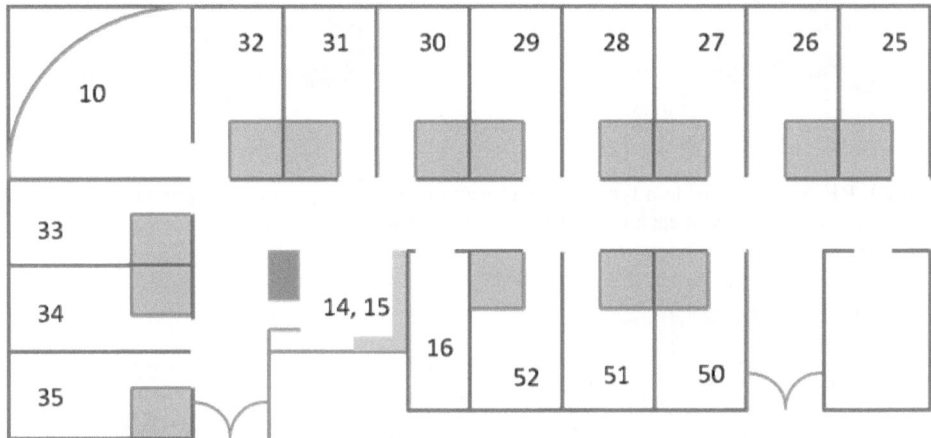

Fig. 1. The top view of the hospital Ward "A" of the Bank of Cyprus Oncology Center. The RTLS system will be installed, on a pilot basis, in rooms 33-35 and around the nurse station (14-15).

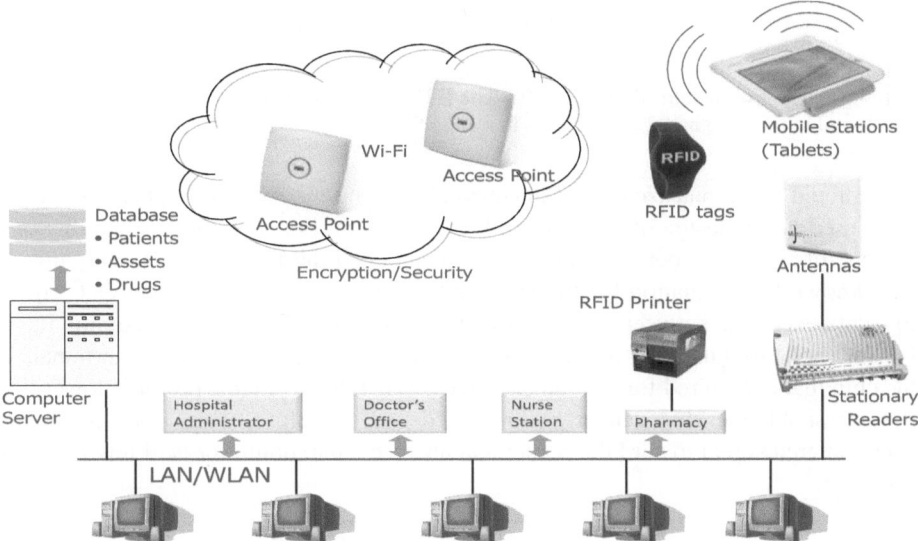

Fig. 2. Block diagram of the RFID system design that is being installed at the Bank of Cyprus Oncology Center

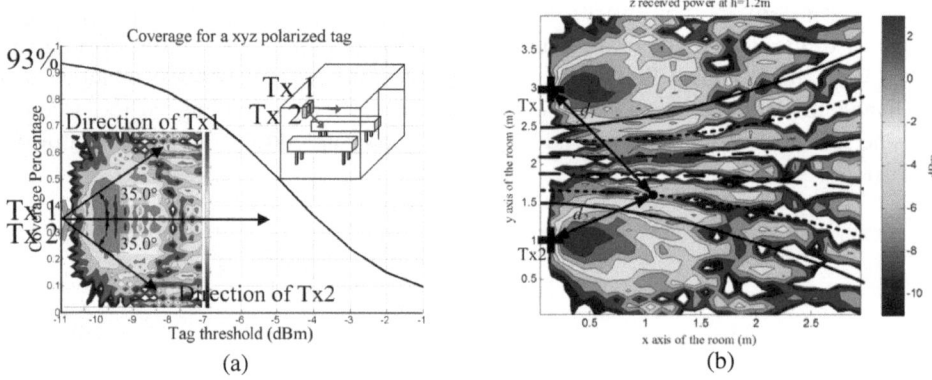

Fig. 3. RF coverage inside a typical patient room using: (a) optimized two-antenna configuration at close proximity to each other; (b) a pair of antennas spaced apart

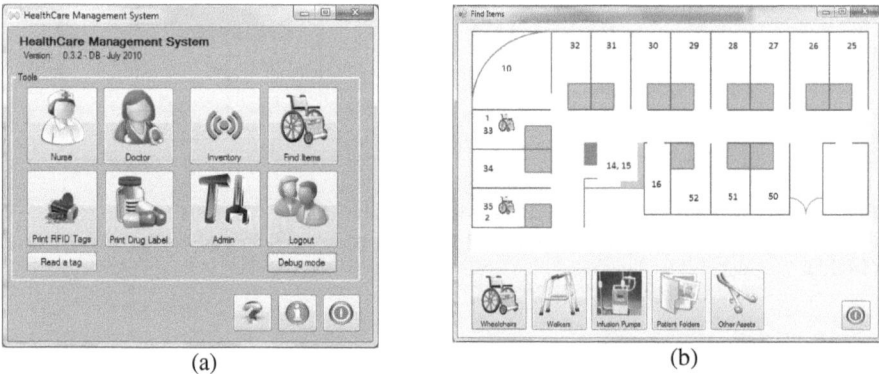

Fig. 4. (a) The Login card of the GUI; (b) The RTLS card where it is shown that 1 wheelchair was found in room 33 and 2 wheelchairs in room 35

It should be emphasized that fundamental antenna theory and propagation models were used in the design of the proposed RFID system. For example, considering only the line-of-sight path between the reader antenna and the RFID tag, one may use the well-known Friis equation [4] to calculate the maximum possible range that will allow data exchange between the reader and the tag (chip). This is the maximum possible forward link budget that corresponds to the minimum power at the terminals of the chip that is required for it to be energized. When the available power is lower than this threshold, the chip cannot be energized and, therefore, there is no modulated backscattered signal toward the reader antenna. This maximum forward link budget is given by

$$r_{max} = \left(\frac{\lambda}{4\pi}\right)\sqrt{\frac{P_{tx}G_{tx}G_{tag}\left(PLF\right)\left(1-|\Gamma|^2\right)}{L_c P_{chip}(min)}} \tag{1}$$

where P_{tx} is the Effective Radiated Power (ERP=2W for Europe), G_{tx}, G_{tag} are the gains of the transmitting and tag antennas, respectively, PLF is the Polarization Loss Factor between the incident field and the tag antenna, Γ is the complex reflection coefficient at the terminals of the tag antenna for a given chip input impedance, L_c is cable loss factor due to attenuation, and $P_{chip}(\min)$ is the minimum power required by the chip (chip sensitivity). The power of the backscattered ASK-modulated signal by the tag is proportional to the differential RCS ($\Delta\sigma$) of the tag antenna terminated to a given chip impedance [5]:

$$P_{received} = \frac{P_{tx}G_{tx}^2(PLF)}{L_c^2}\left(\frac{\lambda}{4\pi r^2}\right)^2\frac{\Delta\sigma}{4\pi}$$

(2)

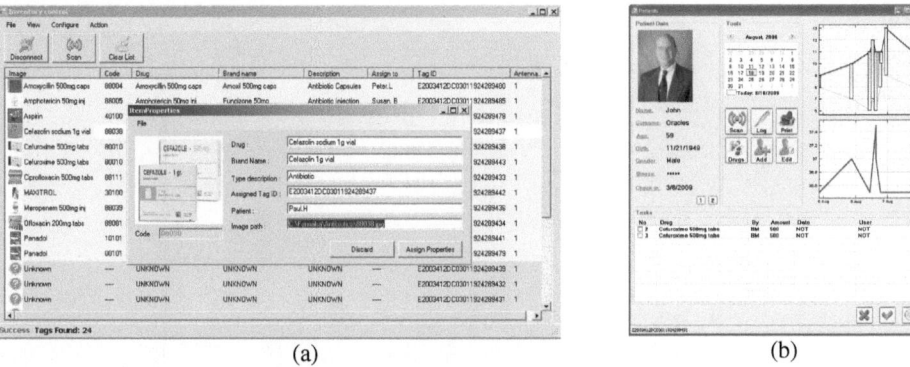

(a)   (b)

Fig. 5. (a) Application card indicating all drugs located in the inventory room/cabinet; (b) patient identification card depicting medical history, patient profile, and routine task icons

Acknowledgments. This research is funded by the Cyprus Research Promotion Foundation grant ΤΠΕ/ΟΡΙΖΟ/0308(ΒΙΕ)/13.

References

1. Institute of Medicine: To Err is Human: Building a Safer Health System. National Academy Press, Washington, D.C. (1999)
2. Glabman, M.: Room for tracking: RFID technology finds the way. Materials Management in Health Care (2004)
3. Saunders, S.R.: Antennas and Propagation for Wireless Communication Systems. John Wiley and Sons, Chichester (1999)
4. Balanis, A.C.: Antenna Theory: Analysis and Design. John Wiley and Sons, Chichester (2005)
5. Nikitin, P.V., Rao, K.V.S., Martinez, R.D.: Differential RCS of RFID tag. Electronics Letters 43(8) (2007)

Poster Session

Real-Time, Remote, Home Based, Non-invasive, Elder Monitoring System

Rajesh Kannan Megalingam, Vineeth Radhakrishnan, Akhil Kakkanattu Sudhakaran, Deepak Krishnan Melepurath Unnikrishnan, and Denny Chacko Jacob

Amrita Vishwa Vidyapeetham, Amritapuri, Clappana P.O., Kollam-690525, Kerala, India
rajeshm@am.amrita.edu, zarbon001@gmail.com, akhil.ase@gmail.com,
mu.deepakkrishnan@gmail.com, dennychakko@yahoo.co.in

Abstract. Real-time monitoring of the physical condition of the elderly people has become mandatory nowadays. The reason for rise in demand of aging services is due to the rise of the elderly population. We need precise, fast and effective transmission of information about their health condition to the concerned. Also there lies a need to transmit more parameters and more data for the convenience and effective response by the concerned people. Since we need an effective response we make use of the voice-call facility apart from the SMS mechanism also. The system proposed here called Noninvasive Elder Monitoring System (NEMS) monitors blood pressure, heart rate, temperature and ECG of the elders. Any critical condition is reported to the medical service center and relatives via an SMS and voice call, to arrange for proper services to the elder at right time. We make use of the GSM modem for the SMS and voice call facility.

Keywords: Voice call, ECG, Heart rate, GSM modem, SMS.

1 Introduction

This fast moving world, where people are in a rat race to make their both ends meet, a very important section of the society which is our elder population has been ignored quite easily. This is a very critical social situation and should be tackled as soon as possible. As the life expectancy of the population in many countries is increasing the elder population is also increasing which increases the responsibility of the young generation to care for these elders. Traditionally elder care has been the responsibility of family members and was provided within the extended family home. Increasingly in modern societies, elder care is now being provided by state or charitable institutions. The reasons for this change include decreasing family size, the greater life expectancy of elderly people, the geographical dispersion of families, and the tendency for women to be educated and work outside the home. Although these changes have affected European and North American countries first, it is now increasing.

Most elders would prefer to continue to live in their own homes. Unfortunately, majority of elderly people gradually lose functioning ability and require either additional assistance in the home or a move to an eldercare facility. The adult children of these elders often face a difficult challenge in helping their parents make the right

J. Lin and K.S. Nikita (Eds.): MobiHealth 2010, LNICST 55, pp. 263–270, 2011.

choices. Usually many bed ridden elders are taken to the hospitals and they spend rest of their life in a hospital bed.

It is this situation which led us to propose an architecture by which old people can be in their home with sensors attached to their body non-invasively. The system is called NEMS – Noninvasive Elder Monitoring System. The vital parameters are monitored continuously and processed by NEMS locally in a computer at their homes. The computer processes the parameter to find critical conditions and report the same to the medical services for timely help. The relatives of the elders are also informed via SMS and voice call facility using GSM modem.

2 Related Work

The ECG monitoring system in [1] only deals with the heart beat monitoring using ECG, which only gives limited information about the present condition of the patient. This system is very costly compared to the system we are proposing here. Paper [2] also deals with the monitoring of heart beat, it does not use any other sensors for monitoring other biological parameters like blood pressure and temperature and it does not make a voice call to the concerned authorities and relatives. Voice call is very important as it can be seen that there are lot of chance that an SMS goes unnoticed, especially during night times. Our system specifically does a voice call along with the SMS messaging. [3] Gives importance to the changes of behavior of patient sensed via camera and force sensors. It does not deal with measuring temperature or heart rate, which are important parameters that should be taken care of especially for elderly people. In [11] authors have proposed the wearable jacket for patients to monitor ECG which might be very uncomfortable for bed ridden elders. Also it is more applicable only for cardiac patients. NEMS uses a wearable glove which is comfortable for elders.

3 Methods and Methodologies

The home based NEMS as shown in Fig.1 consists of the Pair of Gloves, Sensors, Intelligent Wireless Controller (IWC), Receiver and PC module, SMS and Voice Call Gateway (SVCG).

3.1 Pair of Gloves

These are the gloves that the bed ridden elders wear for the vital parameter monitoring. They have the sensors as described in B in this section. The sensors are integrated with the Intelligent Wireless Controller as explained later in this section.

3.2 Sensors

The Sensor Microcontroller module consists of four different sensors for measuring the following four parameters: *Heart rate, Blood pressure, ECG, Body temperature.*

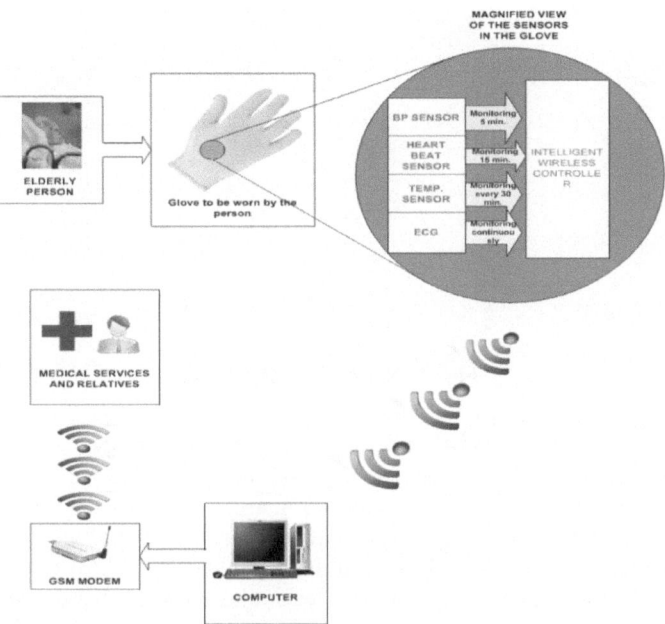

Fig. 1. NEMS Architecture

3.2.1 Heart Rate

Heart rate is the number of heartbeats recorded per minute typically recorded as Beats per Minute (BPM) as in [7]. In the proposed system, we make use of a technique called Photo-plethysmography (PPG). PPG is a simple and low cost optical technique that can be used to detect the blood volume changes in the micro vascular bed of tissues. In this technique, a bright led and a LDR is employed to detect the blood flow at the finger tip or any other peripheral part of the body. The light from the bright led gets reflected from the tissues in the body parts and the amount of light reflected determines the volume of blood flowing. If more blood flows through it, more light is reflected back.

We have to amplify the signal and remove unwanted noise signals. For this purpose we make use of operational amplifiers, LM358. The circuit is shown Fig. 2.

We get the output in the form of analog voltage signal and its peak value is around 3V. We feed this data to IWC.

3.2.2 Blood Pressure

High blood pressure is a common risk factor for heart attacks, strokes and aneurysms, so diagnosing and monitoring it are critically important. However, getting reliable blood pressure readings is not always easy. Traditional blood pressure monitoring requires a cuff, wrapped around the upper arm and inflated until blood flow is completely cut off. The examiner then gradually releases the pressure, listening to the flow until the pulse can be detected.

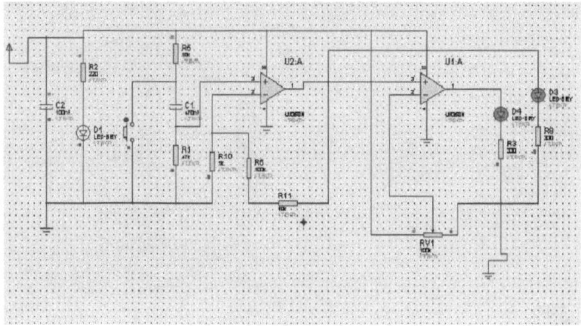

Fig. 2. Noise Filtering Circuit

With the new monitor as in [4], no cuff is required. Instead, the device takes advantage of a method called pulse wave velocity, which allows blood pressure to be calculated by measuring the pulse at two points along an artery. The two points decided are two points of index figure. That posed a challenge because blood pressure in the hand varies depending on its position: If the arm is raised above the heart, the pressure will be higher than if it is below the heart. The researchers solved that dilemma by incorporating a sensor that measures acceleration in three dimensions, allowing the hand position to be calculated at any time. This not only compensates for the error due to height changes, but also allows them to calibrate the sensor for more accurate calculation of blood pressure. As the wearer raise the hands up and down, the hydrostatic pressure changes at the sensor. Correlating the change of pulse wave velocity to the hydrostatic pressure change, the system can automatically calibrate its measurement. The equivalent analog output signal will be fed to IWC.

3.2.3 ECG
An ECG sensor is important for patient monitoring system because their analysis give clear information about cardiac regulation and well insight about pathological conditions. Also, the system should be user friendly, simple, reliable and of affordable cost. The two electrodes of the ECG sensor are connected to the body as in [5] and the signals collected are amplified by means of op-amps (LM358N) so as to interface it with the IWC. The gain of the op-amp is controlled by varying the resistors attached to it. The circuit is shown in Fig. 3.

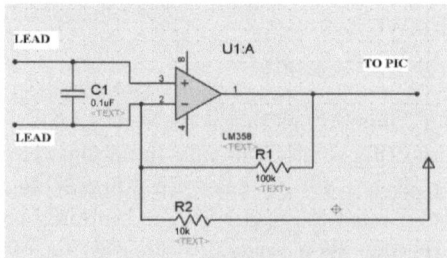

Fig. 3. ECG Sensor Circuit

Here we are using two op-amps so as to reduce the effect of noise generated while sensing.

3.2.4 Temperature

The LM335 series are precision, easily-calibrated, integrated circuit temperature sensors. They are two terminal devices like a Zener and have a break down voltage directly proportional to the absolute temperature at +10mv/°K. The LM335 operates in the range of -40°C to +100°C as given in [6]. LM335Z can measure temperature ranging from -40°C to +100°C. The output from the temperature sensor is an analog signal and is fed into IWC.

3.3 Intelligent Wireless Controller

This consists of a microcontroller to process the analog signals and wireless interface to transmit the processed signals to the PC. The microcontroller and the wireless interface should be a simple and powerful one such that the gloves don't become too heavy for the elders. One option for the wireless interface is to use simple RF TWS 434 Receiver and Transmitter modules. These are light weight and can be easily integrated with microcontrollers. Another option is to use Zigbee transmitters and receivers.

3.4 Receiver and PC Module

The digital data from the IWC is sent to the PC from the wireless receiver module TWS 434, using RS232 cable. The output from the receiver is send to the level shifter MAX232 and interfaced to the PC via RS232 cable as given in [8]. The customized software installed in PC will process the parameters which are measured in the specific intervals as indicated in Fig.1. These timing intervals are based on the enquiry with a local physician. When the parameters exceed critical value in any case of temperature, heart rate, ECG or pressure, the SVCG is activated to SMS and place a voice call to the medical service center and relatives.

3.5 SMS and Voice Call Gateway (SVCG)

A GSM (Global System for Mobile Communication) modem is used to alert the medical service center and the relatives when there is a abrupt change in the measured parameters which exceeds the critical value.

4 Elder Monitor Algorithm (EMA)

The EMA as shown in Fig.4 monitors the elder's heart beat, ECG, blood pressure and body temperature. All the sensors are made compact and integrated into a small unit which could be fit into a glove. It is so convenient for the elderly that they have to wear the gloves in their hands. The sensors monitor the parameters and if it bounces above a critical value it activates the alert mechanism. To avoid the muddling up of the four sensor outputs, we accept the value from each sensor only after a specified amount of time. We send the data of the body temperature in a time interval of 30 minutes; heart beat every 15 minutes and blood pressure every 5 minutes. Since the

ECG being the most crucial one we monitor and send the ECG value continuously. The parameter values from the sensors are given to the intelligent wireless controller and are sent to the computer. All the parameter values are continuously monitored by a custom software and if a critical situation is encountered the computer instructs the GSM modem to send a SMS and a voice call is made to the relatives and medical service center.

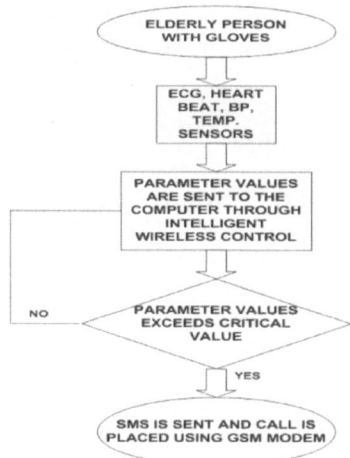

Fig. 4. EMA Flow Chart

5   Modem Control via HyperTerminal

As of now we have conducted simple simulation of sensor circuits. As a preliminary work some simple hardware circuits are also built and tested. Majority of the work is done with the SVCG in successfully messaging and placing a call. The modem which we are using is GPRS/GSM modem. GSM/GPRS modem can be used to send messages and also make a call through computer. HyperTerminal can be used to control the modem. For interfacing HyperTerminal with modem we use the AT commands.

5.1   Setting Up GSM Modem

GSM/GPRS modem is connected to the computer using a RS-232 cable.It is connected to the serial portof the computer. The GSM modem will map itself as a COM serial port in the computer as in [10].

5.2   HyperTerminal Configuration

On the Windows Start menu, Run dialog box is selected. 'hypertrm.exe' is typed in the Open field to open the Connection Description screen as shown in Fig. 5. On the Connection Description screen, for Name, "Cisco" is typed and an icon is selected for the definition. The primary COM port is selected for the Connect in the Connect To dialog box. In the COM Properties dialog box, the following selections are made as shown in the Fig. 6.

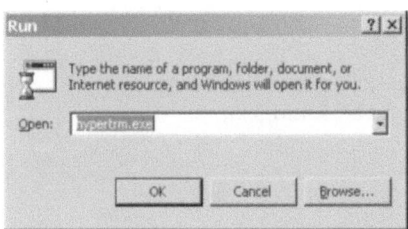

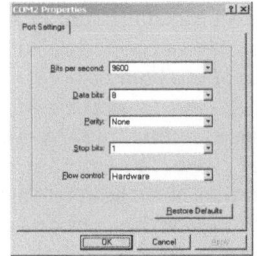

Fig. 5. The Windows Run Dialog Box

Fig. 6. HyperTerminal COM n Properties Dialog Box

Initial setting up of GPRS/GSM Modem, sending SMS through AT commands, and for making call using AT commands we can make use of the reference [9].

6 Conclusion

The system proposed above is simple and cheap that can be used for this purpose. One other beneficiary of NEMS is the doctors who can monitor the physical and medical conditions of the elders from any part of the world and thus can attend to them remotely. Apart from simple circuit evaluations in the preliminary work we have done so far, we are successfully able to SMS and place a call using the SVCG. Obviously the other set of people are the old people who can be monitored from any place with this proposed system.

7 Future Work

Future work involves integrating the entire system as NEMS. The gloves, especially the design and the materials used to make the gloves are yet to be identified and tested. The data can also be stored and used by the doctors to conduct a study and make conclusions. The doctors would be able to give clear and best instructions within the least time. This system can also be used in villages of developing and under-developed countries for remote patient monitoring where there is heavy shortage of doctors.

References

1. Tejero-Calado, J.C., Lopez-Casado, C., Bernal-Martin, A., Lopez-Gomez, M.A.: ECG monitoring system
2. Jubadi, W.M., Mohd Sahak, S.F.A.: Heartbeat Monitoring Alert via SMS. In: 2009 IEEE Symposium on Industrial Electronics and Applications (ISIEA 2009), Kuala Lumpur, Malaysia, October 4-6 (2009)
3. Gaddam, A., Mukhopadhyay, S.C., Sen Gupta, G.: Smart Home Using Optimized Number Of Wireless Sensors For Elderly Care. In: Applied Electromagnetics Conference, AEMC (2009), doi:10.1109/AEMC.2009.5430600

4. Details of Blood Pressure sensor from fingers,
   http://www.coolcircuit.com
5. Details of ECG sensor,
   http://www.sensorsmag.com and http://www.swharden.com
6. Datasheets of PIC 16f877A, MAX232, LM358, LM324, LM 335,
   http://www.alldatasheet.com
7. Information about heart rate monitoring,
   http://www.heartmoniters.com
8. Information on MAX 232 IC,
   http://en.wikibooks.org/wiki/Serial_Programming/
   MAX232_Driver_Receiver
9. Information on serial port,
   http://www.howstuffworks.com/serial-port.htm
10. Modem PC configuration through AT commands,
    http://www.cse.iitd.ernet.in/~cs5050224/GPRS/ATCMDGPRS.pdf
11. Di Rienzo, M., Rizzo, F., Parati, G., Ferratini, M., Brambilla, G., Castiglioni, P.: A Textile-Based Wearable System for Vital Sign Monitoring: Applicability in Cardiac Patients. In: Conference Computers in Cardiology (2005), doi:10.1109/CIC.2005.1588199

Author Index